HEALTH CARE QUALITY MANAGEMENT

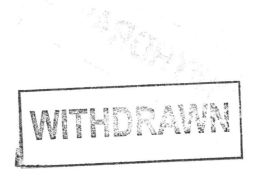

D1323416

HEALTH CARE
QUALITY MANAGEMENT

TOOLS AND APPLICATIONS

Thomas K. Ross

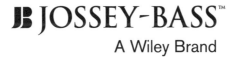

A Wiley Brand

Cover design by Jeff Puda
Cover image by Datacraft | Getty and Yagi Studio | Getty

Published by Jossey-Bass
A Wiley Brand
One Montgomery Street, Suite 1200, San Francisco, CA 94104-4594—www.josseybass.com

Limit of Liability/Disclaimer of Warranty: While the publisher and author have used their best efforts in preparing this book, they make no representations or warranties with respect to the accuracy or completeness of the contents of this book and specifically disclaim any implied warranties of merchantability or fitness for a particular purpose. No warranty may be created or extended by sales representatives or written sales materials. The advice and strategies contained herein may not be suitable for your situation. You should consult with a professional where appropriate. Neither the publisher nor author shall be liable for any loss of profit or any other commercial damages, including but not limited to special, incidental, consequential, or other damages. Readers should be aware that Internet Web sites offered as citations and/or sources for further information may have changed or disappeared between the time this was written and when it is read.

Jossey-Bass books and products are available through most bookstores. To contact Jossey-Bass directly call our Customer Care Department within the U.S. at 800-956-7739, outside the U.S. at 317-572-3986, or fax 317-572-4002.

Wiley publishes in a variety of print and electronic formats and by print-on-demand. Some material included with standard print versions of this book may not be included in e-books or in print-on-demand. If this book refers to media such as a CD or DVD that is not included in the version you purchased, you may download this material at http://booksupport.wiley.com. For more information about Wiley products, visit www.wiley.com.

Library of Congress Cataloging-in-Publication Data

Ross, Thomas K.
    Health care quality management : tools and applications / Thomas K. Ross. — First edition.
      pages   cm
    Includes bibliographical references and index.
     ISBN 978-1-118-50553-3 (pbk.) — ISBN 978-1-118-60364-2 (pdf) — ISBN 978-1-118-60389-5 (epub)
      1. Health services administration—Quality control.   2. Medical care—Quality control.   I. Title.
  RA399.A1R68   2014
  362.1—dc23

                                                  2013027966

Printed in the United States of America

FIRST EDITION

PB Printing   10 9 8 7 6 5 4 3 2 1

CONTENTS

Part 1: The State of Quality Management in Health Care

Chapter 1 Quality in Health Care **3**

Chapter 2 Error and Variation **37**

Chapter 3 Regulating the Quality and Quantity of Health Care . . **63**

Part 2: Quality Management Tools

Part 3: Medical Practice Management

FIGURES AND TABLES

FIGURES

TABLES

Calls for improvement in health care began before the advent of organized medicine and will continue until disease and injury are eliminated. From the Crimean War to *To Err Is Human*, health care reformers have identified major remediable shortcomings in health care delivery processes. Given the life-and-death nature of medicine, it is understandable that we often find the pace of improvement unacceptably slow. Error is the inevitable result of weaknesses in systems and human performance. To improve health outcomes, we must undertake a methodical review of the systems we have created and our performance within these systems. Unfortunately many quality initiatives skip a rigorous systemic review and simply advocate for changes in culture, leadership, teamwork, and communication. These changes are necessary conditions for improvement but they do not instill in people the ability to identify what needs to be changed. A more rigorous application of statistics and data analysis is needed to identify what needs to be improved and how processes can be improved. Some authors tell you what should be done. This text shows you how to do it.

Students taking a course with *management* in its title assume the class will be "soft," except if the course is Financial Management. Management courses rely on common sense and psychology and assume that the appropriate action will be based on the particular individuals present in a situation. A student in a management class may believe the right answer to a question on management style is either theory X or Y, and may expect that either answer will be accepted as correct, as long as it is supported by logical reasons. Conversely, operations research is the application of scientific and mathematical methods to the study and analysis of problems in complex systems. Operations research does not give the impression that answers can be finessed; science and math provide a limited number of correct answers, if not a single answer, and provide clear rationale for rejection of wrong answers. To make that distinction clear, I wanted to include *operations research* in the book title, but marketing considerations led to the current title with emphasis placed on *tools and applications* to distinguish the book from other quality management (QM) texts.

I hope readers will not only come away with a greater understanding of ideas and concepts in quality management and the pressing need to improve quality in health care but also will believe they are qualified to collect and analyze data and develop solutions based on their analyses. Health care is a unique industry because of the dichotomy between its management and medical functions. Physicians and nurses are highly capable individuals trained in the physical sciences, but they often receive little training in business operations (such as QM). The management staff often has little insight into medical processes but understand essential business requirements such as customer and employee relations, logistics, production, billing, and accounting. The text aims to elevate the understanding of all staff, so they can understand how quality data is analyzed and what the analysis indicates about their processes and outcomes. This knowledge will place medical professionals on a more equal footing with the managerial staff, and managerial staff will come away with a greater understanding of the medical decision-making process and the large number of factors that affect medical practice.

Because of the pervasiveness of Microsoft's Excel on workplace computers, this text illustrates how QM tools can be produced using Excel. While dedicated software programs have features exceeding those offered in Excel, there is a "black box" risk attached to using this type of software. The risk is that those entering the data may not be able to recognize problems in the output if they are unfamiliar with the calculations taking place. Developing QM tools in Excel forces users to know the underlying calculations required by the QM applications and to understand the logic behind these calculations. An additional benefit of this approach is that readers will increase their competency in Excel, a useful skill given its widespread use.

Typical textbooks describe techniques and provide examples of their output. This text strives to make QM education a participatory activity by providing data, describing the calculations, and showing the output. Readers can reproduce the examples used in the book, and exercises are provided to apply the newly learned skills to other situations.

QM is a sequential process that starts with identifying problems and discovering the causes of those problems, moves on to formulating potential solutions, and ends with choosing and implementing a solution. The identification of problems and causes is relatively easy. Formulating solutions and successfully implementing the chosen solution is the hard part.

An inability to identify problems or their causes dramatically reduces the probability of improvement. If an organization chases the wrong problem or cause of the problem, the process and its outcomes are unlikely to improve. Action that is based on a misidentified problem or cause may lessen the outward symptoms, but it is unlikely to correct the real problem. When no problem is identified, it is unlikely that any change will be attempted since people must be convinced of the need to do things differently before they will take action.

Once the problem is correctly identified, the second step is the identification of its causes. QM embraces the idea that the primary cause of problems lies in the system or process. QM has moved away from attributing errors to single causes, such as a "bad" employee, and embraced the idea that problems appearing at one point in a system are the result of what came before. There are numerous points before and after a problem appears at which it could be prevented or remediated. Weak systems are susceptible to error regardless of who is operating the system; strong systems do not rely on a single point for control. Solutions that rely on replacing "careless" workers with more conscientious individuals are often unsuccessful. The errors may continue since the rotation of employees does not change the underlying process.

Assuming the problem and its cause have been correctly identified, the more daunting task of choosing a solution arises. There are normally multiple alternatives to improving a situation, and the correct solution is seldom obvious. Because the correct choice may not be obvious, poor choices are often implemented. These choices may have intuitive appeal, but they must ultimately be judged by whether they are capable of changing the system. Teamwork and communication fall into this category. Although failure to communicate or work together frequently results in mistakes, communication and teamwork solutions generally fail to elicit any organizational change.

Likewise, merely relying on better policies and procedures fails to address the root cause of most problems. Bureaucratic responses such as implementing new policies and procedures, training, or additional paperwork are seldom good solutions. These "fixes" do not address how the system operates and generally fail to achieve either temporary or permanent improvement.

Even when the problem, its cause, and a good solution are correctly identified, the hard task of implementing the change remains. Organizations are built on established practices and privileges. Change requires people to move beyond the behaviors they have grown comfortable with and threatens employees by increasing or decreasing their workload, authority, or compensation. Machiavelli noted there is nothing more dangerous than attempting change. Those threatened by change will forcefully oppose it, while those who may benefit will offer lukewarm support, if any.

What the Book Will Not Discuss

QM textbooks devote a lot of space to organizational culture, communication, teamwork, leadership and management, and training and education, among other topics. I recognize the vital nature of people in the quality improvement process; quality initiatives are doomed if they are not supported by the upper management and embraced by workers. But reviewing these topics does not advance or facilitate quality improvement.

I assume that most readers have been exposed to leadership issues, team building, effective communication techniques, and so on through their education and professional careers. On the other hand, the systems, measures, and tools emphasized in this text are ideas with which the reader may be unfamiliar. Rather than cover the general role of management, the text presents readers with specific problems and the tools to analyze them.

The goal of the text is to introduce the reader to concepts and tools they can apply to their work at their discretion. Rather than the top-down approach commonly used in organizations, where upper management or an outside authority initiates or demands quality improvement, the text advocates a bottom-up approach, with the hope that individuals who master the concepts and tools will initiate their own quality improvement programs. A common tenet of quality improvement is that change will only be successful if employees internalize the goals of improvement. The top-down approach is often contrary to internalization and may account for many of the quality fads that have come and gone.

The Central Idea of the Text

The central idea of the text is:

No Measurement → No Management → No Mission

This causal chain recognizes that without measures of performance, an organization cannot know where it stands or whether change is required. Without measurement there can be no management, because managers who change systems without information cannot know when a system requires correction or whether the correction had a positive or negative effect on system performance.

We know that what gets measured is what people focus on. When employees know certain elements of their job are systematically reviewed and their job security or pay is determined by their performance in these areas, they devote extra attention to those processes. The downside of this focus could be that other necessary but less rigorously reviewed operations will be slighted.

The challenge to management is to improve certain elements without creating problems in other parts of the organization. Organizations that cannot envision the totality of their production process or follow through with purposeful action will be unable to compete against those who know how they are performing and have management that can capitalize on the strong points of the organization and minimize or eliminate their weaknesses. In the long run, the ability to measure and manage performance will determine which organizations thrive and which will wither and die.

Overview of the Book

This study of health care quality management is presented in three sections. Part One, The State of Quality Management in Health Care, discusses what quality is and the many ways quality can be measured. The term *quality* is itself misleading; we should discuss *qualities*— the many attributes of a product or service that increase or diminish the value a customer obtains from it. Understanding health care and quality management is advanced by reviewing the lives of the men and women who have contributed to each. The traits shared by these pioneers were observation, analysis, and persistence. They understood what could be done better and devoted themselves to achieving better outcomes. QM is not about individuals and the errors they make but rather about the systems and weaknesses in them that increase the likelihood of error. Chapter Two documents the magnitude of variation in medical practice that characterizes health care treatment. While some of the variation observed is the result of differences in patient preferences, substantial variation results from lack of understanding of medical evidence and the practice of other providers. David Nash's Three Faces of Quality presents a system to move toward evidence-based medicine by specifying the foundation, means, and set of goals on which health care should operate to improve patient outcomes. Chapter Three reviews the economics of health care markets and historical regulatory approaches to ensuring quality.

Part Two, Quality Management Tools, explores the foundation needed for quality improvement. This foundation provides the tools necessary for providers to understand the environment in which they work and the outcomes they achieve. Chapter Four, Process Analysis Tools, introduces ten tools to identify problems, causes, and solutions and to monitor implemented solutions. Chapters Five and Ten cover methods for investigating errors and systems; root cause analysis is a technique for exploring errors after they arise and is required by Joint Commission for errors that achieve the level of sentinel events. Failure mode and effects analysis attempts to review systems and subsystems to identify weaknesses that may allow an error to arise. Both chapters explore ways to improve systems and build safer patient care systems. Chapters Six through Eight introduce statistical process control (SPC). SPC is used to monitor processes in action to determine when a problem has arisen or may arise. In the first case, SPC is used to quickly eliminate problems before more patients are affected. In the second case it is used to modify systems before undesired outcomes arise. Chapter Nine provides formal statistical tests to identify problems and causes and to determine whether corrective actions have substantially improved performance.

Part Three, Medical Practice Management, focuses on how health care practice can be altered to improve patient outcomes. Chapter Eleven explores practice policies that seek to ensure treatment follows the best available medical evidence. Chapter Twelve focuses on case, disease, and outcomes management to demonstrate how specific practice management tools have been developed to achieve specific ends. Chapter Thirteen, Profiling, Economic Credentialing, and Risk Adjustment, tackles the difficult problem of comparing physicians against each other, including the process of risk adjustment. Comparison provides a basis for physicians to understand the performance of their peers and question their own treatment practices in light of the results of others. Risk adjustment reminds us that for comparisons to be useful, equals must match equals. In health care, differences between patients may inhibit direct comparability, so results must be adjusted for these differences and judgment must be constrained, if not reserved. Chapter Fourteen, Benchmarking and Implementation, takes the idea of comparison to the organization level, avoiding the contentious issues surrounding individual comparison. Benchmarking across organizations seeks to improve performance by pushing organizations toward the results achieved by industry leaders. Quality management is only as good as the results it achieves, and results will depend on the ability to effectively implement programs. Effective implementation requires communication of goals and plans, supplying necessary resources, and demonstrating long-term commitment.

Chapter Fifteen, The Future of Quality Management in Health Care, discusses value and what we can do to improve value for patients. The future presents many opportunities to improve services to patients and to produce better health outcomes, but these opportunities require commitment and change. Success requires that we take more deliberative and analytical steps toward understanding our work and what we produce, take effective action when opportunities and problems arise, and put the patient first.

An instructor's supplement is available at www.josseybass.com/go/ross. Additional materials such as videos, podcasts, and readings can be found at josseybasspublichealth.com. Comments about this book are invited and can be sent to publichealth@wiley.com.

ACKNOWLEDGMENTS

This book would not have been possible without the encouragement and support of my students, family, colleagues, teachers, and the publishing staff at Jossey-Bass. Proposal reviewers John T. Cantiello, Leigh Hamby, and Barbara Langland Orban provided valuable feedback on the original book proposal. Elena Capella, Martha Perryman, and Karen Williams provided thoughtful and constructive comments on the complete draft manuscript. The debt I owe all of you can neither be calculated nor repaid. Thank you all.

Thomas K. Ross is a member of the faculty at East Carolina University in the department of Health Services and Information Management. He received his PhD in economics from St. Louis University and BBA in accounting from the University of Cincinnati. He teaches courses on Applied Health Care Research, Quality Management in Health Care, Health Care Financial Management, and Health Care Strategic Planning and Management. Dr. Ross has worked in health care finance as a director of patient accounts, manager of system support, and financial analyst.

HEALTH CARE QUALITY MANAGEMENT

PART 1

THE STATE OF QUALITY MANAGEMENT IN HEALTH CARE

When examining quality in health care, one is immediately struck by the slowness of change. Some companies measure their error rates in millions, while the health care industry continues to measure error rates in hundreds. Dr. David Bates found 1.4 pharmaceutical errors per admission; this is a far cry from the three errors per one million opportunities other organizations pursue. A major difference between health care and other industries lies in defining quality. Health care produces thousands of outputs for patients who vary dramatically in age and condition, so defining what constitutes good medical practice is extremely challenging.

Chapter One introduces the reader to definitions of quality to induce the reader to think differently about the subject. The lives of the early quality pioneers in health care are examined to highlight their goals, challenges, and the impact they had on medical practice. Machiavelli noted, "There is nothing more difficult to take in hand, more perilous to conduct, or more uncertain in its success, than to take the lead in the introduction of a new order of things." The reader will see that those attempting to change medical practice face stiff opposition from those who believe things are as they should be. Chapter One reviews the evolution of production processes and demonstrates how quality control methods have evolved with technology and consumer demand. It is essential that health care providers adopt the perspective and tools of other industries and employ system thinking throughout their work. Only a broad, system perspective will enable health care to adopt changes that will cut across departments and organizations and improve health outcomes. The central idea of this text is: no measurement, no management, no mission. If an organization cannot define and measure what it produces, it will not be able to effectively manage its operations, and without management it will neither fulfill its mission nor endure.

Variation in medical practice and inability to predict outcomes are the main problems in health care. Chapter Two discusses how variability arises from differences in medical knowledge and patient preferences and from the tendency of humans to commit error. Variability arising from treatment choice and ability to carry out the treatment plan is the basis for the observed differences in the use of treatments and resources among patients. If variability is the problem, standardization through practice guidelines is one solution. The chapter concludes by reviewing paradigms for examining health care quality.

Chapter Two describes Nash's Three Faces of Quality, which defines the foundation, means, and goals needed for an effective quality management system. Effective quality management begins with a foundation built on science and statistics and requires the development of tools that will provide medical personnel with information to identify and improve suboptimal processes. Given the unique nature of health care, the industry must recognize the benefit of standardizing treatment while ensuring the ability of providers to respond to unique cases.

Chapter Three examines previous attempts to ensure health care quality and the economic incentives in the current system. It is clear that economic incentives and regulation have altered how health care is delivered, but it is less clear whether either has substantially improved quality. Current programs are reviewed, reminding us that we will get more of what we pay for, and so we must be mindful of how resources are shifted. If we want quality, then we must measure it directly. Half measures and proxies can produce more harm than good.

CHAPTER 1

QUALITY IN HEALTH CARE

Introduction

The most prolific serial killers in the United States are among the least known. While the Green River killer in Washington and the Killer Clown of Chicago are well known, serial killers in health care have been responsible for a higher number of deaths over extended periods of time. What does serial killing have to do with quality management in health care? The issue is, how can health care workers kill dozens of patients without being detected? More to the point, how can highly trained personnel working together to improve the health of their patients realize the worst possible outcome without unleashing an investigative process to identify and understand what was responsible for the deaths of their patients?

The most prolific serial killer in U.S. medical history may be Donald Harvey, who killed between 37 and 87 patients in two hospitals in Ohio and Kentucky over a 17-year period. Harvey was able to continue his murder spree by targeting critically ill patients and changing his method of killing. The death of critically ill patients is not unexpected, and there was no easy-to-identify pattern in Harvey's killings that would suggest something other than natural forces were at work. Harvey's unmasking was rapid when it finally occurred. He targeted a man whose condition was thought to be improving by his family and the hospital staff; his unexpected death sparked an investigation.

The authorities determined the death was a homicide and immediately began investigating the man's family. Satisfied that no member of his family was responsible, the police began investigating his medical providers. Shortly after beginning their investigation at Harvey's employer,

LEARNING OBJECTIVES

1. Set the context for the study of quality in health care

2. Understand the goals of quality management

3. Define quality and health care quality and understand their components

4. Recognize the contributions and challenges faced by health care quality pioneers

5. Understand the evolution of production and quality management processes

6. Apply system thinking to health care processes

they learned from multiple coworkers that Harvey was known as "the Angel of Death" due to his frequent presence when patients expired. Unfortunately, Harvey was no angel. He soon confessed to killing many patients.

Charles Cullen provides a second example. Unlike Harvey, Cullen worked in 10 health care institutions in New Jersey and Pennsylvania. Over 16 years Cullen murdered between 18 and 40 patients. Cullen killed many of his patients by administering overdoses of digoxin. Despite concerns over suspicious deaths, investigations were handled internally by his employers and failed to discover any wrongdoing. Cullen frequently changed jobs, and any concerns, if relayed, did not prevent him from finding continuous employment in the health care field. In the end it was only the dogged efforts of the family of one of his victims that resulted in his arrest for the death of their loved one and in the discovery of the other cases.

The issue for quality management is, how can the worst possible health care **outcome** occur repeatedly without signaling that there is a problem in the **system** that requires investigation? Walshe and Shortell in "When Things Go Wrong: How Health Care Organizations Deal with Major Failures" (2004) note that health care failures differ substantially from failures in other industries. Harvey's case exemplifies the first of these differences: it is not uncommon for critically ill people to die, so questions are not raised when the expected happens. A second difference is that the cost of health care failure is borne almost entirely by patients and their families. Contrast a patient death with a plane crash. In a plane crash not only the passengers die; the flight crew also perishes and a multimillion-dollar aircraft is destroyed. A third difference is that health care is largely a self-governing profession that often works to conceal errors rather than have its shortcomings exposed to public scrutiny (Walshe and Shortell 2004).

The tendency in health care to restrict information and conceal error explains how a person like Cullen could continue to find health care employment despite patient safety concerns. Walshe and Shortell conclude that failures go unrecognized and uncorrected for several reasons: the culture of secrecy and protectionism prevalent in health care, fragmented information, self-deception and ad hoc rationalization, informal mechanisms to deal with problems, nondisclosure legal settlements, multiple investigative bodies, and the high cost of investigation (Walshe and Shortell 2004, 107–108). All these factors explain how malevolent workers can systematically harm patients over an extended period of time without attracting attention. In Cullen's case, a primary factor that allowed him to continue killing patients was the unwillingness of prior employers to perform thorough internal investigations. Instead his employers seemed willing to barter his resignation from their organization for an unblemished personnel record.

outcome
the results of medical treatment

system
a set of interrelated elements assembled to achieve a goal

As Machiavelli noted long ago, "There is nothing more difficult to take in hand, more perilous to conduct, or more uncertain in its success, than to take the lead in the introduction of a new order of things" (Machiavelli [1532] 1992, 25). The question is: Will health care meet this challenge and implement a new order of things for the benefit of patients?

The Goal of Quality Management

The goal of quality management is to ensure that products and services meet customer expectations or generally accepted production standards, or both. If health care were meeting the highest quality standards, patients would be protected from the intentional acts of malevolent persons and the mistakes of well-meaning workers. The challenge facing health care is to improve patient outcomes by changing how care is delivered. While the elimination of harm is not possible, quality management seeks to design and control systems to minimize it to the extent possible.

Perpetrators take steps to avoid detection, so eliminating intentional acts can be difficult. But discovering mistakes is much easier and will improve patient care more than the elimination of intentional acts. The Institute of Medicine estimated in 1999 that medical error results in the death of between 44,000 and 98,000 patients per year (IOM 1999, 1). Many question the validity of this estimate, but even if it substantially overstates the number of deaths due to medical error, it highlights the enormous opportunity for improvement (Hayward and Hofer 2001; McDonald, Weiner, and Hui 2000).

This chapter, after defining quality, begins by demonstrating that the pioneers in quality improvement in health care were those trained in medical science and eager to apply an analytical approach to patient populations (rather than simply review outcomes of individual patients) to achieve better results for their patients. These pioneers stepped beyond the individual patient-doctor relationship to view medical practice from a wider perspective. Interpretation of individual patient results is clouded by the patient's behavior, environmental factors, and luck as well as medical intervention. Each of these factors can increase or decrease the probability of a successful outcome. When we are viewing a single patient, the role of medical intervention in a positive or negative outcome may be difficult to determine. Just as the effect of a medical intervention may be difficult to determine, the performance of a provider, a group of providers, or the health care system is also difficult to judge.

The goal of this text is to provide medical workers with an understanding of the history of quality improvement techniques in health care, improve understanding of quality improvement tools, and review the current state of quality improvement applications. This chapter demonstrates that quality improvement is not new to health care and that those who pioneered the application of statistical tools to health care outcomes did so with the goal of improving outcomes for patients. It is hoped that by the end of the text the reader will understand the tools for assessing performance and be able to apply them for the betterment of patients.

Defining Quality

quality
a measure of the degree to which a good or service meets established standards or satisfies the customer

Quality is a measure of the degree to which a good or service meets established standards or satisfies the customer. Quality according to this measure is judged by two different groups. The first is the customer: is the customer satisfied with their purchase? If the customer is satisfied, a product or service fulfills their definition of quality. Producers, however, should strive for more than simple satisfaction; they should attempt to instill in their customers the belief they are getting the most value for their money. If satisfied customers believe they can get even greater value for their money, they will likely spend their funds elsewhere or on different products or services.

Walter Shewhart noted that quality management should be concerned with *qualities* rather than *quality*. He stated that "every conceptual 'something' is really a group of conceptions more elementary in form" ([1931] 1981, 38). Customers value several elements of a purchase, including the product or service purchased, service (how the product or service is delivered), timing, environment, selection, and price. To flesh out these characteristics, think of yourself in a restaurant (or buying a car, attending an entertainment event, or receiving medical care). Goetsch and Davis (2010) discussed the restaurant industry as one that is easy to evaluate because most people have had multiple interactions with it. The first concern of a consumer is typically whether the **product** meets generally accepted standards: is the meal fresh, tasty, and the right temperature, and does it have an appealing appearance? The portion size also affects satisfaction and provides an example of the interpersonal subjectivity of satisfaction. Many individuals desire large portions and are disappointed if they leave a restaurant hungry, while others are upset with contemporary portions, believing they encourage overconsumption and waste. Although portion size is not a determining factor in everyone's restaurant choices, restaurants consider this factor along with many other characteristics of the meal to determine how receptive the public will be to their product and whether people are likely to go back to their restaurant.

product
something produced to satisfy a human need or desire

A second key factor that affects satisfaction is whether the **service** was acceptable: was the server knowledgeable and competent and did he or she treat the customer with the appropriate amount of respect? Servers walk a fine line between being on-the-spot and overbearing, and they must correctly determine the amount of attention each patron desires so they can provide customers with a satisfying dining experience. Because there is no one-size-fits-all solution, producers must customize their products to the individual tastes and preferences of their customers.

service
(1) what is provided to a customer, for example, health care treatment, haircut, and so on or (2) how a customer is treated in a transaction with a producer

A third factor is **timeliness**: was the meal delivered quickly enough or was there substantial wait between when you arrived and when you were seated, when you were seated and when your order was taken, when your order was taken and when your food arrived, and between finishing your meal and the arrival of the bill? Delays at any point diminish the satisfaction the diner may have gotten from a good meal and good service.

timeliness
an action performed within a time frame that renders it effective or satisfies a customer

Interpersonal subjectivity of satisfaction was discussed regarding the product, but satisfaction may also vary systematically based on gender, age, and other characteristics. The fourth factor, **environment**, often raises different expectations in the minds of females and males. For example, females often prefer a dining atmosphere that can be called romantic, cozy, or stylish. On the other hand, males may prefer rustic or hole-in-the-wall type establishments (especially if they serve large portions). Anyone who works with other people knows the temperature in the workplace can never be set to please everyone. While environmental factors cannot be adapted on a customer-by-customer basis, producers need to be sensitive to the desires of their customers and provide a setting—furniture, color, lighting, temperature—that will appeal to the largest pool of potential customers.

environment
the social and physical factors surrounding an individual

The fifth component is **selection**. Restaurants of all types recognize the need to offer variety: different meats, vegetarian offerings, senior meals, and children's menus. Health care is moving toward capitalizing on the importance of choice by increasingly involving patients in the decision-making process. Research consistently shows higher satisfaction among customers who actively participate in their consumption choices.

selection
the set of options from which a customer can choose

Price is the final factor that affects satisfaction. There is an obvious relationship between price and **value**, but when customers receive the same product for a lower price, their satisfaction usually goes up. Most people enjoy a bargain. However, even here we see the impact of the subjectivity of interpersonal satisfaction. Some consumers enjoy a purchase more if it has a price that others cannot afford.

price
the amount of money that must be given to obtain a good or service

value
the interpersonal satisfaction a person receives from consuming a good or service

Consumer-driven evaluations of quality assume the customer is capable of evaluating the good or service. Customers do not need to be chefs to evaluate the quality of food they consume; nor do they have to be mechanics to judge the performance of their cars. The interesting aspect of a consumer-driven evaluation of quality is that each customer may place different weights on the six measures listed previously, and the weights they place on each measure may change over time. Quality is a dynamic concept, and producers must be sensitive to the differences between consumers and to changes in consumer preferences.

The second evaluator of quality is the producer. Like consumers, producers assess quality by determining whether the product is free from defect or meets generally accepted standards. Some restaurants expect wait staff to greet patrons within two minutes of their being seated and monitor food temperatures to ensure hot and cold foods are stored and served at the appropriate temperature. Producer assessment has been the standard used in health care. Physicians have determined what good or bad care is based on accepted standards of medical practice. The problem with consumer-driven evaluations of health care quality is that patients often lack the training and knowledge to evaluate medical treatment. Moreover, a large part of medical care occurs when the patient is unconscious, anesthetized, in pain, or in a state of high anxiety and is thus incapable of objectively assessing care.

To help patients assess the quality of health care providers, many health care organizations use their Web sites to provide consumers with information about providers' credentials, experience, range of services, participation in research and education, and overall patient satisfaction and outcomes. Credentials address where the provider was educated and trained. Experience addresses how many times the provider has performed a particular operation or type of treatment. Most people believe that practice makes perfect, and evidence suggests that providers who routinely perform care have better outcomes than those who provide a service only on a sporadic basis.

Range of services speaks to the selection of services offered, but in health care it also applies to the ability to handle unexpected complications that may arise. Participation in research and education addresses the idea that organizations engaged in research are on the cutting edge of medicine and will be able to offer their patients the newest and best medical options. Similarly, reporting on participation in medical education seeks to capitalize on the idea that the best provider of care is the one who trains other providers.

Finally, patient satisfaction and outcome return to our original definition of quality: Was the patient satisfied with the care he or she received? As we have seen, satisfaction is a multidimensional concept, and patients' satisfaction with their experiences may be driven by a combination of factors: the interpersonal skills of their care givers, the environment, the wait and recovery time, the cost, and the expected outcome of care. Outcome addresses the results of care—how do the results compare with those of other providers, and with the patients' own expectations? While superior outcomes may lead patients to choose one provider over another or may provide the basis for higher reimbursement, superior average outcomes give little comfort to a patient or their family when an adverse event arises. The elevation of patient expectations may ironically make people less tolerant of adverse outcomes regardless of their source.

The greater knowledge of medical practitioners combined with the lack of consumer ability to evaluate care has led to a system in which providers define and police quality. The problem with any producer-driven system is that producers may place their interests above those of the consumers. Reports of 98,000 preventable deaths lead many people to conclude that producer interests too often supersede patient interests and contribute to the high rate of patient injury.

Defining Health Care Quality

Health care quality is optimal care from the appropriate provider in the most appropriate setting in the most appropriate manner for the patient's unique circumstances (Nash, Coombs, and Leider 1999). There are five aspects to this definition. The first is optimal care, which harkens back to meeting generally accepted standards of medical practice. The definition adds that optimal care should be delivered by the appropriate provider. This requirement simultaneously excludes the untrained and overqualified. Health care systems fail when undereducated or underskilled personnel provide care, but they also fail if rudimentary tasks are performed by highly skilled individuals. In the first case we have the potential for bad care. Through practice such a worker may be able to competently perform routine care, but would the employee be able to respond to an emergency requiring knowledge and skill beyond their experience? In the second case, the patient may receive exceptional care from an overqualified provider, but the service might be overpriced and a poor use of the person's skills.

health care quality
optimal care from the appropriate provider in the most appropriate setting in the most appropriate manner for the patient's unique circumstances

The most appropriate setting parallels the most appropriate provider. Care should be delivered in the setting that maximizes the effectiveness of care, minimizes risk to the patient, and effectively uses resources. Particular types of care require hospitalization; other care can be performed more effectively in outpatient settings, physicians' offices, or the patient's home. Quality care requires that the best setting be identified and used to deliver care.

"In the most appropriate manner" recognizes that patients expect to be treated with respect, and providers must recognize their need to be a part of the medical decision-making process or their desire to delegate decision making to the provider. Finally, the patient's unique situation recognizes that provider fears of "cookbook medicine" are often overstated; the role of the physician will always be to navigate between the standards of medical practice and the unique set of medical conditions a patient has and their preferences for a particular type of treatment.

This definition recognizes that health care quality is a process, but it is less clear on how quality should be measured. The **five Ds of health care quality**—death, disability, disease, discomfort, and dissatisfaction—specify the outcomes that can and should be measured. *Death*, measured by mortality rates, recognizes that given a choice between two providers treating identical patients, the better physician is the one with the lower **mortality rate**. The assumption of identical patients will seldom be met and later chapters will discuss the difficulty of comparing mortality rates, but at this point we will conclude that lower mortality rates are preferred to higher rates.

five Ds of health care quality
death, disability, disease, discomfort, and dissatisfaction

mortality rate
the number of deaths in a population

morbidity
the presence of illness or degree of dysfunction

Disability, or **morbidity**, measures the degree of impairment a patient has after receiving treatment. Again, the idea is straightforward: providers having lower rates of disability or higher rates of functionality should be preferred to those who have higher rates of disability. *Disease*, a different aspect of morbidity, refers to the presence of disease after treatment. Providers achieving higher clearance rates should be preferred to those with lower rates.

Discomfort addresses the process of care rather than the outcome. Did the provider adequately manage treatment to minimize the patient's discomfort or pain? Finally, *dissatisfaction* (or, more accurately, patient satisfaction) is one of the most widely measured factors. Payers and accreditors require organizations to regularly measure patient satisfaction as a key component of their quality programs. Many medical providers are rightly concerned about the use of patient satisfaction scores since patients may not be the best evaluators of medical care. Patients have numerous disadvantages as evaluators of the appropriateness or quality of care due to their lack of medical training, lack of consciousness during major events, physical pain, or emotional distress arising from the uncertainty of illness. In spite of these drawbacks, patients will ultimately decide which providers they patronize, and their voices need to be recognized.

In health care it seems easier to identify poor quality—the death of a young person with no history of medical problems, or the oft-cited reference to 98,000 preventable deaths—than systemic weaknesses, but as we will see, the self-evident may tell only part of the story, and the truth may be very different from what we believe. The single tragic event or the 98,000 preventable deaths statistic have a disproportionate impact on our perception of the performance of the health care industry. The unfortunate result is that too much attention is given to rare events and too little to unsafe practices that may eventually produce a tragic outcome. The goal of this text is to improve health care by making the reader a more sophisticated user of data so that unsafe practices can be identified.

The central idea of the text is:

No Measurement → No Management → No Mission

Measurement provides the foundation for managerial action, and effective management ensures the success of an organization. This causal chain recognizes that without objective measures of performance, an organization cannot know where it stands or whether changes are required, and if so, when they should be implemented. The actions of managers can only be random in the absence of measurement and information. A manager operating without information will not know if a system requires correction or what changes to undertake. In the absence of performance measures, it is also impossible to determine if a change improves system performance since there is no basis for comparison.

We know that what gets measured gets attention. Managers must be certain the critical elements of a system are monitored after measurement is undertaken. When employees know that certain elements of their job will be measured and evaluated and their job security or pay may be determined by their performance, they pay extra attention to these tasks. The downside of this enhanced focus could be that other necessary but less rigorously reviewed operations will be slighted. The challenge to management is to improve elements of a system without creating problems in other parts of the organization. Managers must evaluate and act on information generated from all the vital operations of the organization and should not let themselves fall victim to tunnel vision. The organization could perfect performance in one area (such as timeliness) but lose customers as higher valued activities (such as effectiveness) languish.

The mission of an organization is its reason for being. An organization's mission should state who is to be served and how they will be served. Organizations without direction or purposeful action will be unable to compete with organizations that target the same customers, know how they are performing, and have informed management that can capitalize on the strong points of the organization and minimize or eliminate their weaknesses. A lack of effective management will lead to the production of goods and services that will be less desirable than the offerings of more capable competitors. In the long run, the ability to measure and manage performance will determine which organizations thrive and which will wither and die.

Quality Pioneers in Health Care

Ignaz Semmelweis (1818–1865)

Throughout history physicians and medical workers have been concerned about the quality of care and the well-being of their patients. However, concern and control were left up to the individual provider and there was little formal comparison of results. One of the first physicians to challenge this system was **Ignaz Semmelweis**. Semmelweis, a Hungarian working in Vienna, noticed a substantial difference between the mortality rates for two obstetric clinics operating within the same institution. Mortality rates record the number of patients dying as a percentage of total cases and are one measure of health care quality.

Semmelweis observed that the mortality rate of the clinic staffed by physicians was 9.9% over a six-year period and death was frequently the result of puerperal fever, while the clinic staffed by midwives had a mortality rate of 3.3%. Table 1.1 shows the rate over six years, and Semmelweis noted that actual deaths in the physician-staffed clinic were *higher* than reported, as many dying patients were transferred from the clinic to the hospital and their deaths were not included in the clinic totals (Semmelweis [1860] 1983, 64). The difference of roughly one death in every 10 patients in the physician-staffed clinic versus one death in 25 patients for the patients treated by midwives led Semmelweis to ponder the cause of the radically different outcomes. The high mortality rate in the physician clinic was known among the general public, and Semmelweis stated that he witnessed expectant mothers begging to be treated in the midwife clinic ([1860] 1983, 70). Women also delayed their arrival to the physician clinic for treatment, preferring to give birth outside the hospital.

Ignaz Semmelweis
a Hungarian physician who championed anti-sepsis procedures and demonstrated lower mortality rates due to hand washing

Table 1.1   Clinic Mortality Rates, 1841–1846

	PHYSICIAN CLINIC			MIDWIFE CLINIC		
Year	**Births**	**Deaths**	**Rate**	**Births**	**Deaths**	**Rate**
1841	3,036	237	7.8%	2,442	86	3.5%
1842	3,287	518	15.8%	2,659	202	7.6%
1843	3,060	274	9.0%	2,739	164	6.0%
1844	3,157	260	8.2%	2,956	68	2.3%
1845	3,492	241	6.9%	3,241	66	2.0%
1846	4,010	459	11.4%	3,754	105	2.8%
Total	20,042	1,989	9.9%	17,791	691	3.9%

Source: I Semmelweis, [1860] 1983, *The Etiology, Concept, and Prophylaxis of Childbed Fever,* The University of Wisconsin Press, Madison, WI, 64.

As in the midwife-staffed clinic, the rate of puerperal fever in patients delivering outside the hospital was considerably lower than in the physician-staffed clinic. The prevailing medical opinion was that these deaths were caused by atmospheric-cosmic-terrestrial factors that were beyond human control. Semmelweis demonstrated that these factors could not explain the higher mortality rates in the physician-staffed clinic compared to either the midwife-staffed clinic or street deliveries, as these births were subject to the same atmospheric-cosmic-terrestrial conditions. The different mortality rates, combined with the death of one of his colleagues who was cut with a scalpel during an autopsy and the fact that mortality rates increased when Semmelweis, who performed extensive autopsies, replaced a physician who did not place the same emphasis on postmortem study, led Semmelweis to attribute the higher mortality rates to physicians moving between tasks and patients without washing their hands (Carter and Carter 1994). Semmelweis's chief concern was moving from the autopsy room to delivering babies without washing.

In May 1847 Semmelweis instituted a policy of hand washing in chlorinated lime before delivering babies, and the mortality rate in the clinic staffed by physicians was reduced to 2.38%. This success was short-lived as the mortality rate increased after a new group of medical students was introduced to the hospital. Semmelweis, fearing that the new students were neglecting to wash their hands between tasks, began a program of publicly displaying the names of students and patients so those who neglected to wash could be identified by their higher mortality rates. Semmelweis's efforts again led to a reduction in the mortality rate (Carter and Carter 1994).

The medical community remained skeptical despite his better outcomes, and he was drawn into a power struggle in Vienna that culminated in him not being reappointed to his post. Semmelweis returned to Budapest and was appointed director of a small maternity facility that had recently had a rash of puerperal deaths; again he instituted a policy of washing in chlorinated lime, and mortality rates fell (Carter and Carter 1994). He later replicated his success at the University of Pest, where he was appointed professor of obstetrics. But success in three institutions did not sway the larger medical community (Carter and Carter 1994).

Many physicians were skeptical and dismissive of Semmelweis's conclusion that failure to wash as doctors moved from one medical procedure to another was connected to the higher mortality rates. Physicians were comfortable with their belief that they were doing everything in their power to assist their patients and that these deaths were beyond control. The failure of his colleagues to recognize the fact that the so-called uncontrollable factors producing death had been controlled led Semmelweis to publicly attack his colleagues. His perceived erratic behavior resulted in his forced confinement to a mental institution in 1865. During a struggle with asylum guards he sustained internal injuries and a wound that became infected. He died August 13, 1865. The year of Semmelweis's discovery was 1847, before germ theory was posited. Joseph Lister would later give Semmelweis substantial credit for his development of germ theory, stating "without Semmelweis, my achievement would be nothing" (Lienhard).

Semmelweis's story points out some of the essential ingredients of quality improvement. The first is the ability to quantify outcomes. Semmelweis was trained in statistics, and his training led him to calculate mortality rates. The second is the ability to identify a problem (or opportunity for improvement). The opportunity to compare mortality rates across clinics led Semmelweis to conclude that outcomes were significantly different. After reaching this conclusion, his focus changed to identifying the cause of the difference and determining if outcomes could be improved. Given his hypothesis that it was the actions of the providers that were introducing puerperal fever to patients in the obstetric clinic, he needed only to explore means of avoiding this exposure. Armed with prior outcomes, an identified potential cause, and a remediation method, the next step was to test the hypothesis and avoidance mechanism to determine if the problem had been correctly specified. Unfortunately for thousands of patients, Semmelweis's superior performance was unable to move a medical profession that was not ready to accept that simple hand washing could lead to improved patient outcomes.

Florence Nightingale (1820–1910)

Florence Nightingale
an English nurse known for improving medical services of the British Army, improving conditions of workhouse infirmaries, and formalizing nursing education

Although Semmelweis's contributions were not fully recognized, others began to take a similar approach to medical care. Among the most famous is **Florence Nightingale**. Nightingale noted in the Crimean War the high mortality rate among soldiers brought to the field hospital. However, her journey to the field hospital merits attention. Nightingale was born into an upper-class English family in 1820 and as a young woman struggled against both her family's and society's expectation of the role of a young woman. Her choice of nursing was universally denounced in her family, as hospitals were known as dirty and deadly places and nurses were often characterized as drunken and promiscuous.

Due to her drive, by 1854 Nightingale had established herself as one of the foremost experts in England on hospital construction and operation. She was selected to supervise female nurses in the Crimean War after a series of articles in *The Times* on the treatment of British wounded led to a public outcry. By 1855, Nightingale had cut hospital deaths from 32 percent to 2 percent by improving the food, water, and clothing provided to patients, reducing overcrowding, and ventilating the wards (Winkelstein 2009). Others estimate that deaths fell from 42.7 percent to 2.2 percent (Neuhauser 2003).

One of Nightingale's biographers described the health system of the British army as one that "killed energy and efficiency, crushed initiative, removed responsibility and were the death of common sense" (Woodham-Smith 1951, 99). In this system, Nightingale was given the task of improving the health of the British soldier and the title of Superintendent of the Female Nursing Establishment in the English Military Hospitals in Turkey. This title, however, allowed the military bureaucracy to deny her authority to improve conditions in the Crimea since her authority was limited to Turkey. After the war, Nightingale continued to be impeded by active and passive resistance from policy makers, and even after government officials were replaced with persons sympathetic to her goals, she continued to face resistance from the military bureaucracy.

Like Semmelweis, Nightingale found that the path to improved health care required stirring up vested interests. Nightingale subsequently attempted, with Dr. William Farr, to improve health care service in all English hospitals by publishing mortality rates. In a book published in 1871 Nightingale, like Semmelweis, published mortality rates in maternity wards. She noted that mortality appeared related to the number of patients housed in the same room: 8.0 deaths per 1,000 when there were eight beds per room, 3.4 per 1,000 when four per room. She also documented 193.7 deaths per 1,000 in a hospital in Paris that housed maternity patients with medical and surgical cases (Woodham-Smith 1951, 305).

Nightingale was active in improving sanitary conditions in India, upgrading the conditions in workhouse infirmaries in England, and establishing a nursing school to enhance the skills and status of nurses. Reform in each case struggled against the established order. Hospitals, the military, the infirmaries, and the Indian authorities, who were all used to being accountable only to themselves, did not appreciate seeing their outcomes published for the rest of the world to view. The release of data was met with the only-too-common criticism that the numbers were wrong and the statistical methods were unsound. Fortunately, the attempts of opponents to change the debate from the quality of medical care to the soundness of the statistics were not successful.

While Nightingale often expressed frustration over the pace and extent of improvement, it was clear that her efforts brought great improvements for the often overlooked members of society. Nightingale's work stressed the need to collect data; her work followed the requirements of quality improvement in that she observed conditions and speculated on what would improve outcomes. She wrote, "The most important practical lesson that can be given to nurses is to teach them what to observe—how to observe—what symptoms indicate improvement—what the reverse—which are of importance—which are of none—which are the evidence of neglect—and of what kind of neglect" (Nightingale [1859] 1992, 105). A second lesson that can be drawn from Nightingale's work with the British army is the need to reform the administrative system before quality issues can be addressed.

As in Europe, medicine and medical school training was undergoing a transformation in the United States in the mid-19th century. The rise of science was pushing medical schools to lengthen their degree programs and supplement their basic science requirements (Starr 1982). In 1876 the Association of American Medical Colleges was formed with the goal of standardizing medical education. Restructuring of American medical education reached a threshold in 1893, at **Johns Hopkins**. Hopkins that year required four years of training and an undergraduate degree for admission to its medical school. These changes, combined with licensing changes, put downward pressure on the number of U.S. medical schools. Table 1.2 demonstrates that the number of medical schools continued to increase until 1906 and contracted thereafter.

Johns Hopkins
an American school of medicine credited with establishing rigorous training standards for physicians

Table 1.2 Number of U.S. Medical Schools

1850	42
1870	75
1890	133
1906	160
1910	131
1915	95

Source: P Starr, 1982, *The Social Transformation of American Medicine*, Basic Books, New York, 42, 112, 118, 120.

No discussion of the evolution of American medicine is complete without mentioning **Abraham Flexner's** report titled "Bulletin Number Four" (1910). Flexner, funded by the Carnegie Foundation, issued a scathing report on the quality of medical skills. An earlier AMA report concluded that of the 160 schools existing in 1906, 82 were rated A, 46 B, imperfect but redeemable, and 32 C, beyond salvage (Starr 1982, 118). The AMA report was not published, due to professional ethics, but led to the Flexner report,

Abraham Flexner
educator who reformed medical education in the United States

which judged medical schools more severely. Although this study continues to be heralded as the point of change in American medicine, one can see reform had begun in the 19th century and the number of U.S. medical schools had peaked prior to the release of Flexner's report.

Ernest Codman (1869–1940)

The evolution of medical education introduced into the medical system a new breed of physician who wanted to apply scientific principles to medicine. At the forefront of this group was **Ernest Codman**. Codman graduated from Harvard Medical School in 1895 and immediately began to systematize how he practiced medicine. Codman recorded the number of deaths occurring during anesthesia and believed medical practice could be improved by examining these deaths. To his dismay the primary reaction to these deaths among the surgeons he worked with was that death was an accepted, perhaps inevitable, part of treatment. Undeterred and unwilling to accept operating room deaths as inevitable, Codman began to chart anesthesia deaths and work toward reducing mortality rates. In 1914 he claimed there were no anesthesia deaths at his End Result Hospital (Codman [1914] 1996, 139).

Ernest Codman
an American physician known for championing long-term follow-up of patients, peer comparison, and public release of medical results

His **End Result Idea** became the compelling passion of his life. The End Result Idea was that all patients should be followed long enough to determine the outcome of medical care. In his initial work with anesthesiology, Codman was not satisfied with the conclusion that treatment was unsuccessful; instead, he wanted to know why the patient died and what could be done to prevent future deaths. The End Result Idea required long-term follow-up to determine not simply whether the treatment was successful but also whether the patient's life improved as a result of treatment. Unfortunately, health care has focused on the easier-to-measure treatments than on impacts, and this choice has undermined the drive for health care improvement.

End Result Idea
belief that all patients should be tracked for at least one year to determine the outcome of care

The End Result Idea, in addition to requiring postdischarge patient tracking, included peer comparisons and the public release of results. Peer comparison would allow physicians to understand how their outcomes stood in comparison to other practitioners. Codman hoped peer comparison would lead providers with substandard results to discover the source of outcomes and undertake improvement. Public release of results was advocated to enable patients to make more informed choices when selecting a provider, spurring further improvement. Obviously public release of medical outcomes threatened individual physicians as well as the medical profession as a whole. While Codman is often heralded as the father of outcomes management, none of Codman's ideas was widely accepted by the medical establishment, and he found himself at odds with the generally accepted way of doing things. Codman believed that objective evidence was the only way to evaluate performance and that subjective factors that constituted most performance evaluation systems were merely the outdated remnants of a system that science had rendered obsolete.

Codman's opposition to promotion based on seniority rather than competency led him to quit his job at Mass General; he reapplied based on the superior outcomes he had achieved and was rejected. Undeterred, he opened his End Result Hospital in 1911 in Boston and issued annual reports each year documenting his successes and failures. His hospital closed in 1917 after the Halifax Harbor disaster, which killed roughly 2,000 people, when he chose to go to Canada with his staff to provide medical care to the injured.

Codman never reopened his hospital due to his commissioning in the U.S. Army during World War I. After the war, he would go on to establish himself as an expert in bone sarcoma and publish the definitive study on the shoulder (published in 1934). By the time of his death he was widely recognized for his efforts toward improving health care, and his fame has grown with time. The idea that patients should be tracked after treatment to determine the long-term effectiveness of treatment remains underutilized, however. Codman was concerned that given the emphasis on short-term results, a "physician might dupe a patient with kind words and unnecessary operations without worrying about the ultimate outcomes" (Crenner 2001, 228).

One can see Codman's foresight in reports of the mortality rate of bariatric surgery. Consider the commonly reported bariatric mortality rate of 0.5 percent. When the mortality rate is measured at one year, the rate for men between the ages of 65 and 74 is 12.9 percent, and 51.0 percent for men over 75 (Flum et al. 2005). John Wennberg cites similar statistics in prostatectomy: in-hospital mortality rates are 1.2 percent, 4.0 percent after three months, and 40.0 percent for one subgroup (Wennberg 1984).

These statistics demonstrate that the questions we do not ask often have a significant effect on the information we receive and use. Recent government attempts to publish the outcomes of cardiac surgery were also met by fierce medical opposition, which convinced New York to end its reporting efforts. One can see that the efforts and ideas of Semmelweis, Nightingale, and Codman have been incorporated into routine medical practice and benefited patients, but in a larger sense their ultimate objectives have yet to be fully realized. The ideas of establishing a firm scientific basis for medical practice, standardizing practice, and establishing accountability remain works in process.

Codman is the direct forerunner of the Joint Commission, which accredits many health care organizations. In 1912 the Clinical College of Surgeons of North America formed two committees. The first was to organize the American College of Surgeons. Codman was named chair of the second, to form a Committee of Standardization of Hospitals. The committee was formed to evaluate the quality of medical care and was eventually subsumed by the American College of Surgeons. In 1951, the Hospital Standardization Program merged with groups from the American Hospital Association, American Medical Association, and others to form the Joint Commission on Accreditation of Healthcare Organizations (Mallon 2000), whose standards will be discussed in upcoming chapters. In 2007, the organization shortened its name to the Joint Commission.

Requisite Skills for Improving Health Care

There are two skills required to improve health care delivery. The first is medical. Health care cannot be delivered by those who are unfamiliar with medical science (anatomy, biology, chemistry, and physics) and medical technology (equipment and pharmaceuticals). Health care deals with systems, bodily and medical, and practitioners must understand each. The second set of skills is analytical, which deals with determining how a system should work by examining its performance over time or relative to other systems. Practitioners must be concerned with the processes and systems that are established to perform work and achieve goals. Analytical skill requires the ability to organize data to discover commonalities and to develop plans to improve the performance of systems.

The ability to quantify results derived from groups of patients is essential for evaluation and improvement of care. The first duty of physicians, nurses, and other providers is the care of individual patients, so it is fitting that their education devotes the majority of time to building medical skills. However, it is clear that medical education should devote more time to dealing with patient populations and systems as society demands greater accountability and as insurers and payers increasingly apply quantitative techniques to evaluate patient care. Given the entry of insurers and payers into medical decision making, it is imperative that health care workers become knowledgeable of analytical techniques and capable of applying these techniques to their work. Providers who fear that third-party involvement in medical decision making will detract from individual care must understand that the emerging population perspective is designed to improve the health of patients. Population-based analysis is not a threat to the patient-physician relationship but rather a means of ensuring that patients and physicians have access to the best medical information. Dr. Codman noted that some physicians trust their individual experience more than the history of mankind. Codman, on the other hand, recognized that the basis for knowledge is not a single case but rather accumulated experience (Codman [1914] 1996).

Table 1.3 Essential Ingredients for Quality Improvement

1.	Data collection
2.	Data comparison (benchmarking)
3.	Hypothesis
4.	Testing

The essentials for quality improvement shown in Table 1.3 parallel the elements of the scientific method: observation, hypothesis, prediction, and testing. The scientific method begins with the observation of phenomena and with curiosity; that is, after observing phenomena the viewer asks what accounts for the outcomes observed. Hypothesis arises from curiosity and from attempts to explain the phenomena by building a plausible model of factors that could produce the outcome observed. After a tentative explanation is determined, the third step is to predict future events. If the explanation is valid, it should be able to predict future outcomes; in health care if treatment is effective, future outcomes should improve. The fourth and final step is to build an experiment to test the hypothesis. To improve health care quality, we must implement similar systems to ensure that predicted interventions can be tested to determine if they actually improve patient outcomes.

Evolution of Production Processes

The modern scientific method was developed by the 17th century, coinciding with the rapid transformation of production processes. Understanding this transformation helps us understand the current state of health care and where it may be headed. Four distinct stages have been identified for production processes since the 17th century: **cottage industry, mass production**, **process improvement**, and **mass customization** (see Figure 1.1). In a cottage industry workers use their own tools, production takes place in workers' homes, there is limited capital investment, each product is unique, and workers provide their own direction. This system had significant drawbacks including high cost, low **output**, and poor quality.

The 18th century saw a shift away from home production in many industries. Home production was replaced by factories that were built with large capital investment and that relied on new sources of power (for example,

---

cottage industry
a production system in which workers use their own tools; production may take place in workers' homes, there is limited capital investment, each product is unique, and workers provide their own direction

mass production
a production system designed to produce large volumes of standardized products using standardized and capital-intensive processes

process improvement
a production system designed to improve products by identifying and eliminating errors and defects

mass customization
a production system aimed at producing unique, low-cost, and high-quality products for customers

output
the products produced or the services rendered by a system

Cottage Industry →	Mass Production →	Process Improvement →	Mass Customization
Era: Pre 1800	1801	1931	1974
Innovator:	E. Whitney	W. Shewhart	Burger King
Innovation:	Interchangeable Parts	*Economic Control of Quality of Manufactured Product*	"Have it your way"

Figure 1.1 Evolution of Production Processes

steam and hydraulic). More important than these physical changes was the shift to **accountability**, **authority**, and **standardization**. Workers could no longer set their own hours, determine what they would do, or evaluate their own performance. Integrated mass production systems required work to be performed at certain times. Workers were given a limited set of tasks to perform, and their performance was judged by a third party. Mass production reached its high point with Henry Ford's invention of the assembly line. Mass production greatly expanded output and provided consumers with higher-quality goods and services at lower prices.

As output and quality improved with mass production, the increasing wealth of the United States made consumers more quality conscious. That, combined with Japan's drive to improve the competitiveness of their products on world markets after World War II, led productive processes into a third era: process improvement. The emphasis in process improvement is on improving the performance, durability, and reliability of products. Process improvement shifted producer focus from providing low-cost products to those with both low cost and high quality by instituting processes to identify and eliminate errors and, later, by improving systems to reduce the probability of errors. With the energy shocks of the 1970s, Japanese automobiles began their rapid infiltration into U.S. markets since they were more fuel efficient, had fewer defects per vehicle, and outlasted American-made autos. U.S. manufacturers began to see that their position on world markets was not guaranteed, and they instituted a series of programs—**continuous quality improvement (CQI)**, **total quality management (TQM)**, and Six Sigma among others—to enhance the desirability of their products.

Some producers have evolved from process improvement to mass customization. In mass customization the goal is **efficient** and **effective** customization of products and services that incorporate the features desired by individual buyers and that can be produced at a low cost while meeting quality standards. Customization harks back to cottage industries,

accountability
the obligation to explain one's actions and decisions

authority
the power to make decisions, judge performance, and initiate action

standardization
(1) in products, the production of nearly identical products with interchangeable parts; (2) in processes, the establishment of designated operations

continuous quality improvement (CQI)
a quality philosophy that emphasizes ongoing incremental changes to an organization's products and processes to increase customer satisfaction

total quality management (TQM)
a quality philosophy recognizing customer satisfaction requires superior performance from all aspects of an organization and thus management and improvement efforts must focus on and control the entire range of operations

efficient
utilizing the minimum amount of inputs to produce an output

effective
producing the desired outcome

in which workers would produce a unique product for a particular purchaser. This flexibility, however, came at a high cost in terms of price, ease of repair, and quality. Mass production, with its labor specialization, mechanization, and standardization of components, allowed cost to be driven down dramatically, thus expanding access to products to millions of families, but it was often seen as a one-size-fits-all mentality. Henry Ford famously summed up this attitude by stating that car buyers could have any color they wanted as long as it was black. In his case, the desire to keep Model T costs low trumped the desire of consumers to purchase cars of different colors.

Mass customization combines the best of unique, cottage-industry products with the advantages of mass production to produce custom products for a purchaser at a low cost with consistently high quality. Mass customization allows customers to select the features of the product they wish to purchase. For example, BMW advertises that a customer can select from 10 million options, and the Mars company allows purchasers to imprint M&M candies with their own sayings. The key to success in mass customization is the ability to modify a production process so it can produce high-quality custom products quickly and efficiently.

Where does health care lie along this continuum? Because health care relies extensively on the judgment of physicians, many aspects of health care reflect a cottage-industry model, especially in that medical practice is a profession that establishes its own standards and monitors its own performance. With the rise of medical science in the 19th century and the rapid increase in technology, some aspects of health care shifted to hospital settings, where specialization of labor is practiced and providers use vast amounts of capital in treating patients. The current emphasis on quality improvement in health care grew out of the work of Avedis Donabedian in the 1960s. Donabedian's work (1988) is discussed in Chapter Two. Thus, health care today incorporates aspects of cottage industry, mass production, process improvement, and mass customization. However, I place health care into the cottage industry category. I believe, like Codman, that improvement cannot occur until authority is spread beyond physicians; self-policing does not and cannot work. Mass production requires that someone other than the producer of a good or service evaluate the product. Codman noted that the reported outcomes of medical practice cannot be the sole domain of medical practitioners and suggested that a third party (Codman recommended a lay member of the hospital board) is required to validate the accuracy of these reports.

Quality Control in Industry

Walter Shewhart (1891–1967)

Semmelweis, Nightingale, and Codman highlight the two essential ingredients required to improve quality in health care: the ability to use statistics to identify an area for improvement and medical knowledge to discover solutions. The towering figure in applying analytical skills to quality improvement in industry is **Walter Shewhart**. Shewhart joined Western Electric in 1918 and worked on improving the reliability of their manufacturing processes.

Shewhart realized that all processes are subject to two types of **variance**: natural and assignable. Natural variation is the result of normal fluctuation in performance while assignable variation is due to special causes and signaled a movement away from normal performance. Shewhart's innovation was the creation of a system that could be used by assembly-line employees, workers whose skills lie outside the field of statistics, to distinguish between the two types of variation. Shewhart's **statistical process control** (SPC) charts will be introduced in Chapters Six through Eight to demonstrate how his work can be used to monitor health care processes.

Shewhart demonstrated that performance improvement required workers in a system to be able to differentiate the two types of variance that affect output. Assignable variations—changes in performance away from historical experience that may arise from poor performance or a change in the system—had to be distinguished from natural variance, which is always present in a process. Recognizing assignable variation is essential to knowing when corrective action is required to restore historical performance. Assignable variation signals the operator to investigate why performance is changing and to rectify problems as they arise.

On the other hand, implementing corrections when a system is operating with only natural variance, that is, within the range of performance it has historically operated in, can interfere with performance and reduce quality. Shewhart's work was designed to identify when a system had changed or was moving in a direction that would degrade output. Prompt recognition of assignable variation gives workers a tool to respond quickly to changes that could degrade output and minimize or eliminate problems.

Shewhart also developed the **Plan-Do-Check-Act (PDCA) cycle**, which specifies a definitive approach to problem solving versus ad hoc and random methods (see Figure 1.2).

Plan: Study system, identify problems or opportunities for improvement, and formulate corrective actions for problems or enhancements for improvements.

Walter Shewhart
a pioneer in quality management who distinguished natural and assignable variation, developed statistical process control, and championed the PDCA cycle

variance
the distribution of a variable around its mean

statistical process control
a method of identifying natural and assignable variation based on probability

Plan-Do-Check-Act (PDCA) cycle
a continuous process of examining systems, implementing changes, and evaluating the effect of the change

Do: Implement a small-scale test of proposed correction or enhancement.

Check: Review results of test.

Act: (A) If desired outcome is achieved, implement correction or enhancement across organization; return to Plan and investigate further improvement in same area or focus on new area.

(B) If desired outcome is not achieved, return to Plan: Why didn't the correction or enhancement work? What else can be tried?

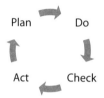

Figure 1.2 The PDCA Cycle

The PDCA cycle is a widely used tool for continuous quality improvement in health care, as workers always return to planning. If improvement or corrective efforts are successful, the PDCA cycle encourages workers to reexamine the system, including other parts of the system, to determine what other improvements can be achieved—improvements that will be valued by customers. If efforts are unsuccessful, a problem continues, or improvement is not achieved, the PDCA cycle encourages workers to return to the original issue and develop other plans to reach their goal.

W. Edwards Deming (1900–1993)

W. Edwards Deming
perhaps the best-known champion of quality improvement, he popularized SPC and PDCA, and identified 14 principles to transform management and the seven deadly sins and numerous obstacles that could derail transformation

inspection
the process of using a second party to review the work of another to determine whether the work meets standards

W. Edwards Deming is among the most recognized advocates, if not the father, of quality improvement. Deming brought Shewhart's SPC work into general use and is widely credited for the economic revival of Japan following World War II. His emphasis on quality led Japan away from inexpensive trinkets to establish it as a world-class producer of electronics and automobiles.

Deming is known for popularizing the PDCA cycle, a Shewhart innovation, and emphasizing the need for continuous improvement. He is also known for his specification of the seven deadly sins that lead to poor quality output. These sins include short-sightedness (focus on short-term profits, counterproductive employee evaluation techniques, and excessive staff turnover) and the lack of discipline or effort (inconstancy and overreliance on easily measured data), all of which inhibit quality work (Deming 1982).

To revive stagnant organizations and improve the quality of output they produce, Deming proposed 14 principles (Deming 1982). Among his principles he suggested moving away from **inspection** toward building quality into the product or service, thus eliminating inspection costs and incorporating everyone into ensuring quality (principles 3 and 14). Deming emphasized that complacency is the enemy; no organization can consider its products to be "good enough," as competitors will perpetually seek advantage in the marketplace by improving products and recognizing changes in customer desires. Organizations must continuously improve to survive (principle 4). Improvement, however, can occur only if employees have the skill required to recognize and act on opportunity. Organizations must institute education programs that can provide the skills needed to maximize the contribution of workers (principles 5 and 13).

Deming suggested that a change in management is required. The function of management should be shifted from oversight to facilitation, and workers should not fear their superiors but see them as partners in the common task of creating the best product for customers (principles 7 and 8). Deming felt slogans should be eliminated; unfortunately the history of quality management has been replete with slogans (for example, "Zero defects") that were unhelpful if not infantile (principle 10). Deming is well known for his assertion that 94 percent of all problems are due to management; that is, to a failure of management to control the system in which employees are working (Deming 1982).

Kaoru Ishikawa (1915–1989)

Kaoru Ishikawa, like Codman, recognized that quality improvement was "too important to be left in the hands of specialists" (Beckford, 1998). Ishikawa is known as the father of the **quality circle**. The quality circle required employees from different operations in an organization to meet to discuss problems. It was designed to break down the silos that develop within organizations, wherein employees are only concerned with what takes place in their area and do not consider the impact their work has on the work of other employees or on customers.

Ishikawa contributed to broadening the view of quality. Quality was not simply the immediate product or service but "after sale service, quality of management, the company itself, and the human being" (Beckford 1998). Like Shewhart and Deming, Ishikawa believed an educated workforce given timely data would be motivated to seek continuous improvement.

Ishikawa also developed **cause and effect diagrams** (also known as Ishikawa diagrams or fishbone charts). The cause and effect diagram is a tool for identifying the cause of problems. Organizations experiencing problems need to identify the problem (that is, the effect) and work backward to identify its cause. The cause and effect diagram guides the examination process and produces an easy-to-understand graphical representation of its conclusion.

Kaoru Ishikawa
quality improvement advocate known for quality circles, cause and effect diagrams, and the view that quality demanded more superior performance in all aspects of an organization and not simply superior goods and services

quality circle
teams of frontline employees assembled to identify production problems and improve operations

cause and effect diagram
a formal means of assembling, displaying, and evaluating the potential causes of a product defect or production problem

The ideas and tools developed by Shewhart, Deming, and Ishikawa are used repeatedly in this book, as the text focuses on the analytical techniques and medical applications that have been used to improve health care outcomes.

Evolution of Quality Management

Ever since people began trading goods and services, craftsmen have sought ways to distinguish themselves from others offering the same products. One way of besting competition is to provide superior quality products. Today we talk of "better, cheaper, faster," but the same three elements of quality, price, and service have always formed the historical basis for competition.

Prior to the industrial revolution, quality was left up to individual craftsmen and customers. The craftsman determined the level of quality he would work to and suffered the consequences of failure if he did not reach the targeted level of quality or if his customers expected a higher level of performance. A more rigorous system to ensure quality was required as the industrial revolution advanced, labor specialization increased, and products became more complex. The production system had to ensure that the work of various personnel seamlessly fit together and that the final good or service met customer specifications.

Inspection was introduced to ensure quality and customer satisfaction (see Figure 1.3). Inspection required dedicated personnel to review the output of a process and determine which products were acceptable to sell and which should be rejected, to be either reworked or scrapped. While inspection is a first step, it has many flaws, the first of which is that accepting or rejecting the final product is very costly. Errors made early in the production process may require substantial reworking of acceptable work to correct the early error, or if the product is scrapped, the organization loses the cost of all resources and effort expended. A second drawback is that inspection is not a value-adding process; it produces nothing. The cost of inspection is part of the total cost of poor quality—this effort and its associated cost would not be required if things were done right. Third, inspection is not perfect; therefore many errors are not caught. Finally, making quality the job of a particular group of employees, the quality control department, often leads other employees to believe that quality is not their responsibility, and to act on that belief.

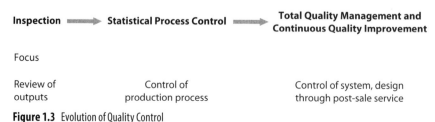

Figure 1.3 Evolution of Quality Control

In the 1920s, Shewhart realized the drawbacks of inspection and developed the more proactive statistical process control. *Process* is a key word, as Shewhart did not want to wait for the completion of a product before determining if it was acceptable or unacceptable. Shewhart's goal was to monitor the production system at various intermediate points to identify when a problem might be arising. If a potential problem is identified, adjustments can be made to the system earlier to ensure an acceptable product is produced and to reduce the number of incorrect outputs and the amount of rework needed to correct the problem. Shewhart's system was designed to be used by personnel on the assembly line. Workers would monitor the system, decide when changes were required, and take the necessary actions to ensure acceptable products were produced without the intervention of supervisory personnel.

Today, quality programs are commonly labeled *total quality management* and *continuous quality improvement*. Quality is now seen as encompassing all aspects of an organization's business, from sales through production and ending with billing and service (versus simply producing an acceptable product). The focus on all aspects of an operation reminds us that it is possible to produce great products and still lose customers. Customers demand more than a good product; they demand to be treated well and want their needs satisfied quickly. Poor service loses customers, and good products are insufficient to ensure success, because other organizations that produce similar products and provide exceptional service will win the battle of the marketplace.

A second major change is that the new quality systems are not content with maintaining quality but strive to continuously improve quality. Statistical process control emphasizes meeting specifications; the new emphasis is to improve products and services to meet changing customer expectations and counter improvements competitors are introducing. Continuous improvement requires an organization to understand its customers, processes, competitors, and evolving technology to ensure its goods and services offer the highest value in the marketplace.

System Thinking

Workers have a tendency to define their tasks narrowly, but quality management requires employees to understand how their performance affects the overall system and the satisfaction of customers. All work is a process, and only by understanding systems will we be able to implement real change—that is, be able to resolve the true causes of a problem rather than merely alleviate the symptoms of problems. This requires **system thinking**.

system thinking
a set of interrelated elements assembled to achieve a goal

input

what enters a system from the external environment; includes labor, supplies, and equipment

throughput

the process of how work is performed or how inputs are transformed into outputs

feedback

information on how a process is performing, which is relayed to the input, throughput, and output processes to improve their performance

Systems are composed of five elements: **input**, **throughput**, output, outcome, and **feedback**, and their performance is affected by what occurs within the organization and by the interaction of the organization with its external environment (see Figure 1.4). Inputs are what enter a system from outside; in health care this includes labor, supplies, equipment, and patients. Hospitals increase the probability of achieving their goals by controlling their purchased inputs (employees, supplies, and equipment) and by extending staff privileges to qualified physicians. Hospitals attempt to identify and use a set of inputs that is most likely to produce the desired outcome. Labor is screened to determine if individuals have the knowledge and skills to successfully complete the tasks they will be assigned. Similarly, supplies and equipment are assessed to determine if they are adequate for the tasks for which they will be used. Inputs that may fail to produce the desired outcome should be identified and eliminated *before* they enter the production system.

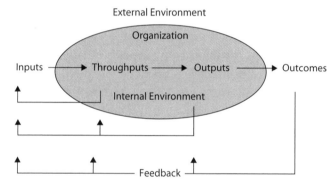

Figure 1.4 The System Model

Unlike labor, supplies, and equipment, a major variable in the production of health outcomes that is less subject to control is the patient. Patients present with a multitude of conditions that affect the probability of successful treatment, but this input and its variability cannot be eliminated. Health care organizations need to identify patient factors that must be incorporated into treatment plans to increase the probability of success. For example, patients allergic to penicillin need to be identified before penicillin is administered and an adverse reaction occurs, or patients admitted with preexisting infections in addition to their admitting diagnosis must be recognized and treated.

Input problems that could prevent the desired outcome from being reached include the use of inferior inputs such as less-skilled labor and low-cost materials or equipment. The use of the wrong inputs in a process may prevent the desired outcome from being achieved and produce harm. For example, in blood transfusions a patient must receive the correct or universal blood type to avoid a hemolytic transfusion reaction, which could result in death. The employment of a spoiled, damaged, or impaired input may similarly have grave consequences. For example, the correct pharmaceutical may have been administered, but its effectiveness could be impaired if it is past its expiration date.

Throughput is the process of how work is performed, or the transformation of inputs into outputs. When a production process is unclear, it is described as a **black box**: an observer can see what enters and leaves the system (the inputs and outputs), but the specifics of the transformation process are unclear. Medicine and education are two black box processes. In medicine, patients enter the system in hopes that they will be released without the problems they had when they began treatment. The process by which a patient is treated is far from a deterministic process and includes dozens, if not hundreds, of tests and procedures. How physicians treat their patient is determined by where they were trained, where they practice, their schedule, the availability of equipment and supplies, the condition of the patient, and the desires of the patients and their families.

black box
a production system
whose internal operation
is unknown

Similarly, students enter the education process with the expectation that they will graduate with more knowledge and new skills, but how knowledge and skills are gained is far from transparent. We see the educator, the textbook, assignments, and tests and student performance on standardized tests, but the process of how a student learns remains unclear. Was learning due to the lectures, reading the textbook, working the assignments, associating with fellow students, or other factors or a combination of factors? The problem in education is that we focus on inputs and outputs and give short shrift to what happens in the transformation process. The educational preoccupation with graduation rates fails to focus attention on what should be the outcome of education: ensuring that students gain the knowledge and skills necessary to be successful in life. This outcome requires educators to assess student postgraduation performance.

Something as seemingly simple as driving an automobile may be described as a black box. A driver may not know how an internal combustion engine works, but he or she knows how to steer, accelerate, and brake. Gas is the input and transport is the outcome, but the driver does not have to understand the working of the pistons or how the transmission operates to move from one place to another. On the other hand, auto production is a white (transparent) box. Each step in the creation of an automobile is sequenced, performance standards are detailed, and performance can be monitored and measured.

Throughput problems include poorly designed processes that may not be capable of producing the desired outcome if followed to the last detail or processes that are susceptible to error. Poorly designed systems increase the probability that employees working within the system will have slips or lapses or make mistakes (Reason 1990). Strong systems reduce the probability that workers will fail to undertake a desired activity, complete tasks, perform to standard, or use the correct process.

Organizations should monitor transformation processes to determine if they are operating in a manner likely to achieve the desired outcome. Monitoring a **white box** process is easier than a black box, as the steps are sequenced and performance standards are clear. In black box systems, such as health care, there is wide variability in how similar patients are treated. Because health care transformation processes vary based on who is operating the system and who is being treated, monitoring performance is a challenge. The difficulty of instituting effective monitoring increases with variability in the system.

white box

a production system whose internal operations are known and can be monitored

Output refers to the products produced and services rendered, for example, tests, procedures, patient days, or discharges. Output is the result of the combination of inputs and how the inputs are manipulated (the transformation process). Potential output problems include bad design, such as that which occurs when the correct inputs are used and they are transformed as expected (the system functions to specifications) but the output fails to meet the use for which it was designed. The output either does not fit with subsequent processes or it is unsatisfying to the customer. A second problem would arise if the wrong output is produced, that is, if the wrong process is used.

Outputs are generally easy to measure and often become the end point in quality control processes. Measuring what is produced is easier than monitoring how it is produced. Health care billing systems generate on a daily basis the number of patients seen, the type and number of tests performed, the type and number of drugs dispensed, and so on, but these outputs do not tell us how many people were involved in the production process, how long production took, or the quality of the output. Did the physician identify and treat the patient's problem? Was the right test ordered and was it performed correctly? Was the right medication prescribed and delivered appropriately? The purpose of medical care is to improve patient health; the purpose is not the production of outputs.

Outcome refers to what is taken away from the system and is the proper measure of performance; for example, has the health status or function of a patient improved? Outcome is the performance of the outputs outside the production process. Did the set of products and services have the desired effect on the patient? When poor health outcomes arise, they may be the result of the care provided to the patient or the result of patient issues, such as an untreatable condition or a lack of patient compliance. In health care poor outcomes arise even if everything is performed according to generally accepted standards. Treatment may be flawless, yet a poor outcome may arise due to idiosyncrasies in how a patient responds.

A prime issue in assessing outcomes is the time frame used for evaluation. Codman pointed out that one year might be the minimum time frame to determine if treatment was successful. Unfortunately most health care organizations evaluate outcomes on much shorter and more arbitrary time frames, typically at discharge. A discharge focus allows providers to assess immediate outcomes but fails to determine if treatment improves a patient's long-term quality of life.

In a properly functioning system, acceptable inputs enter the production system and are effectively transformed into outputs that satisfy a human need or desire. When the desired outcome is not achieved, the problem may have arisen from poor inputs, a flawed transformation process, producing the wrong output or set of outputs, or a combination of these factors.

The fifth element, feedback, is designed to keep a system operating effectively and efficiently by monitoring performance and generating signals to alert those operating the process when the system is not performing as desired. Effectiveness is judged by whether goals are achieved, and efficiency measures whether excessive or unnecessary resources are consumed in the production process. The three feedback loops demonstrated in Figure 1.4 highlight the need for effective and timely feedback. While we would like to think all systems perform in the desired manner all the time (versus according to how they were actually designed and operated), the fact is that errors arise in all parts of a system.

We would like to think that all controllable inputs meet minimum standards, but experience shows that substandard inputs routinely enter systems. Before throughput begins, workers should evaluate the inputs to determine if they are appropriate for the task at hand. If an organization's resources are inadequate for the task, the feedback loop should be used to change the input function: what changes are required to ensure only acceptable inputs are allowed to enter the transformation process in the future?

The transformation process, however, may begin and finish before input deficiencies are recognized. In this case, the defect must be fixed or the product discarded, and a signal must be relayed to the intake process so similar problems are recognized and avoided in the future. The first feedback loop, between throughputs and inputs, is required when problems can be identified in the transformation process. Obviously the sooner a defect is recognized the better.

When problems arise due to inadequate inputs entering the system, the goal is to either screen out substandard inputs or, for those problems that cannot be eliminated, to accommodate them in the transformation process. Accommodation requires the transformation process to be altered to rectify the deficiencies in the incoming inputs. For example, when a patient is admitted with an infection in addition to the primary reason for the admission, additional pharmaceutical orders to treat the infection should be triggered, the patient may have to be placed in isolation, and universal precautions to prevent the spread of the infection to other patients should be implemented.

The second feedback loop connects output to throughputs and input. This feedback loop recognizes that problems may not be detectable until a product or service is produced. Early detection of problems may not be feasible. A physical product or a service may need to be created before problems can be identified, so operators must wait until the end of the production cycle to evaluate the process. In this case the error was not or could not be identified by those performing the work during the transformation process. For example, an x-ray technologist could shoot an x-ray and not recognize that the x-ray does not meet the requirements of the ordering physician or the radiologist. Since early detection is always more desirable, if the x-ray technologist recognizes the x-ray does not meet the required clarity standard, he or she can immediately reshoot the x-ray. If the error is discovered later, the patient must be retransported, the x-ray set up a second time, and a second reading of the x-ray must be performed by the radiologist. These costs can be avoided if the x-ray problem is discovered by the radiology technologist in the transformation process.

When a product or service is lacking or defective, the problem may have arisen from poor inputs, a faulty transformation process, or the production of the wrong output. We may assume that since substandard inputs were not detected during production, we should begin by examining the transformation process. But the question must be asked: Is the product defective as a result of an error made in combining inputs, or perhaps because the wrong output was produced? The problem could be due to any of the three causes, but at this stage the questions are: Why didn't the workers operating the process recognize and correct the defect before completing their work? Why was the process completed and the product passed forward even though there was a problem?

The third feedback loop connects the outcome produced—the ultimate goal of an organization—to all parts of the system. Poor outcomes may result from producing the wrong set of outputs, that is, from delivering the wrong set of services. Errors may also still emanate from problems with throughputs or inputs that were not discoverable until the outcome could be observed. Discovery at the point of outcome raises the question of who discovered the defect: Was it an employee or a customer? When defects are discovered outside the organization, the organization risks alienating and losing customers, who may seek more reliable suppliers. The goal of system thinking is to discover problems as early as possible in the production process to initiate prompt corrective action, avoid poor outcomes, and prevent the problem from appearing in future cases.

The delineation of internal (within the organization) and external (outside the organization) environments emphasizes the fact that organizations should be able to exercise a high degree of control over activities that occur within their system: the intake of input, the transformation process, and the outputs produced. Failure to control these basic components is the basis of malpractice suits. Health care organizations cannot control the external environment, such as patients' behavior before and after they arrive for treatment (input and outcomes), however.

The challenge of controlling systems that function on a case-by-case basis, in which production decisions are made by individual physicians and patients, is substantially higher than those facing a production process in which large lots are produced at a scheduled time with detailed procedures, performance standards, and dedicated quality management staff. Effectiveness and efficiency require control of personnel, maintenance of equipment, availability of supplies, monitoring of output and outcomes, and initiation of corrective action as necessary. Health care has yet to fully incorporate system thinking into its operations, and this failure partially explains why the health care industry measures error rates per hundred while other industries expect rates of less than three errors per one million opportunities.

Summary

This chapter introduced the goals of quality management and how to define quality. Quality was conceptualized as a set of characteristics in which a deficiency in any element is sufficient to undermine the value of a good or service, demanding that producers recognize and control their entire production process. The pioneers in quality management in health care—Semmelweis, Nightingale, and Codman—demonstrated that data collection, data comparison, identifying causes, and developing and testing improvements are essential to improving patient care and showed that one of the largest obstacles to overcome is inertia.

Quality pioneers outside of health care have created multiple techniques to document and improve outcomes, and these advances have led to a rapid improvement in production processes and quality control in other industries. The bedrock of quality improvement in other industries is system theory, which is the ability to view processes as a set of inputs, throughputs, outputs, and outcomes controlled by effective feedback that always keeps in view the goal of the system. It is insufficient to focus on how parts of a system are operating; all parts of a system must be coordinated to achieve a desired outcome. Judgment of system performance should be based solely on how well a system serves its customers or patients. The chapter included a quote from Machiavelli pointing out that change occurs within the confines of existing systems and that change, however well intentioned, will be met with fierce resistance even by people who benefit from the system being challenged. Change will occur only if we can make a compelling case for it, identify what parts of a system need improvement, introduce improvements, and monitor the system to ensure that the new order of things is followed.

KEY TERMS

Accountability	Health care quality
Authority	Input
Black box	Inspection
Cause and effect diagram	Ishikawa, Kaoru
Codman, Ernest	Johns Hopkins
Continuous quality improvement (CQI)	Mass customization
	Mass production
Cottage industry	Morbidity
Deming, W. Edwards	Mortality rate
Effective	Nightingale, Florence
Efficient	Outcome
End Result Idea	Plan-Do-Check-Act (PDCA) cycle
Environment	Price
Feedback	Process Improvement
Five Ds of health care quality	Product
Flexner, Abraham	Quality

Quality circle	System thinking
Selection	Throughput
Semmelweis, Ignaz	Timeliness
Service	Total quality management
Shewhart, Walter	Value
Standardization	Variance
Statistical process control	White box
System	

REVIEW QUESTIONS

1. Define health care quality.

2. Describe the various components that may increase or decrease the quality of a good or service in the eyes of the consumer.

3. What were the common elements that characterize Semmelweis's, Nightingale's, and Codman's attempts to improve health care quality?

4. What two skills are required to improve health care quality?

5. At what point in the evolution of production processes does the health care industry reside? Explain your answer.

6. Explain the five components of a system.

References

Beckford J, 1998, *Quality: A Critical Introduction*, Routledge, New York, NY.

Carter KC and Carter BR, 1994, *Childbed Fever: A Scientific Biography of Ignaz Semmelweis*, Greenwood Press, Westport, CT.

Codman EA, (1914) 1996, *A Study in Hospital Efficiency*, Joint Commission on Accreditation of Healthcare Organizations, Oakbrook Terrace, IL. Citations refer to JCAHO edition.

Crenner C, 2001, Organizational Reform and Professional Dissent in the Careers of Richard Cabot and Ernest Amory Codman, 1900–1920, *Journal of the History of Medicine and Allied Sciences* 56 (3): 211–237.

Deming WE, 1982, *Out of the Crisis*, Massachusetts Institute of Technology, Cambridge, MA.

Donabedian A, 1988, The Quality of Care: How Can It Be Assessed, *JAMA* 260 (12): 1743–1748.

Flexner A, 1910, *Medical Education in the United States and Canada: A Report to the Carnegie Foundation for the Advancement of Teaching*, Bulletin No. 4, The Carnegie Foundation for the Advancement of Teaching, New York, NY.

Flum DR, Salem L, Broeckel Elrod J, Dellinger EP, Cheadle A, and Chan L, 2005, Early Mortality Among Medicare Beneficiaries Undergoing Bariatric Surgical Procedures, *JAMA* 294 (15): 1903–1908.

Goetsch D and Davis S, 2010, *Quality Management for Organizational Excellence*, 6th ed., Pearson Prentice Hall, Upper Saddle River, NJ.

Hayward RA and Hofer TP, 2001, Estimating Hospital Deaths Due to Medical Errors: Preventability is in the Eye of the Reviewer, *JAMA* 286 (4): 415–420.

IOM (Institute of Medicine), 1999, *To Err Is Human: Building a Safer Health System*, National Academy Press, Washington, DC.

Lienhard JH, Engines of Our Ingenuity: Ignaz Philipp Semmelweis, http://www.uh.edu/engines/epi622.htm.

Machiavelli N, (1532) 1992, *The Prince*, Alfred A. Knopf, New York, NY. Citations refer to Martino edition.

Mallon WJ, 2000, *Ernest Amory Codman: The End Result of a Life in Medicine*, W. B. Saunders, Philadelphia, PA.

McDonald CJ, Weiner M, and Hui SL, 2000, Deaths Due to Medical Errors Are Exaggerated in Institute of Medicine Report, *JAMA* 284 (1): 93–95.

Nash, DB, Coombs, JB, and Leider H, 1999, The Three Faces of Quality, American College of Physician Executives, 1999 Winter Institute.

Neuhauser D, 2003, Florence Nightingale Gets No Respect: As a Statistician That Is, *Quality and Safety in Health Care* 12 (4): 317.

Nightingale F, (1859) 1992, *Notes on Nursing*, JB Lippincott, Philadelphia, PA. Citations refer to Lippincott edition.

Reason JT, 1990, *Human Error*, Cambridge University Press, New York, NY.

Semmelweis I, (1860) 1983, *The Etiology, Concept, and Prophylaxis of Childbed Fever*, The University of Wisconsin Press, Madison, WI. Citations refer to University of Wisconsin edition.

Shewhart, WA, (1931) 1981, *Economic Control of Quality of Manufactured Product*, ASQ Quality Press, Milwaukee, WI. Citations refer to ASQ edition.

Starr P, 1982, *The Social Transformation of American Medicine*, Basic Books, New York, NY.

Walshe K and Shortell SM, 2004, When Things Go Wrong: How Health Care Organizations Deal with Major Failures, *Health Affairs* 23 (3): 103–111.

Wennberg JE, 1984, Dealing with Medical Practice Variations: A Proposal for Action, *Health Affairs* 3 (2): 6–32.

Winkelstein W, 2009, Florence Nightingale, Founder of Modern Nursing and Hospital Epidemiology, *Epidemiology* 20 (2): 311

Woodham-Smith C, 1951, *Florence Nightingale*, McGraw-Hill, New York, NY.

CHAPTER 2

ERROR AND VARIATION

Introduction

Is medicine a science or an art? Patients who have suffered through a misdiagnosis or a delayed diagnosis wonder how a capital-intensive industry staffed by some of the most educated people in the world can make such mistakes. The prevalence of **overuse**, **underuse**, and **misuse** in the U.S. health care system strikes hard at the idea that medicine is a science. Brent James (1993) notes only 10% to 20% of health care practice is based on scientifically sound studies and therefore 80% to 90% is based on the traditional approach. James is quick to acknowledge this does not mean 80% to 90% of medical practice does not benefit patients. In fact history shows most of these practices help patients. The point is that the lack of scientific validation encourages different practice styles, which may not result in all patients receiving optimal care.

The source of many problems in health care is treatment variation. Too many health care providers approach medical problems in different ways, resulting in too much care, too little care, poor performance of necessary care, injury to patients, and high costs. This chapter begins by examining the medical decision-making process and **small area variations**, then reviews the quality paradigms of Donabedian and Nash, and concludes with an examination of variation and how it can be managed.

The Medical Decision-Making Process

David Eddy (1990), in the first of a series of articles on clinical decision making, succinctly summarized the key issues and developed a well-known model of the medical decision-making process (see Figure 2.1). He also explored the medical,

LEARNING OBJECTIVES

1. Define the medical decision-making process

2. Understand why and how humans produce error

3. Understand small area variations and their impact on quality assessment

4. Explain the quality paradigm of Donabedian

5. Explain the quality paradigm of Nash

6. Distinguish underuse, overuse, and misuse of care

7. Understand the means to control variance

overuse
the delivery of care when the medical risks exceed the expected benefit

underuse
the failure to deliver medical services when benefits exceed risk

misuse
occurs when a proper medical treatment is selected but a delivery error occurs

small area variations
the variation in the per capita use of medical services within a small area with a relatively homogenous population

David Eddy
author of a series of articles on clinical decision making emphasizing the roles of medical evidence and patient preferences

economic, social, and political implications of medical decisions, which will be further discussed in Chapter Eleven. Health care quality is determined by the decisions made by physicians regarding what actions to take and their execution.

High-quality health care requires selecting the best treatment for a patient and delivering the required care in a timely and effective manner. The desirability of health care interventions should be determined by the benefits and harms of treatment, the expected outcomes and costs, and opportunity costs. While the benefits, harms, and expected outcomes of treatment are standard inputs into a medical decision, providers have not had to deal with larger societal issues such as the cost of treatment or opportunity costs. According to the *Statistical Abstract of the United States*, 2012, in 1960 the U.S. spent 5.3% of gross domestic product (GDP) on health care, roughly one in every $20 earned in the country. In 2009 we spent 17.6%, one in every $5.68 earned. As private and public insurance programs face increasing financial pressure, the issue of limited resources and what will be sacrificed to fund health care will increase public scrutiny of medical processes. The bottom line is that medicine must become more proactive to convince the public that appropriate treatments were chosen and provided. Understanding Eddy's medical decision-making framework is essential for anyone concerned with individual patient care decisions or health policy at the national level.

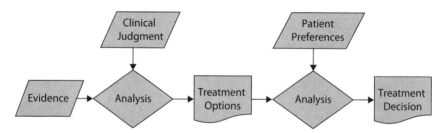

Figure 2.1 The Medical Decision-Making Model

According to Eddy, a practice policy—which treatment should be selected—is the outcome of a process with three distinct inputs and two sets of analyses that produce two conclusions involving providers and patients. The first two inputs to the process start with the physician and concern the existing evidence on disease and injury and the physician's clinical judgment. Information on disease and injury predates recorded history and has grown over the millennia. As of March 17, 2011, PubMed included over 20 million citations (http://www.ncbi.nlm.nih.gov/books/NBK3827). The challenge to providers is to understand the existing body of evidence and stay abreast of new developments while maintaining a practice.

The second input is the providers' clinical judgment. Clinical judgment begins with medical training, where they trained and what they studied, and expands with experience. Where providers practice has a large impact on their clinical judgment as they interact with other providers and adapt to the health care processes used in the organizations in which they practice. The job of physicians is to analyze the evidence and determine, based on their experience, treatments options and possible outcomes of those treatments. At this point they reach their preliminary conclusion.

Once the treatment options and outcomes are determined, a second analysis begins by incorporating the patient's goals and desires. In this process, the physician communicates the possible outcomes, with risks and benefits, to the patient, and the patient and physician evaluate the desirability of each outcome. The process highlights the expansive role that physicians play in arriving at a treatment plan. Physicians must comprehend the medical literature, integrate this knowledge with what they have learned in practice, and combine their medical knowledge with their understanding of each patient. After compiling this information the physician must communicate it to the patient so that the patient can fully understand the implications of his or her treatment decision.

The patient adds the final input, his or her preferences, to the decision-making process. Patient preferences complicate the decision-making process by introducing physiological factors (**comorbidities** and age) that may reduce the likelihood of success of certain treatments and psychological factors (their preference for one type of intervention or nonintervention over other treatments) that reduce the desirability of certain treatments. Psychological factors must be incorporated into the decision-making process as these factors have a direct impact on patient compliance and medical outcomes.

comorbidities
medical conditions unrelated to the primary diagnosis

The outcome of this data collection and analysis process is the medical treatment plan that will be pursued. While the model presents the optimal way to arrive at medical decisions, it is clear the process could not be economically implemented for every case. The problem with this process is it is extremely time consuming. First, there is a huge amount of evidence to weigh and, second, the evidence is often contradictory. Ioannidis (2005) found that 16% of research in frequently cited journals was contradicted by subsequent studies, and another 16% reported stronger effects than could be replicated by other studies. In addition to the existing data reserve, the flood of new articles published monthly is increasing.

In addition to the arduous task of data collection, the physician must weigh the various data sources. Physicians are heavily influenced by where they received their medical training and the peers with whom they interact—both factors expedite the decision-making process. Instead of arriving at a decision on a case-by-case basis, providers often rely on established rules. If Eddy's model were followed for every case, an enormous amount of time would be consumed by physicians describing treatment options to patients and patients attempting to explain their preferences to their doctors. The culmination of the process—attempting to distill the view of the medically trained provider and subjective views of patients into a treatment decision—would be not only time consuming but also difficult. While this process is impractical on a case-by-case basis, it clarifies the essentials of medical decision making. First, decisions should be based to the degree possible on existing medical evidence and, second, the decision should be based on what is important to the patient.

Eddy's model highlights where errors can arise in the process. Misunderstandings of clinical evidence or patient preferences can lead to suboptimal decisions. Practice policies, such as options, guidelines, and standards, are attempts to facilitate the decision-making process by centralizing the data collection and analysis tasks. A centralized body could monitor the literature and distribute practice policies rather than each doctor having to perform these functions. The goal of practice policies is not to usurp physician authority but rather to minimize or eliminate tasks that reduce the time that providers could otherwise devote to treating patients.

Human Error and James Reason

"To err is human." Anyone can observe on a daily basis multiple examples of human error. Understanding *why* humans err is a more interesting pursuit, and understanding why we continue to repeat previous errors is vitally important to quality management. Health care is a labor-intensive industry: it relies on human beings to plan and undertake action to drive treatment. Given health care's reliance on human beings, a review of human error is required. **James Reason** (1990) identifies three types of error: **planning errors**, **storage errors**, and **execution errors**. A planning error is the selection of inappropriate means to pursue an end. That is, the plan of action is unlikely to lead to the desired outcome. A storage error could arise because of interruptions in the production process when there is a lag between the formulation and execution of a plan. Last, an execution error is an effective plan that is incorrectly implemented.

Reason's types of error extend Jens Rasmussen's skill-rule-knowledge model of human behavior. Rasmussen defines skill-based behavior as performance governed by preprogrammed instructions. Reason considers **skill-based errors** to be storage and execution errors and labels these *slips* and *lapses*. Slips and lapses arise from the inattention of workers and may

---

James Reason

author of *Human Error* known for his classification of error types, description of how they arise and may be prevented, and discussion of how people respond to error

planning errors

an error arising from the selection of inappropriate means to pursue an end

storage errors

an error arising from a lag between the formulation and execution of a plan

execution errors

an error arising from the improper implementation of an effective plan

skill-based errors

performance governed by preprogrammed instructions

include double-capture slips (two routines running simultaneously), omissions after interruption, reduced intentionality (forgotten goal), perceptual confusion, and interference. On the other hand, slips and lapses can arise from overattention, leading to omissions, repetitions, and reversals.

Rule-based behavior is performance governed by the classification of a situation. Production in this case requires a worker to categorize a situation and, based on his or her assessment, select a course of action from a menu of choices. The if-then statement is an example of rule-based behavior. If a statement is true, one course of action should be pursued; if a statement is false, an alternative plan of action is appropriate. Performance failure is labeled a mistake, that is, the wrong rule was selected and used for a situation (Reason 1990, 53). **Rule-based errors** arise from misapplication of good rules or application of bad rules. Misapplication of good rules includes first exceptions, countersigns and nonsigns, rule strength, general rules (which are stronger than exceptions), redundancy, and rigidity. Applying wrong, inelegant, or inadvisable rules results from encoding or action deficiencies.

Rule-based errors
misapplication of good rules or application of bad rules

Knowledge-based behavior is performance that is based on the absence of rules and on the ability of a decision-maker to analyze and evaluate a situation and devise action. Knowledge-based behavior is required in rare or unique situations. Similar to rule-based errors, **knowledge-based errors** are labeled mistakes. But knowledge-based behavior is not supported by the level of certainty available to rule-based action. Knowledge-based behavior should be seen as unstructured decision making or operating in uncharted territory. Knowledge errors arise from selectivity, workspace limitations, out-of-sight/out-of-mind, confirmation bias, overconfidence, biased reviewing, illusory correlation, halo effect, causality problems, complexity problems, and delayed feedback (Reason 1990, 69). Knowledge-based errors are problems of bounded rationality; individuals' decision-making processes are limited by the capacity of their minds, the information they possess, and the amount of time they have to work on a problem, which can be severely tested by rare or complex medical conditions.

knowledge-based errors
the inability to analyze and evaluate a situation and devise an effective action plan

A primary difference between rule- and knowledge-based error is information flow. Feed forward—what should be done—is needed to prevent rule-based errors. Feedback—what was done and its outcome—are the control mechanisms required to prevent future knowledge-based errors. To prevent knowledge-based errors, the knowledge base must be continually expanded while good rules, known by the actors, must be in place to reduce rule-based errors.

Understanding types of error and how they arise is an important step toward controlling error. Knowledge of error rates should affect where, when, and how error-reduction initiatives are undertaken; that is, improvement activity should first be focused on areas where the greatest improvements are possible. Reason notes that the absolute number of skill- and rule-based errors exceed knowledge-based errors (1990, 58). This is unsurprising as the vast majority of human activity is based on following instructions and applying rules rather than identifying novel solutions to problems. However, when errors per opportunity, or relative error, is examined the result is opposite: people operating in ill-defined areas produce more knowledge-based errors than skill- and rule-based errors.

Quality management has evolved from attributing error to individuals. The focus is now on the performance of systems rather than blaming one person for a mistake. The system perspective asks whether an error or failure was the result of a single, isolated mistake or whether it arose from a series of problems within the system. Reason defines errors as active (operator) and latent (system) errors and states that latent errors pose the greatest threat to desired performance. Identifying a single error is straightforward, but seldom will correcting a single error prevent reoccurrence. Without systemic change, problems often reoccur with a different set of actors, at another place, or at a different point of time.

Having dissected error, Reason summarizes how people deal with failure; reactions to failure include denial, repair, and reform. Denial involves the refusal to accept the reality of the situation and may involve suppression of facts or encapsulation of the event to minimize its significance, for example, by saying that the error was a rare or special case. A more positive reaction to failure is repair, which recognizes the problem and attempts remediation. Unfortunately, repair often takes the form of fixing the perceived problem rather than the actual problem, for example, a public relations change versus fixing the process. Another inadequate approach is repairing a system problem on a local basis; for example, the remediation is implemented only at its point of origin. The problem with local solutions is that the error can arise in other locations or may arise at the same location at a future point of time.

Quality management requires the third reaction: reform. Reform requires fundamental rethinking and modification of processes. Reason includes reorganization and dissemination under reform. Reorganization requires heeding Einstein's advice: "the significant problems we face cannot be solved at the same level of thinking that created these problems." Dissemination is the second aspect of reform. Instead of preventing the discussion of errors (suppression), organizations must ensure that others are made aware of errors. Dissemination of information may be the minimum obligation we owe to each other as members of the human race, but this minimum requirement is often trumped by fears of embarrassment or a malpractice claim. As noted by the Institute of Medicine (IOM) in *To Err Is Human* (1999) a more conducive environment is needed to encourage health care providers to identify, analyze, and report errors. Dissemination of health care errors will be impeded until a legal environment is developed that fairly compensates patients for injury sustained due to medical error, rather than viewing compensation as an arbitrary, big-money lottery.

Small Area Variations and John Wennberg

One of the earliest attempts to determine if there was an objective standard of medical practice was undertaken by the American Child Health Association in 1934 (Wennberg and Gittelsohn 1973). The association chose 1,000 school children to determine if their tonsils should be removed. The prevailing medical opinion was that approximately 50% of children should have their tonsils removed. The association found 600 of the 1,000 children had already undergone a tonsillectomy. Based on the prevailing medical opinion, one could assume none of the remaining 400 children would require a tonsillectomy.

To test the validity of the prevailing medical opinion and whether there were objective signs indicating the need for a tonsillectomy, the 400 children with tonsils were sent to school physicians for a tonsil assessment. The doctors concluded 45% or 180 of these children should have a tonsillectomy. After this assessment, the remaining 220 children with intact tonsils were sent to other doctors for a third assessment, and these doctors determined that 46% or 101 children required a tonsillectomy. The remaining 119 children with intact tonsils were sent for a fourth assessment, and 45% were identified as needing a tonsillectomy. At the end of the study only 65 of 1,000 children had not been recommended for surgery.

This study demonstrated that medical practice based on established rules of thumb are inefficient and potentially dangerous, exposing patients to unnecessary invasive procedures. In the case of tonsillectomies, it was clear that no objective standard existed to determine when a tonsillectomy was required. In the 1934 study the rate of surgery reached 93.5%.Van Den Akker et al. (2004) reported a tonsillectomy rate in 1998 of 50 per 10,000 persons between the ages of 0 and 14 in the United States. Van Den Akker and colleagues were concerned with differences in the use of medical care across countries. Their study found wide differences in tonsillectomy rates, with a high of 118 per 10,000 persons in Northern Ireland versus only 19 per 10,000 in Canada. Their findings lead to the question raised at the beginning of the chapter: Can medicine be a science when utilization rates for tonsillectomies vary by a factor of six (118 ÷ 19 = 6.21) across countries and when one considers the wide variation in use observed for many types of treatment?

John Wennberg

John Wennberg
medical researcher known for documenting wide differences in utilization of medical treatment across relatively homogeneous populations

John Wennberg is responsible for much of the attention given to differences in the utilization of health care services. His groundbreaking article with Alan Gittelsohn on differences in medical practice patterns did not appear in a medical journal but in *Science* (1973). Wennberg and Gittelsohn learned what earlier pioneers experienced: critical assessment of medical practice is not welcomed with open arms by the medical profession. Wennberg's research destroyed the illusion that medical practice was grounded in science and proved that medical practice was often based on the subjective evaluation of individual providers.

Wennberg and his colleagues set out to determine why medical procedures were used at different rates in different areas. The first article with Gittelsohn documented vast differences in utilization rates, hospital beds, manpower, physicians, and expenditures in Vermont in 1969. Table 2.1 summarizes their findings on the rate of surgical procedures per 10,000 persons.

Table 2.1 Variation in Surgical Rates

Procedure	State Average	Average of Two Lowest Areas	Average of Two Highest Areas	Ratio of Highest to Lowest Areas
Tonsillectomy	43	22.5	118.0	5.24
Appendectomy	18	12.5	29.5	2.36
Hemorrhoidectomy	6	3.0	9.5	3.17
Hernioplasty	41	33.5	47.5	1.42
Prostatectomy	20	12.0	33.0	2.75
Cholecystectomy	27	18.0	51.5	2.86
Hysterectomy	30	21.0	47.0	2.23
Mastectomy	18	13.0	30.5	2.34
Dilation and curettage	55	36.0	124.5	3.46
Varicose veins	12	6.5	26.0	4.00

Source: J Wennberg and A Gittelsohn, 1973, Small Area Variations in Health Care Delivery, *Science* 182: 1105.

Vermont was selected for study due to the availability of data and its relatively homogeneous population. A homogeneous population was sought to minimize differences in health need. Table 2.1 demonstrates that there was substantial variation in the use of surgical procedures despite similar health needs. Tonsillectomy had the greatest variation between high and low utilization; there was more than a fivefold increase in use between the two lowest use areas and the two highest use areas. The magnitude of difference illustrates considerable disagreement among practitioners on the necessity of this procedure. Wennberg and Gittelsohn use correlation to show surgical utilization increased with the number of general surgeons performing the procedure and decreased with the number of physicians who did not perform the surgery. They conclude that variation is an indicator of the uncertainty within the medical profession over the effectiveness of health services. The high variation in the use of tonsillectomies and surgery for varicose veins indicates a lack of medical consensus, while the lack of variation in hernioplasty displays the consensus over its utility.

In 1982, Wennberg and Gittelsohn examined six surgical procedures—tonsillectomy, appendectomy, herniorrhaphy, prostatectomy, cholecystectomy, and hysterectomy—in Rhode Island, Maine, and Vermont. Interviews with patients determined that there was little difference between patients in the number of episodes of acute and chronic illness, income levels, proportion with insurance, or utilization of physician office visits.

They observed that the rate of tonsillectomy varied by a factor of six, which they attributed to the fact that some practitioners performed tonsillectomy for minor inflammation (Wennberg and Gittelsohn 1982). Hysterectomy and prostatectomy rates were about four times higher in high-utilization versus low-utilization areas. Rates of herniorrhaphy clustered between 25 and 35 per 10,000 people and displayed the least variation. The lack of variation was attributed to the fact that inguinal hernia is easy to recognize and treatment is clear. They conclude that utilization and the cost of medical treatment was influenced by the number of physicians, their medical specialty, the medical procedures they prefer, and the number of available hospital beds in addition to the health needs of patients.

This article attributes some of the variation in surgical rates to **practice style**, meaning local surgical patterns exert a strong influence on how physicians practice. Physicians tend to practice medicine similar to the peers with whom they work. Practice style has the largest effect on physician practice when the risks and benefits are least established. Physicians look to their peers for guidance in the absence of medical consensus. On a positive note, Wennberg and Gittelsohn demonstrate that distributing utilization rates to physicians can lead to reduction in use. The effect of peer comparison data can be seen in the rapid decline in rates of tonsillectomy for patients under the age of 20, which fell from 60% to 10% from 1969 to 1973 (Wennberg and Gittelsohn 1982).

practice style
the impact of medical education and colleagues on choice of treatment a physician selects for a patient

Wennberg and Gittelsohn's conclusion, that procedure rates were strongly correlated with the number of surgeons and beds in the area, was controversial due to its insinuation that medical care was based on the desires of providers rather than the needs of patients. Their work is integral to the ideas of **supplier-induced demand** and the **target income hypothesis**. Both ideas hold that medical demand can be created by providers. The target income hypothesis states that providers can increase demand for their own services by influencing patient perceptions of the need for care. Under the target income hypothesis, providers set a desired income level and increase demand if their target income is in jeopardy of being missed due to insufficient demand or reimbursement reductions. The idea that providers may manipulate demand is not new; Shain and Roemer (1959) contended that a hospital bed built is a bed filled. Nevertheless, the idea that health care utilization is determined by anything other than patient need remains a controversial subject.

It is fashionable to criticize the U.S. health care system for its failures, such as supplier-induced demand, but critics often fail to acknowledge that other health systems experience the same or similar problems. In 1982, McPherson et al. decided to determine if other countries experienced the same rate of variation as the United States. Similar to Wennberg's earlier study, they decided to analyze rates of tonsillectomy, appendectomy, hernia repair, hemorrhoidectomy, prostatectomy, and hysterectomy in 18 hospital services areas in New England, 21 districts in England, and 7 hospital service areas in Norway.

McPherson et al. (1982) found appendectomy was the only procedure where average utilization was lower in the United States than in England or Norway. Appendectomy was also the procedure with the lowest rate of variation within a country. More typical was prostatectomy. New England had the highest use per 100,000 population, which was similar to Norway, but England had significantly lower rates. On the other hand, hysterectomy rates were lowest in Norway, English rates were twice that of Norway, and New England rates were five times higher.

While the rates of use in England and Norway were lower than New England for six of the seven procedures, large variation in use was seen in all countries. Variation was independent of how health care systems were organized and how services were financed; that is, there was no difference in variation between national health systems and a decentralized system (McPherson et al. 1982).

In "Dealing with Medical Practice Variations: A Proposal for Action," Wennberg (1984) examined the medical and surgical admissions that account for more than 50% of all admissions. Table 2.2 classifies admissions by their level of variation across 30 hospital markets, documents the number of conditions in each class, and provides an example of one type of admission. Table 2.2 demonstrates that medical admissions are more variable than surgical cases, but in both categories the number of high and very high variation conditions substantially exceeds low or moderate variability conditions.

Table 2.2 Variation and Hospital Admissions

	Medical Admissions	**%**	**Surgical Admissions**	**%**
Low variation	0	0.0	6	17.1
	None		Atherosclerosis	
Moderate variation	3	7.5	4	11.4
	Acute myocardial infarction		Major bowel surgery	
High variation	23	57.5	12	34.3
	G.I. obstruction		Foot operations	
Very high variation	14	35.0	13	37.2
	Chronic obstructive lung disease		Knee operations	
Total admissions	40	100.0	35	100.0

A second contribution of this article was the comparison of Boston, Massachusetts, and New Haven, Connecticut, which documented that utilization and expenditures increased as per capita beds and personnel increased. Boston had 4.5 beds per capita versus 2.7 in New Haven. The number of medical personnel was almost twice as high in Boston (18.2 per 1,000 residents) versus New Haven (9.5). The result of Boston's greater investment in medical personnel and equipment was that the average Bostonian consumed more than twice as much health care measured in expenditures. More recent studies (Fowler et al. 2008; Sirovich et al. 2006) have not found that higher health care expenditures increase patients' or physicians' assessment of quality, and Baicker and Chandra (2004) conclude that areas with higher Medicare spending had lower quality of care.

When expenditure differences arise, the key question is whether the additional expenditures produce a commensurate benefit; that is, do people who consume more health care services have better health? "Hospital Use and Mortality among Medicare Beneficiaries in Boston and New Haven" (Wennberg et al. 1989) explored the effect of variation on outcomes and health quality. Did Boston, with its higher utilization rates, have better health than New Haven? Wennberg and Gittelsohn in their 1973 paper recognized that differences in health utilization were in fact income transfers from low-utilization to high-utilization areas since both areas paid similar premiums for health care but consumed dramatically different amounts of care.

Wennberg et al. demonstrated that the use of health services was higher in Boston than in New Haven. Per capita admissions were 47% higher, length of stay was 15% higher, Medicare reimbursement per case was 22% higher, and per capita reimbursement was 70% higher. In Boston 65% of all patients were admitted for high-variation conditions, versus 59% in New Haven. Boston admissions also required more days of hospitalization. Despite the higher use of medical services, Wennberg et al. conclude that "there was no discernible difference in survival associated with an 80% difference (adjusted for age, sex, and race) in Medicare reimbursement" (1989, 1172). While there was no difference in mortality rates between the two cities, the authors recognize that mortality is not the sole determinant of quality and that functionality could be higher and quality of life better in the high-expenditure city. On the other hand, quality and functionality could also be lower in the higher-expenditure city.

Wennberg's work highlights many of the issues that should be addressed when health care is evaluated: what is the evidence base for medical practice, what effect does medical training and location of practice have on medical decisions, what is the right level of care, how much overuse and underuse is in the system, what type of care should be closely monitored, does more care equal better care, and should one group of patients subsidize other groups? Part of the problem, according to system theory, is that in an open system there are many paths to reach an outcome, and medicine has many routes to improved health. Figure 2.2 presents a treatment continuum. For some conditions, the only appropriate medical choice is either surgery or medicine. On the other hand, for many conditions there is a large gray area, in which a patient could be successfully treated either way. In the gray area, clarity regarding medical evidence, physician experience, and patient preference is needed to determine which treatment the physician and patient should select.

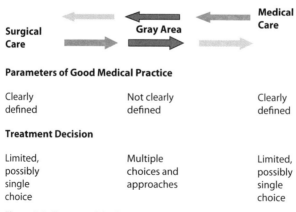

Figure 2.2 Treatment Selection

The issue for quality management is to identify inappropriate use: patients who require medicine but are treated surgically, or patients who require surgery but are treated medically. Understanding medical knowledge and current practice is vital before any change to medical practice can be suggested. The magnitude of the task of understanding current practice is one of the largest factors impeding the establishment of quality standards and systems that have been successfully used in other industries for decades.

Practice Guidelines and Brent James

It remains to be seen if quality management techniques can be instituted on a national, state, or even multihospital basis. Some believe the development of integrated delivery systems will provide a means of instituting quality improvement across institutions. However, as Wennberg and colleagues have demonstrated, the use of medical procedures varies greatly within small geographic areas and physicians located within miles of each other can have distinctly different practice styles. **Brent James** (1993) provides a succinct case study on an attempt to establish clinical guidelines in a single pulmonary ICU department.

Brent James
physician known for advocating greater standardization of medical practice

James describes the process of developing a guideline for adult respiratory distress syndrome (ARDS). This work was motivated by a mortality rate of two-thirds for ARDS patients, a somewhat defined ventilator therapy treatment process that identified high-risk patients (those with a 10% chance of survival), and the development of a new treatment ($ECCO_2R$). One of the first contributions from examining the treatment process was the realization that physicians on the unit did not treat ARDS patients the same. In addition to differences in practice styles between physicians, James noted individual clinicians provided different care for similar patients on different days, and treatment differed between morning and evening rounds.

Inconsistency in treatment rendered it impossible to identify the causes of different outcomes or when modification of treatment improved outcomes. The **randomized controlled trial** (RCT) was developed to avoid this problem. An RCT attempts to hold all variables, save one, constant and evaluate what effect changes in the single variable have on outcomes. When multiple variables are changing, the effect of one variable cannot be distinguished from the effect of the others. The stringent requirements of an RCT cannot be implemented in clinical practice, but James recognized that his first task was to increase the consistency of treatment for ARDS patients.

randomized controlled trial
a study design that assigns subjects to experimental or control groups by chance to minimize selection bias and compare outcomes

James reports that after the differences in treatment were identified, the physicians worked together to standardize the process. The process included reviewing the literature, developing a protocol, reviewing the protocol with all parties, establishing measures, placing the protocol at the bedside, and undertaking retrospective reviews of exceptions. The standardized protocol was subsequently presented to the ICU physicians as a recommendation that they were free to modify as necessary based on their own clinical judgment. As a result, ventilator protocol compliance rose from approximately 50% to 80% or more.

The effect of this initiative was enormous. Patient survival rates increased to 38% compared to 9% to 15% in other institutions (James 1993). Physicians discovered that their time to manage ARDS cases fell as the standardized treatment process reduced the need for individualized and ad hoc decisions. Patients benefited from faster discharges from ICU, and the cost of treatment fell by $40,000.

James's study highlights the fact that variation is the core problem in clinical practice. Variation will always be a major component of clinical practice, but providers need to minimize unnecessary and inappropriate variation. System theory highlights the difficulty that health care professionals have controlling inputs to health care processes and patients' behavior after they leave the provider's care. In addition to exchanges with the external environment, health care has an enormous amount of variation in what is delivered and how it is produced. Assuming that the right diagnosis and treatment are determined, health care must deal with the tremendous variation in how human beings, subject to mistakes, lapses, and slips, complete their work. The point that James emphasizes is that patients, providers, and payers all benefit when inappropriate practice variation is reduced.

The Structure-Process-Outcome Paradigm

Avedis Donabedian receives much of the credit for the current emphasis on quality improvement in health care and is known for his **structure-process-outcome** paradigm. The structure-process-outcome paradigm, first presented in 1966, was a logical attempt to describe the resources and processes needed to produce desirable health outcomes.

Structure identifies the resources available to produce health care; these resources are often things that can be seen and touched. Structure records the attributes of the existing physical and human capital and how these resources are organized. Typical structural measures include the age of the equipment and facilities, the number of employees, the ratio of physicians to nurses, how lines of authority are structured, and how decisions

---

Avedis Donabedian
health care quality advocate known for the structure-process-outcome paradigm

structure-process-outcome
model for examining health care quality by focusing on resources, what is done, and the effects of care

structure
identifies the context in which health care is delivered, what resources are used, and how decisions are made

are made. Donabedian's idea is that organizations with a wider range of more abundant resources, for example, higher-skilled employees and newer equipment and facilities, will be more capable of producing higher-quality health care. Structure deals with the attributes of the health care delivery setting: human resources, materials, equipment, buildings, organizational structure, and so on.

Process examines what is actually done in delivering care, including patient and practitioner activities. Process seeks to determine whether providers are performing their duties according to generally accepted standards: are diagnoses accurate and is effective treatment rendered? Credentialing, board certification, and Joint Commission accreditation are attempts to determine if providers are following generally accepted methods. The logical chain is self-evident: providers who make accurate diagnoses and deliver effective care are likely to produce better patient care.

Process
assesses whether care is delivered according to generally accepted standards

Outcome is concerned with the effects of care on the health status of patients and populations. Outcome attempts to measure the change in a patient's condition following treatment. Typical outcome measures include morbidity and mortality and can include changes in the patient's behavior and satisfaction with care (Donabedian 1988).

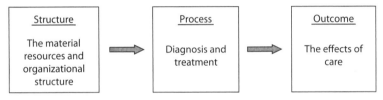

Figure 2.3 Donabedian's Structure-Process-Outcome Paradigm

The weakness in this causal chain is that an abundance of resources does not mean these resources will be effectively used. Similarly, credentialing and accreditation systems can be gamed or can fail to detect questionable practices and providers. Donabedian (1988) recognizes the weak causal relationships among structure, process, and outcomes. Process measures are readily assessable in the medical record but they document mainly medical facts or outputs, whereas outcome is the primary concern of patients, providers, and third-party payers. The outcome is usually known only after an extended period of time, is difficult to obtain, and is determined by many factors that are not under the control of the provider.

David Nash
physician and developer of the Three Faces of Quality that provides a road map for quality improvement in health care

The Three Faces of Quality

Dr. **David Nash** of Jefferson Medical College recognized the weaknesses in the structure-process-outcome paradigm and developed a new paradigm

Three Faces of Quality
system for health care improvement focusing on quality management theory, medical practice tools, and outcomes

in the 1990s, focusing first on the skills and knowledge required for quality improvement and ending with health outcomes. Nash's system consists of three main components, known as the **Three Faces of Quality** (see Figure 2.4): quality management theory, medical practice tools, and outcomes (Nash, Coombs, and Leider 1999a).

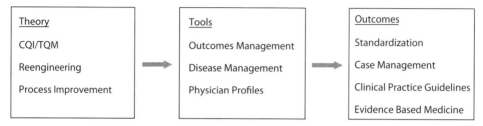

Figure 2.4 Nash's Three Faces of Quality

Quality management theory
body of knowledge that supplies the foundation for quality improvement efforts

Quality management theory emphasizes the need for workers pursuing quality improvement to understand the bodies of knowledge that constitute statistics and quality improvement. Statistics is a field of study dealing with the collection, organization, summarization, and analysis of data and with drawing inferences about a body of data when only a part of the whole is observed. Statistics provides a quantitative foundation for evaluating the performance of systems to determine when change is desirable and recognizes that effective management is possible only with measurement. Different providers will have different outcomes, but at what point do the differences suggest that a treatment process may be flawed and producing suboptimal outcomes for patients? While statistics may never be able to identify poor quality, statistics can suggest which processes or providers should be investigated to determine whether they are producing the greatest benefit for patients. Any determination of inappropriate care must be made by medical providers who understand the medical, biological, and chemical implications of a chosen treatment plan. The use of statistics allows us to focus on those things that may need attention, such as processes or providers with high variation, and not waste time or resources on low variation processes that do not need improvement or alteration.

When statistics identify high and potentially inappropriate variation, they must be confirmed by medical science. The medical staff must investigate the statistical finding of high variation to conclude whether it is inappropriate and could harm patients. Personnel entrusted with ensuring quality must be familiar with the methodology of process improvement. They must know when incremental changes to existing systems should be undertaken, as well as be able to recognize when incremental changes are undesirable and when wholesale change is required.

Quality management incorporates statistics to identify system changes and includes methods to improve the functioning of systems and a set of ideas and tools to diagnose problems. Continuous quality improvement (CQI) emphasizes organization, systems, and processes (versus individuals), recognizes internal and external customers, and emphasizes continuous learning and improvement. Total quality management (TQM) emphasizes the need to monitor and control every transaction, starting with the receipt of resources from suppliers and ending with the delivery of a good or service to a customer. TQM is built on recognizing which aspects of products and services are important to customers and putting systems in place to ensure these features are consistently provided. Benchmarking, the comparison of one organization's processes and outcomes to those of other organizations, is often used to ensure that an organization's product is comparable to those of its competitors or industry leaders.

Medical practice tools are designed to put into the hands of providers information that will allow them to assess their performance vis-à-vis other practitioners and assist them in making medical decisions. Similar to Donabedian, Nash recommends specific instruments such as **outcomes management**, **disease management**, and **physician profiles**. Outcomes management requires establishing systems and standards for monitoring and measuring the quality of patient care based on targeted patient outcomes (Nash, Coombs, and Leider 1999b). Disease management documents generally accepted treatment practices and is designed to inform physicians. Disease management is based on the idea that when large groups of patients suffer from the same disease, taking the time to discover best practices and standardize practice across providers will yield better patient outcomes. Treatment choices that lead to definitive improvements in patient health should be prescribed and not left to decisions of individual physicians and patients. Physician profiles document the use of medical services and compare physicians against other practitioners serving comparable populations. Profiles allow physicians to evaluate their practice and assess whether they are providing too much or too little care relative to their peers.

The goal of medical practice tools is to provide physicians with information to illuminate and guide the health care delivery process. Nash's tools are designed to provide health care providers with information on how they are practicing, best practices, and expected outcomes. With process information, providers will be more capable of assessing their practice and determining when improvements can be made.

The final component of Nash's system is concerned with outcomes of care. Nash again advances our understanding of how better outcomes can be achieved by clearly defining the means to be used to achieve the ends. He

medical practice tools
set of tools to document how care is delivered, provide comparisons to other providers, and supply information to assist medical decision making

outcomes management
a system to monitor and adapt health care treatment to achieve desired, specific patient outcomes

disease management
a system to improve health outcomes for people with specific diseases involving practice guidelines, process and outcome measurement, and patient self-management

physician profiles
a set of measures and benchmarks to evaluate physician performance

evidence-based medicine
the use of the best available medical research to inform medical decision making and treatment

clinical practice guidelines
a scientifically determined set of specifications for the provision of care to typical patients in given disease or injury categories

case management
a system to improve health care treatment for specific patients, typically high-risk or high-cost patients

seeks to establish **evidence-based medicine** (EBM) using **clinical practice guidelines**, **case management**, and standardization. In the evolution of production systems, standardization led to lower-priced and higher-quality products. Standardization is the idea that once the best method for production is determined, it should be followed until a superior process is identified; otherwise standardization will not produce the desired outcome. Standardization is the polar opposite of variation. Although some variation can lead to better outcomes, in many cases excessive variation is the enemy of quality.

Standardization will be achieved by doing the right things in the right situation at the right time. EBM seeks to apply the knowledge gained from randomized clinical trials to medical practice. Nash recommends the use of guidelines and case management to facilitate EBM in practice. His definitions of each tool are aimed at specific actions for specific conditions. Clinical practice guidelines are defined as "a scientifically determined set of specifications for the provision of care to typical patients in given disease or injury categories". Similarly, case management is "an outcomes-driven patient care approach that involves all appropriate health professionals in planning the course and direction of the care program for specific patients and disease or injury conditions" (Nash, Coombs, and Leider 1999b, 17–18). Nash's *outcomes* component also addresses how to implement change and the barriers that must be overcome to change medical practice.

This book follows the Nash paradigm as I believe that without a sound foundation of science and statistics, health care workers will not be able to systematically improve quality. The *tools* component of Nash's system recognizes that even with a firm foundation in statistics and quality management, information must be delivered to individual providers to allow them to compare themselves with their peers and identify where their performance can be improved. The *outcomes* component involves pursuing the goals of standardization and accountability. In the presence of strong evidence of the most effective treatment, society should demand that providers deliver treatment according to the standards of evidence-based medicine. We must develop better systems for capturing the long-term outcomes of care. The simplistic measures now in place, mortality and patient satisfaction, do not do justice to the complex world of medicine, and better measures are overdue. There is a plethora of information available to facilitate many mundane consumer decisions (booking a hotel room, purchasing a car, or selecting a restaurant) but questions of medical treatments and selection of providers are still made with minimal information.

Underuse, Overuse, and Misuse

Dr. Mark Chassin, while at Mount Sinai Medical Center, popularized the widely used categorization scheme for quality problems of underuse, overuse, and misuse; in other words, doing too little, too much, or performing poorly (Chassin 1991). These problems can be viewed from a medical or an economic perspective. According to Chassin, underuse is the failure to deliver medical services when benefits exceed risk. Medical risks include pain and suffering and potential adverse consequences. Examined from an economic perspective, underuse occurs anytime the cost of treatment is less than the benefit of treatment. Economically speaking, underuse arises when preventive care is not undertaken, when prevention is cheaper than curative care, or when restoring the health of a person allows him or her to reenter the workforce and generate income exceeding the cost of treatment.

Overuse is the delivery of care when the medical risks exceed the expected benefit. Prescribing antibiotics for a virus (a cold) is overuse, because antibiotic treatment is ineffectual against viruses, and the overprescribing of antibiotics leads to antibiotic-resistant bacteria. Similarly, exposing patients to surgery or radiation entails real costs that must be balanced against the expected medical benefits of the procedure. When the risk of adverse effects exceeds the expected benefit, overuse has occurred. From an economic point of view overuse occurs when the cost of care exceeds the expected benefit of care. For example, when considering an organ transplant for an advanced-age patient with multiple comorbidities, the probability of success and how long the patient will survive after a successful treatment should be considered.

Misuse occurs when a proper medical treatment is selected but a delivery error occurs. Misuse may diminish or eliminate the expected benefit from the treatment or may harm the patient. Economically, misuse results in the squandering of scarce resources. If the expected benefit is diminished or eliminated, the treatment may have to be redone, essentially doubling the cost of treatment. If remediation of harm is required, in addition to repeating the treatment, the cost may be many times higher than the cost of treatment. The IOM (1999) reports that medication errors resulted in 7,391 deaths in 1993 and increased the cost per case by $4,700.

What is a good measure of quality? Lab tests are judged on their **sensitivity** and **specificity**. A high-sensitivity test produces a positive result given the existence of the disease, and a high-specificity test produces a

sensitivity
the probability of a positive test result given the presence of disease

specificity
the probability of a negative test result given the absence of disease

negative result in the absence of disease. Similarly, a good quality indicator should signal a quality problem, issue, or defect when a medical error has occurred and should rule out a quality issue when no error has arisen. Chassin states that we should not expect perfect measures given the abundance of factors other than medical care that can contribute to poor outcomes. Second, if measuring a process as an indicator of quality, the process must have a proven relationship to a desired outcome. That is, if we improve the process, it will lead to better outcomes. If there is little relationship between the process and the desired outcome, it makes little sense to track the measure. Third, if measuring an outcome to assess quality, the outcome must have a proven relationship with a health care process. In this case good or bad outcomes should be related to the health care delivery process. For example, are poor outcomes related to when the condition was discovered and are screening programs available that could have provided earlier detection and superior outcomes? If screening could have improved outcomes and was not undertaken, we have a legitimate quality issue. If earlier detection would not have improved the patient's prognosis, there is no quality issue.

McGlynn et al. (2003) conclude that only 54.9% of patients received recommended care and that underuse of medical services is a threat to the health of U.S. citizens. Their study documents wide differences in the use of recommended services based on the type of care. One of the chief contributions of the study was its technical appendix (available online). This appendix detailed 30 conditions, beginning with alcohol dependence and ending with prenatal care, and 439 quality indicators. For example, 25 quality measures are provided for asthma. Providers treating patients with asthma could use their indicators to assess their performance: Are they providing these services? If they provide the service, is their performance better than average? (A mean score for each indicator is provided.)

The laudable attempts by the IOM to mandate reporting standards, equality of care, and patient-centeredness overlook fundamental implementation difficulties. In spite of the best intentions of the IOM, a top-down approach seems unlikely to elicit the necessary changes to processes required to improve health care outcomes. The hope that computer systems will somehow overcome information flow difficulties ignores the fact that improved information systems have not been widely implemented within or between health care providers. One of the weaknesses in the IOM approach is its emphasis on national or state-level reports that cannot address issues at the individual or institutional level, where changes to processes must be made.

Controlling Variation and Improving Outcomes

The theme of this chapter is variation. Wennberg and colleagues documented the pervasiveness of variation across time and health systems, and Nash developed a quality paradigm identifying the tools that providers should use to identify and control inappropriate variation in their practices. The final discussion of this chapter will briefly explore how variation can be tackled.

A first step is to identify high-risk patients. These could be patients who have multiple comorbidities or a history of noncompliance. The goal is to identify, before treatment begins, patients who may contribute to high and variable resource use and be at high risk of having a poor outcome. Second, providers should recognize high variability medical conditions and treatments. Medical treatments that have high-variability should be monitored more closely than care that has less variation. Both sources of variability, patient and treatment, can be tackled using a combination of case, disease, and outcomes management techniques.

Third, high-variability providers should be identified. Nash suggests physician profiling so providers can understand how their practice patterns differ from those of other providers. Are there providers whose rates of admission, surgery, and medication are so much higher or lower than those of their colleagues that their patients may be harmed? If the answer is yes, it is the duty of their colleagues and the institutions they work in to determine whether the variation benefits or harms their patients. Wennberg and James were successful in changing provider practice patterns by providing information and collegial dialogue.

A fourth mechanism is to identify outliers. While the first three mechanisms could identify situations in which variation could arise (prospective analysis), the fourth focuses on identifying when excessive variation is already occurring (retrospective analysis). We need outcomes management and clinical variance analysis to recognize when desired outcomes are not being realized or when excessive resources are being consumed. Organizations must have systems in place to identify outliers, to collect, analyze, and learn from patient data the cause of high resource use, and to implement change that reduces the probability that unwarranted variation will reoccur.

Fifth, providers must be given credible and easy-to-use information. The information must not add to the provider's workload but rather must make the practice of medicine easier. Information must supply relevant guidance to providers at the point it is required. Sipkoff (2003) identified nine ways to reduce variation, shown in Table 2.3.

Table 2.3 Controlling Variation

1.	Identify high-risk patients
2.	Provide resource use incentives
3.	Identify and act on outliers
4.	Continuously improve
5.	Implement disease management programs
6.	Provide provider-level information technology
7.	Encourage the practice of evidence-based medicine
8.	Involve patients in care process
9.	Control capacity

Source: M Sipkoff, 2003, 9 Ways to Reduce Unwarranted Variation, *Managed Care*, November 2003.

Variation is a primary determinant affecting patient outcomes and the cost of health care. While the health care industry should be applauded for great strides in medical science, it continues to lag behind other industries in its ability to implement widely used management techniques. Public and political impatience with medical outcomes and costs is increasing. The ability to manage variation will be an important factor in determining whether medicine will continue to direct its own future or be controlled by external forces such as payers or politicians.

Summary

The chapter began with Eddy's model of medical decision making, emphasizing that medical decisions must be technically sound, based on medical evidence and practitioner experience, and incorporate patient preferences. This medical decision-making process parallels the first definition of quality introduced in Chapter One—a measure of the degree to which a good or service meets established standards or satisfies the customer. The vast amount of medical knowledge and the need to incorporate a myriad of patient preferences presents higher challenges to medical providers than those faced by producers of other goods and services. The second topic explored in this chapter was why people make errors. This discussion illuminated the challenges of processes that rely heavily on human behavior and provided a transition to the discussion of variation in health care.

Wennberg and colleagues have documented the wide differences in the use of health care services and challenged the medical profession to justify the differences in use. As James noted, excessive variation makes it difficult, if not impossible, to gauge the effectiveness of health care treatment; when all factors are changing, the positive or negative effect of any one factor on outcomes cannot be determined.

The chapter concluded by foreshadowing the remainder of the text. Donabedian provided one of the earliest attempts to systematize how quality issues should be examined. His structure-process-outcome paradigm identifies key issues and the factors that should be measured and monitored to improve patient outcomes. Nash builds on this model by identifying specific bodies of knowledge that must become part of a practitioner's core competencies and provides a set of tools to facilitate the incorporation of evidence-based medicine into medical practice. Recognizing and responding to variation is critical to quality improvement. Future chapters will expand on quality management theory and tools (Chapters Four through Ten) and medical practice management tools (Chapters Eleven through Fourteen). Before these issues are discussed, Chapter Three will explore various economic and legal issues around health care and health care quality.

KEY TERMS

Case management	Process
Clinical practice guidelines	Quality management theory
Comorbidities	Randomized controlled trial
Disease management	Reason, James
Donabedian, Avedis	Rule-based errors
Eddy, David	Sensitivity
Evidence-based medicine	Skill-based errors
Execution errors	Small area variations
James, Brent	Specificity
Knowledge-based errors	Storage errors
Medical practice tools	Structure
Misuse	Structure-process-outcome
Nash, David	Supplier-induced demand
Outcomes management	Target income hypothesis
Overuse	Three Faces of Quality
Physician profiles	Underuse
Planning errors	Wennberg, John
Practice style	

REVIEW QUESTIONS

1. Using Eddy's decision-making model, what errors can arise to produce an inappropriate or ineffective treatment plan?

2. What are the two essential inputs to a treatment decision?

3. Describe the difference among planning, storage, and execution errors.

4. Provide an example of a skill-, rule-, and knowledge-based failure.

5. Describe the three ways people deal with failure.

6. What is a small area variation?

7. What causes have been identified that contributed to small area variations?

8. Briefly summarize the three major components of Donabedian's structure-process-outcome paradigm.

9. Briefly summarize the three major components of Nash's Three Faces of Quality.

10. What steps can providers take to control variation?

References

Baicker K and Chandra A, 2004, Medicare Spending, the Physician Workforce, and Beneficiaries' Quality of Care, *Health Affairs* (April 7, 2004) doi: 10.1377/hlthaff.w4.184.

Chassin M, 1991, Quality of Care: Time to Act, *JAMA* 266 (24): 3472–3473.

Donabedian A, 1988, The Quality of Care: How Can It Be Assessed? *JAMA* 260 (12): 1743–1748.

Eddy, DM, 1990, Clinical Decision Making: From Theory to Practice: Anatomy of a Decision, *JAMA* 263 (3): 441–443.

Fowler FJ, Gallagher PM, Anthony DL, Larsen K, and Skinner JS, 2008, Relationship Between Regional Per Capita Medicare Expenditures and Patient Perceptions of Quality of Care, *JAMA* 299 (20): 2406–2412.

Institute of Medicine, 1999, *To Err Is Human*, National Academy Press, Washington, DC.

Ioannidis JP, 2005, Contradicted and Initially Stronger Effects in Highly Cited Clinical Research, *JAMA* 294 (2): 218–228.

James BC, 1993, Implementing Practice Guidelines through Clinical Quality Improvement, *Frontiers of Health Services Management* 10 (1): 3–37.

McGlynn EA, Asch SM, Adams J, Keesey J, Hicks J, DeCristofano A, and Kerr EA, 2003, The Quality of Health Care Delivered to Adults in The United States, *New England Journal of Medicine* 348 (26): 2635–2645.

McPherson K, Wennberg JE, Hivind OB, and Clifford P, 1982, Small-Area Variations in the Use of Common Surgical Procedures: An International Comparison of New England, England, and Norway, *New England Journal of Medicine* 307 (21): 1310–1314.

Nash DB, Coombs JB, and Leider H, 1999a, The Three Faces of Quality, American College of Physician Executives, Amelia Island, FL.

Nash DB, Coombs JB, and Leider H, 1999b, Pre-Course Reading for the Three Faces of Quality, American College of Physician Executives, Amelia Island, FL.

Reason JT, 1990, *Human Error*, Cambridge University Press, New York, NY.

Shain M, and Roemer MI, 1959, Hospital Costs Relate to the Supply of Beds, *Modern Hospital* 92 (4): 71–73.

Sipkoff M, 2003, 9 Ways to Reduce Unwarranted Variation, *Managed Care* (November 2003): 27–28, 30.

Sirovich BE, Gottlieb DJ, Welch HG, and Fisher ES, 2006, Regional Variations in Health Care Intensity and Physician Perceptions of Quality of Care, *Annals of Internal Medicine* 144 (9): 641–649.

Statistical Abstract of the United States, 2012, http://www.census.gov/compendia/statab/.

Van Den Akker EH, Hoes AW, Burton MJ, and Schilder AG, 2004, Large International Differences in (Adeno)tonsillectomy Rates, *Clinical Otolaryngology and Allied Sciences* 29 (2): 161–164.

Wennberg JE, 1984, Dealing with Medical Practice Variations: A Proposal for Action, *Health Affairs* 3 (2): 6–32.

Wennberg JE, Freeman JL, Shelton RM, and Bubolz TA, 1989, Hospital Use and Mortality among Medicare Beneficiaries in Boston and New Haven, *New England Journal of Medicine*, 321 (17): 1168–1173.

Wennberg J and Gittelsohn A, 1973, Small Area Variations in Health Care Delivery, *Science* 182, 1102–1108.

Wennberg J and Gittelsohn, A, 1982, Variations in Medical Care among Small Areas, *Scientific American* 246 (4): 120–134.

CHAPTER 3

REGULATING THE QUALITY AND QUANTITY OF HEALTH CARE

Introduction

More health care does not necessarily produce better health, but society often equates more with better. This incongruence is a good way to view the dilemma over health care quality. The health care quality problem is often portrayed as too little care being delivered to patients. On the other hand, overuse of tests and procedures subjects patients to unnecessary and risky treatments, longer stays expose patients to hospital-acquired infection and decubitus ulcers, and overuse of medications leads to dependency and to antibiotic-resistant bacteria. Less can be better.

Medical decision making was discussed in Chapter Two. This chapter begins by contrasting medical and economic decision making. When patients go to a doctor, they expect the physician to engage in **need-based decision making**. Need-based decision making is concerned with the type and amount of care required to treat a condition. This is a technical problem, and we do not expect the physician to introduce into his or her decision the cost of resources that will be consumed, who will pay for these resources, and who will reap income. The **Hippocratic oath** supports this approach by requiring physicians to apply *all* measures necessary for the benefit of the sick.

Economic decision making is based on choice and the explicit recognition that consuming more of one good or service means that less of other goods and services can be consumed. The economist must consider if the value created by a health care expenditure is greater than or less

LEARNING OBJECTIVES

1. Distinguish the difference between medical and economic decision making

2. Identify the role and effects of licensure, accreditation, and credentialing

3. Understand the role and effect of medical malpractice

4. Understand the economics of health care markets

5. Explain how reimbursement influences medical practice

6. Recognize the impact of pay for performance

need-based decision making
medical decision making centered solely on what treatment is necessary for a patient's illness or injury

Hippocratic oath
an oath taken by many physicians and other health care providers to uphold professional standards

opportunity cost
the alternative forgone

than the value of other goods and services including alternative health care services that could be consumed. Economists consider **opportunity cost** rather than need. The crucial question is, what must be forgone when a course of action is taken? A second point of departure between the decision-making processes of physicians and economists is that the physician asks, what is best for my patient? The economist asks, what is best for society?

A physician should decide to use an extremely high-cost medical procedure even if it has a low probability of success. The economist would not evaluate this use of resources by asking if it could benefit the patient but rather if the same expenditure of resources could create larger benefits by being used to produce other goods or services for the patient or other people. Economists ask questions such as, should the use of high-cost curative services be reduced in order to increase the delivery of low-cost preventive services, or should less be spent on health care to expand access to education, improve nutrition, and upgrade housing? The economic question is, will society be better off with a different allocation of resources?

The industrialized countries have debated health care cost, access to services, and quality for decades. The United States spends more on health care than other countries, spending $8,099 per person in 2009 or 17.6% of gross domestic product (*Statistical Abstract of the United States*, 2012). This expenditure means one dollar is spent on health care for every $5.68 of income earned by U.S. citizens. The OECD reports in 2006 the United States spent 15.8% of GDP on health care versus 10.0% in Canada and 8.5% in the United Kingdom (OECD 2009). It is partially due to this massive investment in health care that U.S. citizens question whether the system produces a benefit equal to or greater than the amount of income it consumes. Reports of 46 million uninsured, 44,000 to 98,000 preventable deaths, and international rankings that place the United States in 20th place raise questions as to whether society is receiving its money's worth.

This chapter reviews how the United States has attempted to regulate the quality and quantity of health care services delivered to its citizens. Health care has historically relied on professionalism to guarantee the quality of medical services. Professionalism relies on the members of an occupation to establish standards of behavior and performance, monitor performance, and take corrective action when customers do not receive appropriate service. The underlying assumption of professionalism is that professionals do not need outside oversight and are capable of policing themselves.

The problem with professionalism is that professions often act to improve the welfare of their members rather than the people they should serve. The failures of professions to serve their public result in calls for external review to reduce the possibility that professionals will fail to deliver quality products or harm their clients. The result is that government is petitioned to issue regulations specifying performance and is tasked with monitoring the activities of organizations and individuals to ensure that standards are met. The assumption underlying the **public interest theory of regulation** is that the goals of the public and government regulators are the same.

The **capture theory of regulation** holds that external regulators may be co-opted by those they are supposed to police and fail to serve the public. Part of the problem facing regulators is that they must often rely on information generated by the regulated parties to do their jobs. Regulated parties have an incentive to skew information to their advantage, and regulators may be hard-pressed to identify biased or fraudulent information. A second problem is the revolving door of employment between regulatory agencies and industry. There are many cases in which regulators have been employed by the firms they previously regulated, often receiving salaries many times larger than their public service salaries. The capture theory of regulation holds that regulators work for the benefit of the regulated industry (by restricting competition, for example) rather than the public.

Three main regulatory tools—**licensure**, **accreditation**, and **credentialing**—have been developed to buttress professionalism and enhance quality. The underlying assumption of these tools is that there are measurable standards individuals and organizations should meet that demonstrate their ability to deliver safe and effective care.

public interest theory of regulation
the idea that regulation is instituted for the protection of society and not particular interests

capture theory of regulation
the idea that over time regulation ceases to protect society and is continued in order to serve the regulated entities

licensure
the process by which an individual or organization obtains a permit to provide a good or service

accreditation
the process of determining whether hospitals and other health care entities are complying with professional standards

credentialing
a process used by hospitals to determine whether physicians are qualified to perform the tasks for which they seek staff privileges

Licensure, Accreditation, and Credentialing

Occupational Licensing

States have the legal right to restrict access to occupations such as medical practice and nursing. State occupational licenses are designed to protect consumers from harm caused by unqualified practitioners. The goal of professional licensing is to prevent harm to patients by restricting the ability to perform defined medical activities to providers who demonstrate minimum standards of competence. States have the ability to establish standards, require minimum levels of qualifications and competency, collect license fees, and impose other requirements for the safety of the public (Pozgar 1996).

For example, as of 2011 North Carolina lists 194 jobs requiring licensure, starting with acupuncturist and ending with well contractor. While many occupations are health care–related, there are many others, including barber, cemetery salesperson, cosmetologist, manicurist, and taxidermist, for which the necessity of licensing to protect the public is unclear (NCDOC).

One problem with licensing is that states typically delegate responsibility for setting standards and testing competency to the profession. In medicine, state medical boards set the standards, determine which individuals demonstrate minimum competency, and authorize physicians to practice. Although the state issues the license, those who receive licenses are regulated by the profession.

Another drawback of licensing is that it is mainly an entry-level restriction. Once licensed, few lose their license. Medical science continues to leap forward at an astounding rate, and providers' knowledge may be outdated in spite of mandatory continuing education requirements. An economic argument can also be made against licensure: In restricting the **supply** of providers does licensing enhance quality, or does it merely increase incomes? Licensing will improve the quality of health care if it increases the competency of providers by ensuring that only the best and brightest practice medicine. On the other hand, if licensing simply reduces the number of providers without improving the quality of the pool of practicing physicians, it could be simply a tool to increase price.

supply
the amount of a good or service that will be produced at various prices

Suspended Licenses

Morrison and Wickersham (1998) report that approximately 10,000 complaints are lodged against California physicians each year, or slightly less than one complaint for every ten physicians. About 80% of claims do not survive an initial review, after investigation another 15% are eliminated from further action, and prosecution is only recommended for one in four of the remaining cases. Five hundred cases are subsequently referred for prosecution, and roughly 250 cases (or 2.5% of the total complaints filed) eventually result in disciplinary action. Given the ratio of complaints to physicians (slightly less than 1:10), approximately 0.24% of physicians were disciplined.

Morrison and Wickersham found that board certification reduces the likelihood that a physician will be subject to disciplinary action. On the other hand, the number of years of practice and specializing in anesthesia increased the probability that a physician would be subject to disciplinary action. Disciplinary actions were deemed the result of negligence or incompetence in 34% of cases, drug or alcohol abuse in 14%, mental or physical impairment in 13%, inappropriate prescribing in 11%, and inappropriate contact in 10% of cases. The most common penalty was revocation or suspension of the practitioner's license, which was subsequently stayed in 45% of cases. Actual revocations were 21% and actual suspensions were 13%.

The study found that roughly 53 physicians had their medical licenses revoked out of the 10,000 complaints, a revocation rate of 0.53%.

A study by Kohatsu et al. (2004) on professional disciplinary action found that males, older practitioners (measured in 20-year increments), international medical school graduates, the non-board-certified, and those practicing in family practice, general practice, obstetrics and gynecology, and psychology were more likely to be disciplined by their state board. The causes of disciplinary action paralleled those found by Morrison and Wickersham: negligence 38%, drug or alcohol abuse 19%, and unprofessional conduct 10%. The most common action taken by the board was probation 34%, followed by public reprimand 22%, surrender of license 21%, and revocation 16%.

Cardarelli and Licciardone (2006) found that years of practice and practicing in the fields of anesthesia, general practice, and psychiatry were associated with higher rates of license revocation. The authors also found having more than one violation doubled an individual's probability of license revocation. Occupational licensing has not been totally effective in satisfying the public's demand for quality or accountability, and state medical boards continue to restrict the information the public can access regarding licensure actions.

Licensing of Facilities

Health care facilities are among the most extensively regulated organizations in the United States (Miller 2006). State governments have police power and therefore the right to regulate health care facilities operating within their state. To ensure that regulations are enforceable, states must provide public notice and an opportunity for comment, and some states require other criteria, such as an economic impact statement. Facility licensing, similar to occupational licensing, focuses on personnel but also covers issues of organizational structure, services offered, equipment and facility standards, safety and sanitation, and record keeping. Multiple states initiated certificate of need (CON) laws to control health care capacity. CON laws require state approval to expand bed count in order to avoid overcapacity, which could stimulate unnecessary **demand** for health care services.

demand
the amount of a good or service that is purchased at various prices

In Texas, the Department of State Health Services defines what a hospital is: a facility with the capability to provide round-the-clock medical care for two or more persons, and a minimum set of medical services, including lab, x-ray, and surgery. The department has developed rules defining minimum standards for procedures, fees, operational requirements, inspection and investigation procedures, construction, fire prevention and safety requirements, and potential licensure actions, including denial, probation, suspension, and revocation (Texas DSHS).

The act of applying for a license is viewed as consent to reasonable searches and gives the state the right to conduct facility inspections. Institutions found deficient must be provided due process; that is, they must be notified of the deficiency and given opportunity to correct it. If the deficiency threatens life or health, a state can immediately revoke a facility's license. Penalties can range from license revocation for serious deficiencies to monetary penalties for lesser violations.

Actions against institutions, such as financial penalties or license suspension or revocation, are rare. The Nevada State Health Division on June 9, 2009, announced that a 95-bed psychiatric facility faced closure due to a patient suicide and three other events over the prior six months. A settlement was announced July 17, 2009, that required the facility to hire a manager to oversee hospital operations and patient safety. A financial penalty of $5,500 was assessed, but it was later credited toward hiring the manager and undertaking training and correction (NSHD 2009). Revoking a facility's license is a last resort, as revocation will have a major impact on the facility's patients and the local community.

Accreditation

External nongovernmental evaluation of hospitals began with the American College of Surgeons (ACS) in 1917 and evolved into the Joint Commission. Accreditation received a large boost when Medicare was enacted and required "deemed status" for hospitals to be eligible for reimbursement. Joint Commission accreditation rendered a hospital eligible to participate in the Medicare program. In addition, Joint Commission accreditation is used by 45 states in their hospital licensing decisions. In 2000, over 96% of hospital beds were accredited by the Joint Commission (Schyve 2000).

The Joint Commission establishes standards and audits health care organizations' compliance with these standards. The standards cover provision of care, treatment, and services (PC); ethics, rights, and responsibilities (RI); surveillance, prevention, and control of infection (IC); medication management (MM); improving organizational performance (PI); leadership (LD); management of the environment of care (EC); management of human resources (HR); information management planning (IM); medical staff (MS); and nursing (NR). The goal of the Joint Commission is to "help organizations identify and correct problems and to improve the safety and quality of care and services provided" (Joint Commission 2009). Historically, the Joint Commission scheduled site visits, giving hospitals time to study the standards and refine their operations, but surveys are now performed unannounced, emphasizing that compliance must be standard operating practice rather than a periodic event. The levels of accreditation are accreditation, accreditation with follow-up survey, contingent accreditation, preliminary denial of accreditation, and denial of accreditation. Institutions receiving accreditation with follow-up survey or contingent accreditation are given 30 days to six months to resolve issues. Institutions receiving preliminary denial of accreditation and denial of accreditation have significant issues that justify denial. In cases of preliminary denial the decision may be appealed (Joint Commission 2012).

The effect of accreditation on quality is subject to debate. Chen et al. (2003) sought to answer the question: Is Joint Commission accreditation associated with compliance to commonly accepted treatment guidelines and patient outcomes? The authors evaluated the treatment variables of the use of aspirin, beta blockers, and reperfusion on mortality. The researchers found no statistical difference in the treatment variables, but mortality rates were lower in hospitals accredited at the highest level and they were higher in hospitals that were not surveyed. Mortality rates were equivalent for hospitals accredited without recommendation, with recommendation, and conditional, according to the pre-2011 accreditation-level categories.

The authors conclude that accreditation had "modest ability to assess the quality of AMI [acute myocardial infarction] care" and "a higher accreditation level was not necessarily a guarantee of higher-quality care or better outcomes in the management of AMI" (Chen et al. 2003). The authors note that the lack of effect could be expected due to a number of factors; the first is standards do not assess day-to-day patient care. How people act while being monitored may differ greatly from how they behave unsupervised. Second, accreditation levels cover substantial differences in performance; for example, hospitals with a single recommendation or many recommendations are accredited "with recommendations." Finally, audits may be influenced by surveyor discretion; that is, different surveyor teams could bestow a different level of accreditation on an institution.

Miller et al. (2005) sought to determine if Joint Commission scores (0–100) were correlated with 15 quality indicators, including various mortality, cesarean section, laparoscopic cholecyestectomy, appendectomy, and cardiac catheterization rates and 18 safety indicators including complications, deaths in low-mortality **diagnosis-related groups** (DRGs), and decubitus ulcers. None of the 15 quality indicators was found to be correlated with the accreditation score.

diagnosis-related groups
a system of reimbursement that pays hospital based on the type of care provided and the severity of a patient's condition

The authors found that 14 of 18 safety indicators were uncorrelated with the Joint Commission score. Two indicators, postoperative respiratory failure and technical difficulty, were positively correlated with accreditation score; as organizational performance improved, accreditation scores were higher. Opposite results were seen for the two remaining indicators, iatrogenic pneumothorax and OB trauma; lower organizational performance was associated with higher accreditation scores. The authors concluded: "at best, we can say that there appears to be no relationship between JCAHO survey results and these evidence-based measures of health care quality and safety" (Miller et al. 2005, 246).

A third study, Thornlow and Merwin (2009), found that infection and bedsores were lower in institutions with higher accreditation scores, while failure to rescue and postoperative respiratory failure were uncorrelated with accreditation level. The authors conclude that infections and bedsores were easy to identify and amenable to commonly known corrective actions and that the need for improvement could be easily conveyed to staff. Failure to rescue and postoperative respiratory failure were not correlated with the institution's accreditation score and require multifaceted strategies that may not be effectively conveyed by standards. The authors divided health care operations into four processes: surveillance capacity (reassessment procedures, safety plans, and assessment of staff competency), assessing patient needs (initial assessment, availability of patient information, medication use), care procedures (infection control, planning and providing care, operative procedures), and measuring processes (education, measurement systems) to assess organizational capacities and their impact on outcomes. The authors found that the rate of decubitus ulcers declined with higher care procedure scores and infections declined with higher assessment scores.

The conclusion that can be drawn is that accreditation does not effectively differentiate health care organizations based on quality. This does not mean that accreditation does not improve quality of care and patient safety but suggests that more effective controls should be developed and implemented.

Credentialing

Assessing the competency of physicians and granting them staff privileges are two ways hospitals regulate the quality of care delivered in their facility. Hospitals are legally responsible for determining that individuals in their facility are duly qualified to perform the tasks for which they are granted privileges. The task of granting staff privileges falls to the credentials committee of the medical staff. Physicians seeking medical staff privileges must provide information on their medical education, internships, residencies, medical licenses, board certification, malpractice coverage, privileges requested, and other data (Pozgar 1996). While hospitals can be sued for failure to exercise due diligence in granting practice privileges, they are also subject to litigation and potential damages if they restrict medical staff membership for reasons other than patient safety. Hospitals can be sued for restraint of trade by physicians who believe their denial of privileges is an attempt by the institution to limit the number of providers offering services to the market.

The key question is: Does credentialing, with its standards for certification, reappointment, and modification of privileges, improve outcomes? Sloan, Conover, and Provenzale (2000) examined hospital credentialing processes across nine measures, including board certification, investigation of complaints, and review of objective performance measures, and assigned a high stringency score to institutions meeting eight or more conditions, medium to those meeting five to seven, and low to those with four or less. The goal of their study was to determine if deaths, complications, and excessive lengths of stay across six medical procedures declined as the stringency of the credentialing process increased.

They found evidence for three procedures in which quality improved with stringency: hip replacement outcomes were significantly better in hospitals with high and medium stringency scores, open cholecystectomy outcomes were better in high stringency institutions, and hysterectomy outcomes were better in medium stringency organizations. The outcomes for three other conditions—laparoscopic cholecystectomy and stomach and intestinal operations—were uncorrelated with the stringency score. The authors conclude that the stringency of credentialing does "not improve outcomes on average."

Malpractice

While accreditation, licensure, and credentialing attempt to prospectively improve the quality of health care delivery, they are not always effective. Malpractice exists to address quality problems when patients are injured. Legal action serves two purposes: first, to compensate patients for wrongful harms and second, to deter similar actions in the future. The threat of a lawsuit and large financial settlement should encourage providers to pay greater attention to their craft and benefit future patients. In 2010, 10,195 malpractice cases were filed in the United States. There has been a strong downward trend in suits filed since 2001, as shown in Figure 3.1.

To prevail in a malpractice case, a patient must demonstrate that there was a duty to care, a standard of care, a breach of the standard, and injury resulting from the breach. A duty to care requires a recognized relationship between a provider and a patient; that is, the provider must have an obligation to treat the patient. A standard of care is the expected conduct

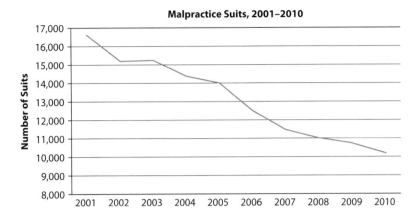

Figure 3.1 Malpractice Suits, 2001–2010

Source: U.S. Department of Health and Human Services, National Practitioner Data Bank 2010 Annual Report, 2012.

of a provider in a similar situation. As noted previously, there is substantial variation in medical practice between geographic areas, so the acceptable diagnostic process and delivery of treatment may be based on a community standard rather than on a national standard. A breach of standard is the failure of a provider to meet the standard of care. Finally, the patient must prove that injury was sustained as a direct result of the failure to meet the standard and was not the result of the natural progression of the disease or injury.

premiums
the payment made in the advance of an undesirable event to insure the payer from loss should the event occur

The high cost of medical malpractice **premiums** has sparked a heated debate between physicians and malpractice attorneys. Attorneys contend that they provide a vital policing function over medical practice and that legal reform would reduce the quality of medical care delivered in the United States. Physicians argue that medical malpractice is reducing the availability of medical services and increasing the cost of health care.

To evaluate these competing claims, we must understand the malpractice process. Localio et al. (1991) reviewed 31,429 hospitalizations and found 1,133 adverse events, an adverse event rate of 3.6 per 100 admissions. Failure rates of this magnitude are not acceptable in other industries, but adverse events cannot be attributed solely to medical malpractice since numerous factors contribute to poor medical outcomes.

Negligence, the failure of a provider to exercise ordinary, reasonable, usual, or expected care, prudence, or skill, was found to the cause of the adverse event in 280 cases, a failure rate of 0.89%. In spite of the fact that the failure rate is documented at less than 1%, it is reasonable to demand better health care from medical providers. It is important to recognize that less than 25% of adverse events, 280 out of 1,133 adverse events, were due to provider negligence. The point requires emphasis: according to Localio et al., more than 75% of adverse events are due to factors other than provider negligence.

A total of 47 malpractice claims were filed, roughly 0.15% (47 ÷ 31,429) of all cases; 39 of these claims were not linked to negligence. Only 8 claims were filed for injury caused by negligence. The probability of being sued for negligence—when a provider should be held responsible and the patient compensated for injury—is very small: 2.9% (8 claims out of 280 negligent events).

Localio et al. found there were almost five times as many claims that involved no negligence as there were for negligence (8 claims filed when negligence was present versus 39 claims against nonnegligent providers). The overwhelming number of malpractice claims filed, 82%, were against nonnegligent providers. The number of unwarranted claims is a major problem. To compound the problem, many of these unwarranted claims prevail in court as sympathetic juries wish to compensate injured patients and ignore the cause of the injury. Localio et al. suggest that the probability of winning a case when no negligence is present is equivalent to the probability of winning when negligence has occurred.

According to this study, the malpractice system is arbitrary; it does not hold negligent physicians accountable, and it penalizes physicians and other medical providers who are not guilty of malpractice. A system that rewards the undeserving, penalizes the innocent, fails to compensate negligently injured patients, and does not hold negligent providers accountable is not meeting the objectives of deterrence or of compensating the injured. Existing systems—licensing, accreditation, credentialing, and malpractice—have not achieved the level of health care quality that patients and society expect.

The Economics of Health Care Markets

The continuing failure of health care to satisfy society's performance expectations and the failure of regulatory and legal systems to enhance quality have elevated economic factors. Health care reimbursement has had a significant effect on how much health care is produced and how it is delivered, but can economic incentives improve quality?

Demand and Supply of Medical Services

People often claim that health care is different from other goods and services. Whether this is true is moot, because society treats it as such. Many say that health care is essential and must be treated differently, but food, which is more vital on a day-to-day basis, is primarily transacted through private markets. If we ask what goods and services are needed or desired to have a "good" life, many people rank education, housing, clothing, and transportation above health care. The result of treating health care as special is that there is little differentiation in health services; we all consume roughly equivalent care. Physicians would be offended if we suggested they treat patients differently based on their **insurance** or payment status. Due to government regulation, patients do not have multitiered consumption opportunities where trade-offs can be made between the price and quality of care such as are available for food, education, housing, clothing, and transportation.

insurance

a contract by which one party in exchange for a premium indemnifies another for loss in the event a specified, insured event arises

Consumers have little choice over how much quality they consume (since physicians act as gatekeepers to services) and because of third-party payment, they generally want the best care. Part of the explosive growth in health care expenditures since 1965 is attributable to the fact that patients use a high level of services and demand top-quality care. Patients would make far different choices if they bore the full burden of their consumption choices. The quality problems in health care involve overuse, underuse, and misuse, and each problem requires a different solution. The systems developed to control the delivery of health care have been strained by attempting to simultaneously manage three interrelated but distinct problems.

The belief that health care is different from other goods and services has created a system in which the purchase of health care goods and services occurs in a substantially different marketplace than other purchases. This chapter will demonstrate that health care consumers and producers face the same constraints on their decision-making processes as consumers and producers of other goods and services. The existence of information asymmetry and third-party payment, however, produces incentives to overconsume and overproduce health care goods and services.

People consume goods and services to improve the quality of their lives; economists say people act to maximize their satisfaction. When the benefits of consumption are separated from payment for the goods and services consumed, individuals can increase their satisfaction by shifting cost to other members of society. Health insurance encourages individuals to overuse health goods and services because the consumption cost is subsidized by employers and taxpayers. Similarly, people produce services to increase their incomes and consume more goods and services. The power physicians have over medical decisions provides them with considerable power to determine the amount of services they produce.

The Decision to Purchase

The question a consumer must answer when making a purchase is not whether the good or service provides greater benefit than the amount of money that must be paid to obtain it but rather whether the good or service provides more or less benefit than other things that could be purchased. When consumers recognize that purchasing one good or service means they must forgo another purchase, they are recognizing opportunity costs. There are an unlimited number of goods and services that consumers believe are worth more than the price they must pay, but they cannot purchase them all with the money they have available. Given a consumer's **budget constraint**, he will buy the set of goods and services that provides him the highest satisfaction (recognizing that if he had more money he could purchase more or better things). The relevant comparison is not goods and services versus money but goods and services versus other goods and services—money is only the medium of exchange.

budget constraint
the amount of money a consumer has to purchase goods and services

Health insurance insulates patients from the total cost of their decisions and encourages excessive utilization of health care goods and services. Economists call this **moral hazard**; consumers who do not have to pay the full price for goods and services will be encouraged to overconsume these items because others are subsidizing their purchase. To understand moral hazard, let us look at a simple market in which consumers must pay the full cost of their purchases and judge the value of goods and services to maximize their satisfaction. The purchase decision made by consumers who must bear the entire cost of their consumption choices is then compared to the purchases made when insurance covers all or part of the cost of consumption.

moral hazard
the tendency for people to demand more of a good or service when the cost of acquiring it is subsidized by others

Demand is the amount of a good or service that a consumer is willing and able to purchase at a particular price. The **law of demand** states that due to opportunity costs and limited budgets people will purchase more of a good or service as price declines. Since economic decisions are based on choice, the buyer asks whether the purchase of one good or service is more important than other possible purchases.

law of demand
consumers will purchase more of goods or services as their price decreases

A **demand curve** displays the relationship between an individual's consumption of a good or service and his or her evaluation of the value of the good or service. The **marginal benefit** received from consuming one unit (or one more unit) of a good or service defines the demand curve. Many people have difficulty with the somewhat nebulous concept of value and are uncomfortable with the idea that what an individual is willing to pay for a good or service is an adequate measure of its value. But price reflects value; people are unwilling to pay more for a good than they believe it is worth. If a good is overpriced, consumers will forgo purchasing the good to increase their consumption of other goods.

demand curve
a graph showing the relationship between the number of units purchased of a good or service and its price

marginal benefit
the additional satisfaction received from consuming one more unit of a good or service

When people are able to obtain a good for less than they are willing to pay, they consider it a bargain. When offered a bargain, consumers often reduce their consumption of other goods to increase the number of units of the bargain good they can consume. People frequently claim that a value cannot be placed on health care, but this assertion is refuted every day when consumers evaluate and purchase the goods and services that provide them with the greatest satisfaction, some of which may not be the healthiest choices. Some contend that everyone should be given all the health care they think they need. The claim that health care should enjoy an uncontested position in society is untenable; individuals and societies routinely restrict their use of health care to increase their consumption of more highly valued goods and services.

A demand curve shows a negative relationship between a good's price and the number of units a consumer will purchase, reflecting the fact that higher quantities of a good or service are valued less by an individual than the prior units consumed. This is logical since the first unit of a good or service is used to satisfy an immediate need or desire. Additional consumption may provide increased satisfaction but is unlikely to be valued as highly as the first unit consumed. Carl Menger (1871) illustrated this idea with water. The first unit of water would be devoted to maintenance of life, that is, meeting one's thirst; additional units would be used to sustain meat- and milk-providing animals; any additional available units would be used for washing; and finally, if any water remained, it would be expended on flowers or companionship-providing animals. Individuals allocate water to their meet their most important need, quenching their thirst, and with a sufficient supply of water will allocate any remaining units to less important uses. The lower perceived value of additional units consumed is called the **law of diminishing marginal utility**.

law of diminishing marginal utility
the decrease in satisfaction from consuming an additional unit of a good or service as more units are consumed

As mentioned earlier, limited budgets are another reason individuals reduce purchases when prices increase. Most consumers have a defined amount of money to spend for a basket of goods including food, clothing, shelter, and health care. When prices increase, purchases must be reduced. Individuals do not want to consume only a single good (or type of good) and so must distribute their budget between goods to maximize their satisfaction. The benefit arising from consuming additional health care must be balanced against other goods that could be consumed with the same dollars. Consumers determine the optimal mix of goods and services to maximize their satisfaction given their tastes, preferences, and budget. The combination of satisfied needs and fixed budgets means that price reductions are required to encourage individuals to consume additional units of a good or service they have already obtained.

The value individuals place on goods and services varies dramatically. One individual may place high value on fashionable clothing, whereas another settles for secondhand clothes and uses their budget for other things. The value of goods varies based on an individual's situation; young, single people may place high value on entertainment, food, clothing, and stylish transportation while older people with families seek safe and comfortable transportation, housing, and health care. Although consumption generalizations may apply to a large percentage of a group, there are always exceptions to the rule, individuals with unique tastes and preferences that vary dramatically from those of other members of their group.

The Demand Curve

A demand curve (D) is the graphical representation of the relationship between the number of units consumed (quantity, Q) and an individual's evaluation of the worth of each unit (price, P). The demand curve shows how an individual's demand for a good changes with price and the maximum price the consumer would pay for additional units of the same good (the marginal benefit, MB). Figure 3.2 shows the demand (or value) an individual places on physician visits in a year. Time is an important element in any consumption decision. As indicated earlier, people's tastes and preferences change over time based on their situation (age, health, income) and alter their consumption patterns. How often a particular good or service is consumed is another important element involving time.

To personalize this example, assume that Figure 3.2 represents the value placed on physician visits by a 30-year-old female without chronic health problems. The demand curve indicates that this individual is willing to pay up to $100 for her first visit to the physician (point A). During the first visit she may receive tests and x-rays to uncover unknown problems, receive medical advice, inquire about any health concerns that have arisen in the last twelve months, and maintain her relationship with the physician.

When a second physician visit is contemplated, the patient may believe the value is lower since many of her concerns were addressed during the first visit. During the second visit, new concerns that have arisen since the first visit may be raised and progress on health and lifestyle goals may be recorded, but the overall value is unlikely to be as great as the first visit. We'll assume the patient places a value of $67 (point B) on her second visit. The demand curve defines how much a consumer is willing to pay to consume a good or service. The value of a third visit, $33, is less than either the first or second visits, and finally, the fourth visit is valued at zero. The demand curve slopes downward, indicating that reductions in price are required to encourage this individual to consume additional units.

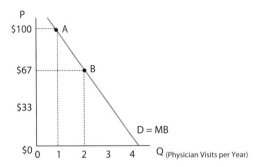

Figure 3.2 Demand for Physician Visits

Some argue against the application of economics to the evaluation of health care, noting that one can neither quantify the value of health nor the value of a visit to the doctor. This is nonsense; people continually make judgments on the value of life and health in their personal lives when they engage in high-risk behavior and in purchasing decisions. Does everyone purchase the safest automobile, or do some buy economy cars and use the money saved for other goods? As members of society, we empower legislators to determine the appropriate trade-offs between safety and cost in the design and construction of highways, acceptable environmental quality, and funding of police, court, and prison systems.

Arguing that every health intervention is vital to maintaining one's health is similar to arguing that water is used only to quench thirst and maintain one's life and thus is priceless. Water is used for trivial purposes; similarly not every health care purchase is vital. If we focus on the value of physician visits, statistics show that not every physician visit is a life-or-death situation. The primary reason for seeking a physician visit is for a general medical exam (59,796,000 visits per year in the United States), followed by progress visits (28,583,000). The third most cited reason was cough (25,735,000 visits). The low-urgency nature of these visits speaks to the fact that these services can be forgone at the discretion of the patient (Woodwell 1999). Patients will evaluate the benefit of a first or additional visit to the doctor against the other goods and services they could consume and select the goods and services that provide the highest benefit.

An elderly person or a person with a chronic condition may place higher value on physician services, thus shifting the demand curve outward (to the right on Figure 3.3). An elderly person with a chronic condition may value his first visit at $150 (point B) versus the $100 that the 30-year-old female was willing to pay (point A). The 70-year-old man may also be willing to pay more for the second, third, and fourth visits and believe it beneficial to consume five or more visits.

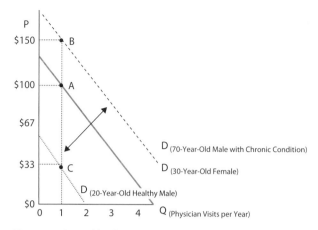

Figure 3.3 Demand for Physician Visits by Different Individuals

Likewise, males, the young, and the healthy may see little advantage to consuming physician services and would rather use their funds to purchase other goods and services. Woodwell (1999) again provides statistical support: 20.7% of males do not seek physician care during the year versus 11.3% of females. Similarly the need for care varies with age and health status: 21.6% of people between the ages of 18 and 44 do not seek care versus 7.3% of those over 65. Of those who described their health as good to excellent, 16.6% do not seek care versus 9.7% of those who describe their health as fair to poor. For the young and healthy the demand curve shifts inward (to the left); this third demand curve shows that a 20-year-old healthy male would not be willing to pay more than $33 for his first visit (point C), would visit a doctor a second time only if the visit was free, and would not consume any additional visits.

Although systematic differences are observed in the utilization of health care services by different members of society, it is impossible for any centralized body to prescribe the correct level of care. Individuals differ greatly in their health needs and in their attitudes toward health care and other goods and services, rendering it impossible for anyone but the individual to define the optimal mix of goods and services that will maximize his or her satisfaction.

The Decision to Produce

So far, the discussion has concentrated on the value a patient places on physician visits. To complete the market, we must consider how physicians decide how much care to produce. Physicians weigh the cost of providing a visit against the income received from providing care. The physician must earn sufficient income to compensate her for her time, training, and practice expenses (staff, rent, supplies, malpractice insurance, and utilities).

As long as what the physician earns equals or exceeds the value she places on her time and what she pays in practice costs, she will provide care. In the extreme case, when reimbursement does not cover her time or practice expenses, she may seek other lines of work. In a less extreme case, the physician may evaluate the cost of additional office hours and, having obtained a reasonable income and met her practice expenses, may choose to engage in leisure activities rather than provide additional care.

The Supply Curve

Assume a physician visit costs $80 to produce, and additional visits neither increase nor decrease in cost. Cost defines the minimum price for the service; hence $80 defines the cost of production and the price to be charged to the patient. The cost and price charged are assumed to include the physician salary, practice costs, and the cost of any tests or procedures incidental to the physician visit. We will assume that $80 is sufficient compensation to induce the physician to provide a normal caseload, typically 107.2 patients in a 52.8 hour week (*Statistical Abstract of the United States*, 2003, 120). Cost defines the **supply curve**. It is assumed that a physician will not produce or sell any visits at a price under her cost of production. The supply curve (S) is horizontal, indicating that the physician will provide additional visits as long as they do not exceed her expected work week. As with other workers, hours in excess of 40 per week may have to be compensated at higher levels to induce the individual to work more. At the point where the provider demands additional compensation to expand her work week, the supply curve would slope upward. We will assume that as long as fewer than 107 patients are seen per week, the price will remain $80.

Figure 3.4 demonstrates the complete market, incorporating the preferences of the consumer and the producer. The demand and supply curves allow us to determine how many visits our hypothetical patient will demand and how many visits the physician will provide at a price of $80.

According to supply and demand, consumers will purchase and producers will sell the number of units defined at the intersection of the supply and demand curves, which establishes the **equilibrium price**. In this case, our patient will purchase and consume one visit per year (demand is rounded down to the nearest whole unit). The value placed by the patient on the first visit is $100 and the physician charges $80; a good or service will be purchased anytime its benefit exceeds or is equal to the price the consumer must pay. The patient is very satisfied since she must pay an amount less than

---

supply curve

a graph showing the relationship between the number of units of a good or service a seller would offer for sale at different prices

---

equilibrium price

the price at which the quantity demanded of a good or service equals the quantity supplied

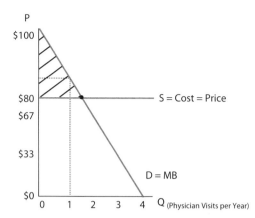

Figure 3.4 The Supply and Demand for Physician Visits

what she is willing to pay to obtain the service, $80 versus $100. Economists call the difference between what a consumer would pay and what they actually pay **consumer surplus** (the cross-hatched area in Figure 3.4).

A second visit will not be purchased, because the price that the patient must pay to consume the service, $80, is higher than its value to the patient, $67. The consumer forgoes the second visit and can now purchase other goods or services that will provide her with greater value. Consumers do not purchase goods and services that cost more than their perceived marginal benefit. The physician could induce the purchase of a second visit by reducing her price to $67, but she would have no need to do so if other consumers are willing to pay $80. Even if there are no additional patients willing to pay $80 for an office visit, the physician might still decline to cut her price and opt instead for more leisure time (a smaller patient load) rather than produce an additional visit and earn $67.

Table 3.1 summarizes the consumer's decision-making process. She will purchase a physician visit anytime value (marginal benefit) is greater than or equal to the price she must pay; each unit of consumption must provide positive net benefit. Conversely, she will not purchase a visit if it provides negative net benefits.

consumer surplus the difference between what a consumer is willing to pay to obtain a good or service and its market price

Table 3.1 Self-Pay, No Health Insurance

Visit	Value	minus	Price	equals	Net Benefit	Purchase?
1	$100	–	$80	=	+$20	Yes
2	$ 67	–	$80	=	–$13	No
3	$ 33	–	$80	=	–$47	No
4	$ 0	–	$80	=	–$80	No
Total	$100	–	$80	= Total Net Benefit	+$20	

Table 3.1 demonstrates that an individual spending her own money will elect to visit a physician one time per year. The second, third, and fourth visits provide less (and declining) benefit than the individual must pay to obtain the service and thus will not be purchased.

Health Insurance and Moral Hazard

The problem with the standard market model is that most patients do *not* purchase health care using their own funds but rely on health insurance to defray the cost in whole or part. How does insurance affect an individual's consumption decisions? If an individual has **first dollar coverage**, insurance pays 100% of the cost of care, and the patient does not have to make any contribution to the services she consumes, other than any premiums she pays. Under first dollar coverage, the patient will choose to consume health care as long as it provides any benefit. In Figure 3.5, the patient chooses to consume four physician visits where her out-of-pocket price, $0, is less than or equal to her perceived benefit.

first dollar coverage
insurance pays all costs for a contracted event; insured pays zero

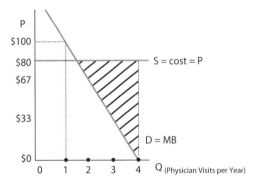

Figure 3.5 Overutilization of Physician Visits

Under first dollar coverage, each visit produces a positive benefit for the patient. She receives $200 in total benefits ($100 + $67 + $33 + $0) with no out-of-pocket cost. However, the costs associated with the four physician visits she consumes must be paid; society pays $320 (4 visits @ $80) to secure our patient's $200 of benefits. This level of utilization produces a $120 loss to society. The problem is clear: if patients do not have to pay for services, they will consume too much care. A fully insured patient will elect to visit her doctor four times and may recognize, but be unconcerned, that the value of consuming these services, $200, is less than their cost of production, $320. It is only because the patient does not have to pay for the services that this level of consumption is rational. A person spending her own money would never purchase a set of goods for $320 that she thought was worth only $200.

The difference between the value to the consumer and the cost of production, −$120, is called a **deadweight loss**. In Figure 3.5 this is the cross-hatched area lying under the supply curve and above the demand curve. The supply curve defines the amount of resources consumed to produce a service while the demand curve represents the value of the service to the consumer. When our patient consumes more than one visit, the cost of production exceeds the benefit received. Deadweight loss is the opposite of consumer surplus. Consumer surplus represents a benefit received without cost to others; deadweight loss is the consumption of resources without the creation of corresponding benefit to the patient or others.

deadweight loss
the excess cost of production over the value created for a consumer

Copayments

One method for controlling utilization is **copayments**. Copayments require patients to pay a percentage of the price of service they consume. In the next example we will assume a 20% copayment; the patient must pay $16 (20% of $80), her out-of-pocket cost, every time she visits the doctor. Unlike Table 3.1, which showed a patient who had to pay the entire price for services received, the net price in Table 3.2 has declined by 80% and increased the net benefit of consumption to the patient.

copayments
a percentage of the price of a good or service that a consumer must pay to consume the product

Table 3.2 Health Insurance with 20% Copayment

Visit	Value	minus	Out-of-Pocket Cost	equals	Net Benefit	Purchase?
1	$100	−	$16	=	+$84	Yes
2	$ 67	−	$16	=	+$51	Yes
3	$ 33	−	$16	=	+$17	Yes
4	$ 0	−	$16	=	−$16	No
Totals	$200	−	$48	=	+$152	

Table 3.2 demonstrates that our patient will purchase physician visits as long as her marginal benefit exceeds 20% of the purchase price. When subsidized at 80%, the patient would choose to consume three physician visits. The copayment continues to encourage overutilization (the total benefit to patient is less than the total cost of production), but it reduces total utilization. The second visit provides less benefit to the patient ($67) than its cost of production ($80) but since the out-of-pocket cost is only $16 and the marginal benefit is $67, the patient will visit her doctor a second time. The fourth visit, however, is not purchased as its value ($0) exceeds her out-of-pocket cost ($16). Copayments discourage patients from seeking low-value care.

Copayments force consumers to recognize part of the consumption cost and consequently they reduce use of services. The unwillingness of the patient to spend $16 to receive the fourth visit saves her $16 and reduces total health care expenditures by $80. Without a copayment, the dead-weight loss imposed on society was −$120 ($200 benefit less $320 production cost). The copayment reduces this loss to −$40 ($200 benefit less $240 production cost), since the fourth and lowest-valued visit is forgone.

The advantage of copayments is they make patients responsible for part of the purchase price and discourage them from consuming to the point where the last unit provides little or no benefit. Table 3.2 demonstrates that individuals will overconsume health care (the value of services received is less than their total production cost) when consumption choices are subsidized by others. This phenomenon is seen in the clockwise rotation of the demand curve in Figure 3.6 that occurs when 80% of the cost of medical care is subsidized by insurance. If an individual believes a service is worth $100, and another party is willing to subsidize 80% of the purchase, the patient would be willing to purchase the service at any price up to $500; the patient's out-of-pocket cost would be $100 or less (20% of $500). Insurance influences **elasticity**, making demand more inelastic: increases in price do not substantially reduce demand (note change in Y scale in Figure 3.6).

elasticity
the percent change in demand divided by the percent change in price

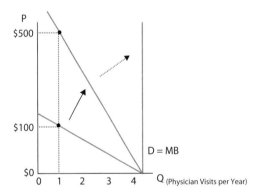

Figure 3.6 The Effect of Third-Party Payment on Demand

Figure 3.6 demonstrates that if an individual has first dollar coverage (is not responsible for any payment toward her medical utilization), the demand curve would be vertical. A fully insured individual would demand the first visit or any subsequent visit, even if it costs $500 or more. When price is no object, neither the patient nor the physician has any economic incentive to restrict health care use. The provider serving a patient with first dollar coverage has an incentive to increase her production costs, price, and number of visits since these costs can be passed on to insurers.

Caveats

The preceding analysis discussed only out-of-pocket costs. In the real world other costs are recognized by patients before they seek care, including how much time is required to locate and obtain care. Longer search and wait times reduce the value of care to the patient and the demand for care and explain why consumers will not demand an infinite amount of a good or service even if their out-of-pocket price is zero. Universal health systems that do not regulate access to care through price, such as the United Kingdom and Canada, rely on waiting lines to reduce their citizens' demand for care. Another cost patients consider in their decision making is the cost of transportation to and from the provider. These other costs reduce the demand for care and explain why our 30-year-old female would refuse to consume more than four visits even if she incurred no out-of-pocket cost.

Recognizing that health care services may create benefits for people other than the patient would justify public subsidies to encourage patients to seek more care. A positive **externality** is generated when one person is vaccinated and his treatment reduces the possibility of passing a disease to other members of society. When positive externalities are present, the social benefits of care exceed the individual's benefit and the demand curve should be shifted outward, increasing the price that consumers (or society) should be willing to pay for care.

externality
a cost or benefit imposed on or received by a person or group that is not a party to a transaction

Supplier-Induced Demand and the Target Income Hypothesis

It is important to remember that one person's use of health care services provides income to another set of people. Under voluntary exchange, the buyer and the seller believe they are better off as a result of the transaction. Buyers purchase goods only when they perceive that the value of the good exceeds the value of the resources they must forgo to obtain it. Similarly, sellers aim to sell products and services for more than their cost of production. Sellers lose money if they overestimate what buyers will be willing to pay and have to sell their product for less than their cost of production.

We have seen that insurance, by separating consumption from payment, encourages patients to overutilize health care services. The second departure from a typical market occurs when patients are not the decision-makers in health care purchases. The problem arises from the technical nature of health care services and the patient's lack of medical knowledge, or **information asymmetry**. The lack of knowledge leads patients to delegate purchasing decisions to their physicians, creating a **principal-agent relationship**. The patient, the principal, recognizes that he does not have

information asymmetry
a situation in which one party in a transaction has superior knowledge to the other

principal-agent relationship
a situation in which one party, the principal, delegates decision-making authority to a more informed party, the agent

sufficient information to make medical decisions, so treatment decisions are delegated to his physician, the agent.

The physician, when acting as a patient's agent, is supposed to make the same decisions the patient would make if he were knowledgeable of the effectiveness of the proposed treatments and any side effects. Medical decisions should not be made based on the preferences of the physician but rather should reflect the values and preferences of the patient. Information asymmetry between the principal and the agent creates another force that creates excessive demand for medical services. The issue is whether a provider will exploit her position as an agent by encouraging patients to undertake treatments to increase her income.

Supplier-induced demand is the label given to actions of agents that exploit their superior knowledge over principals to advance their own interests. The discussion of small area variations in Chapter Two provides support for the supplier-induced demand thesis. Wennberg and others demonstrated in multiple studies that utilization of health care increases as the supply of medical resources increases. Arguments against supplier-induced demand contend that health care resources were concentrated in high-need areas (supply follows demand) or that areas receiving more services had better health (low-utilization areas were underserved), but neither of these possibilities appears to be supported by evidence.

Evidence suggests that health care supply may create its own demand. Areas with a high ratio of beds to population have high admissions rates, areas with a plentiful supply of surgeons have higher surgery rates, and new drugs are developed for the real or perceived needs of the population. The problem is that many patients are not qualified to judge their medical needs or how much health care they should consume. A recent report concludes only 12% of U.S. adults have sufficient health literacy to effectively use medical information (Kohl et al. 2012). Medical questions therefore must be answered by providers, who may benefit from higher health care utilization.

Provider control over demand weakens attempts to control health care expenditures. Typical regulatory attempts to control health care spending involve reducing reimbursement, assuming that the quantity of services will remain constant. But the influence that suppliers exert over demand provides ample opportunity for providers to offset reimbursement reductions. The target income hypothesis holds that a provider wishes to enjoy a certain level of income and will adjust the volume of services he or she provides to generate this income.

Assume that a physician wants to earn an income of $200,000 per year and his sole service is office visits, which are reimbursed at $100 by Medicare. We will also assume that every patient is covered by Medicare.

The physician sees 100 patients per week, has office expenses of $300,000 per year, and works 50 weeks per year. Column 2 in Table 3.3, Baseline, shows that after practice expenses are paid, the physician takes home the desired $200,000.

Now assume that Medicare wants to reduce physician outlays by 10%, so they reduce the reimbursement for office visits to $90. Column 3, 10% reduction in reimbursement, shows our physician's income will be reduced by $50,000 if everything thing else remains constant.

Table 3.3 Impact of Supplier-Induced Demand on Health Expenditures

	Baseline	**10%↓ Reimb**	**10%↓ Reimb w/SID**
Total revenue	$500,000 (100 patients × 50 weeks × $100)	$450,000 (100 × 50 × $90)	$499,500 (111 × 50 × $90)
Office expenses	$300,000	$300,000	$300,000
Physician income (residual)	$200,000	$150,000	$199,500

Column 4, 10% reduction in reimbursement with supplier-induced demand (SID), shows that if the physician can increase by 11% the number of visits delivered, he can essentially eliminate the impact of the reimbursement reduction. The physician could increase visits by seeking additional patients (expand his practice) or by counseling existing patients to have more frequent visits. The regulatory problem is offsetting behavior; the reduction in medical outlays sought by regulators will not occur if producers can take counterbalancing actions.

The problem of controlling utilization in health care markets is largely due to moral hazard and supplier-induced demand. The forces of supply and demand in a typical market work in opposite directions to limit consumption. In normal markets, consumers attempt to limit their expenditures by seeking the lowest-priced good that will meet their needs or desires and purchase only the number of units they deem essential. When purchases are subsidized, consumers become less sensitive to the price and quantity of goods they consume. In many cases, insured patients demand the most expensive care as well as services that may provide little benefit.

Suppliers in normal markets recognize the price sensitivity of consumers and compete for customers by lowering price. Advertising is built on the idea of inducing additional demand by capturing additional customers and reducing price sensitivity. In health markets we have the same tendency to encourage demand, but the desire to hold down prices is absent as providers know that the majority of the cost of care will not be borne by the patient.

A Brief History of Health Care Financing in the United States

In 1960, total U.S. expenditures for health were $28 billion and consumed 5.3% of gross domestic product. In 2009, spending was $2,486 billion and consumed 17.6% of the economy output. In 1960, patients bore 46.4% and government 25.0% of total health care costs. By 2009, out-of-pocket spending had fallen to 12.0%, and government payment accounted for 43.4% of total health expenditures. The massive increase in spending is directly attributable to the ability of patients to obtain subsidized care and to how health care providers are reimbursed for their services.

cost reimbursement
reimbursement system that pays providers for services rendered based on their cost of production

In 1965 Medicare introduced **cost reimbursement** for hospital services delivered to those over 65 years of age. While Medicare was implemented as an outlay-saving measure—the government would not have to fund hospital profits but only the costs of care incurred for their patients—the unintended consequence of this policy was a dramatic run-up in health care costs. Physicians who previously had been circumspect in ordering tests and procedures were encouraged to order freely since Medicare would pick up the cost of care. Medicare in 1967 had expenditures of just under $3.4 million ($3,395,000). By 2009, expenditures stood at $471.3 billion, or nearly $73.4 billion in 1967 terms, an increase of approximately 21,614 times (adjusted for inflation). The rush of revenue into the health system increased access and demonstrated the effectiveness of economic incentives on changing consumer and producer behavior.

The 1960s were an era of unprecedented growth in demand driven by increased access to care and an expansion in the amount of services delivered. It can be called the era of quality, if more testing and services equal higher quality. There is evidence to support this argument as life expectancy in the United States increased from 73.1 years in 1960 to 78.1 in 2006 (OECD 2009), and one can argue that patients who had previously limited their use of care due to out-of-pocket costs now benefited from more tests and procedures and longer hospital stays. Even tests run to rule out disease could be seen as improving medical diagnoses, in addition to alleviating the concerns or fears of patients.

The rapid increase in medical outlays led Medicare to implement diagnosis-related group (DRG) reimbursement in 1983. Under DRG reimbursement, hospitals are paid on a per case basis for inpatient care based on what care should cost versus actual cost. Under cost reimbursement, two hospitals treating a patient with heart failure could receive vastly different payment for the care they delivered, based on their cost. Under DRG reimbursement hospitals should receive comparable payment for comparable care.

The expected cost of care (and reimbursement) in the DRG system was determined by what care was delivered, whether treatment was surgical or medical, the presence or absence of comorbidities or complications, and patient age. Additional payment was given for hospitals situated in high cost of living areas, those treating a high percentage of poor patients, and those training physicians. The primary aim was to pay roughly equivalent amounts for the same care and shift emphasis from input use under cost reimbursement to output under DRG reimbursement. Table 3.4 provides a simplified example of the effect of DRG reimbursement on hospitals.

Table 3.4 Objective of DRG Reimbursement

Cost Reimbursement	Hospital A	Hospital B	Average
Cost	$6,000	$4,000	$5,000
Reimbursement	$6,000	$4,000	$5,000
Net income	$0	$0	$0
DRG Reimbursement	**Hospital A**	**Hospital B**	**Average**
Cost	$6,000	$4,000	$5,000
Reimbursement (based on average cost)	$5,000	$5,000	$5,000
Net income	−$1,000	$1,000	$0

As seen in Table 3.4, hospitals before DRG reimbursement would be paid whatever it cost them to treat a patient and would break even. After DRG reimbursement, hospitals could make or lose money for treating Medicare patients and were incented to reduce the amount of inpatient care provided and its cost; that is, they had an incentive to operate efficiently. Under cost reimbursement, hospital A had no incentive to reduce its costs, whereas under DRG reimbursement the hospital would lose $1,000 per case if it did not improve its care processes.

Medicare was attempting to constrain the explosive growth of inpatient payments by reducing the incentive to overtreat patients. Under DRG reimbursement if too many tests are ordered or patients are retained too long, hospitals will incur a loss on treatment. The effect of DRG reimbursement was a dramatic reduction in length of stay (LOS) and an increase in the reported number of comorbidities and complications treated, which increased reimbursement as more serious cases warranted higher payment.

The shift of Medicare away from cost reimbursement to a methodology designed to control expenditures led other payers to adopt more restrictive

capitation
a reimbursement system that pays providers a flat fee for anticipated treatment; payment is not determined by actual treatment rendered

reimbursement policies, including per procedure, per diem, per case, and **capitation** arrangements. The difficulty for providers is that the different reimbursement mechanisms present different and often conflicting financial incentives, and efforts to achieve higher quality or more efficient operations (or both) could reduce a provider's income.

Reimbursement Methodologies and Operating Incentives

Prior to 1929, patients were expected to pay for the services they consumed at the prices charged by the provider. This pricing system parallels the arrangement between buyers and sellers in most markets. The patient's obligation to pay for the services he consumed created a natural brake on the use of health care services. Rationing care based on willingness or ability to pay encouraged providers to keep their costs low to attract patients.

The problem in an ability-to-pay system is lack of access to required care. With the emergence of Blue Cross in 1929 (Starr 1982) and expansion of employer-provided health insurance during World War II, many workers gained hospital coverage. Hospital coverage was an appropriate event for insurance; it is a low-probability, high-cost event that patients generally do not control. Lack of patient control over use was the direct result of patients being unable to judge their needs or gain access to health care services without the intervention of a physician. Separation of decision making did not unleash high demand until third-party reimbursement reduced or eliminated patient copayments, and insurance expanded to include a range of higher-probability events such as office visits. The expansion of health insurance benefits created an environment in which providers could increase prices and demand for their services without driving away patients, and patients could obtain services at little or no cost.

charge reimbursement
a reimbursement system that pays providers based on the price they charge for services rendered

Under third-party **charge reimbursement**, providers desiring higher revenue simply had to increase prices. Because of advancing medical science, providers could also encourage patients to expand their use of care or render more services per admission or visit. Charge reimbursement encouraged providers to be efficient because any reduction in the cost of delivering care (with constant revenue) would increase the provider's net income. While providers may have felt some compulsion to keep prices low when their patients paid a substantial part of the price of services, this incentive was significantly weakened as third-party payment grew.

Price became less relevant when Medicare introduced cost reimbursement because payment would be based on how much it cost to deliver care.

Under cost reimbursement, provider incentives changed dramatically; raising prices had little impact because cost was the predominant factor affecting revenue. Providers continued to have an incentive to increase demand through higher utilization and to increase the intensity of care provided as each led to higher costs and reimbursement. Cost reimbursement had a negative effect on efficiency because providers had little incentive to lower costs by holding down input costs or reducing unnecessary care. Providers did not have to be concerned with how long it took to perform services (labor hours), wages (the cost per hour), or the number of services performed because increases in any factor increased cost and reimbursement.

When Medicare shifted to DRG reimbursement in 1983, other third-party insurers adopted new payment mechanisms to limit their medical outlays. These payment systems sometimes adopted a Medicare-like system for paying providers on a per case basis while others used a per diem or capitation system. **Per diem reimbursement** pays hospitals on the number of inpatient days used per admission. The goal of this system was to reduce the overuse of inpatient days, tests, and procedures by restricting payment to a set fee per day. Per diem reimbursement encouraged providers to increase efficiency and reduce costs below their per day payment by lowering their use of resources.

Per diem reimbursement
a reimbursement system that pays hospitals a flat fee for every medically necessary day a patient is hospitalized

Hospitals under per diem reimbursement have no incentive to increase prices because the fee per day is fixed and price increases would not increase their revenue. The per day payment was set by periodic (often annual) negotiation between the provider and payer. The only ways to increase revenue in a per diem system are to increase admissions or extend length of stay. Payers were aware of this risk and instituted utilization review to determine if admission was warranted and if continued hospitalization was medically necessary. Insurers would pay for any admissions and inpatient days they deemed medically necessary but denied payment for unnecessary admissions and days and did not permit providers to bill patients for these services. Per diem reimbursement encourages efficiency because reductions in the number of services provided and the amount of time required to produce the service, and lower input costs such as wages would increase provider net income.

Capitation was a more radical break from prior reimbursement systems in that it does not pay providers based on the delivery of care but rather on the basis of a predicted level of care. Under capitation, providers agree to a fixed fee per enrollee (often called per member per month, or PMPM) based on the expected utilization of service during a contract period. The provider of care receives the agreed-on payment whether a patient presents for treatment or does not receive care.

Capitation shifts emphasis from stimulating demand and focuses on reducing care. Capitation rewards providers for achieving health rather than treating the sick. It was hoped that this type of reimbursement would encourage providers to expand preventive services and reduce the need for curative care. This shift in care would be financially advantageous for the insurer if the negotiated PMPM payment was less than the historical cost of treatment and for providers if the cost of preventive care was less than the cost of curative care. Under capitation, providers have two ways to improve their financial performance: reduce cost by improving efficiency or reduce the quantity of services provided.

The problem for a provider is to incorporate reimbursement systems with conflicting incentives into a coherent operational plan. Increasing the intensity of services delivered increases revenue under charge- or cost-based reimbursement but reduces net income in per diem, per case, or capitation systems, since expenses increase but revenue is constant in the latter three. Reducing demand (admissions and visits) improves provider financial performance in capitation systems but reduces revenue from charge, cost, per diem, and per case payers. Table 3.5 summarizes the actions that providers can take to improve their financial performance; the reader should note there is no action, such as increasing the number of patients served, that has a consistently beneficial effect on net income.

Table 3.5 Provider Incentives under Different Reimbursement Systems

Reimbursement (Price)	Quantity	Intensity	Cost/Efficiency
Charge	↑ prices ↑ admissions	↑ LOS, ↑ tests	↓ cost (↑ efficiency)
Cost	↑ admissions	↑ LOS, ↑ tests	↑ cost (↓ efficiency)
Per case	↑ admissions	↓ LOS, ↓ tests	↓ cost (↑ efficiency)
Per diem	↑ admissions	↑ LOS, ↓ tests	↓ cost (↑ efficiency)
Capitation	↓ admissions	↓ LOS, ↓ tests	↓ cost (↑ efficiency)

Reimbursement and Overuse, Underuse, and Misuse

History demonstrates the power of revenue. Health care expenditures soared as patient out-of-pocket costs fell and government assumed responsibility for payment. As Table 3.5 shows, restraining prices, limiting admissions, and reducing LOS and number of tests are absent under charge- and cost-reimbursement systems. Even under charge reimbursement, which provides some incentive to keep costs low, providers were now encouraged to increase costs. The ability to raise prices to offset any detrimental impact of higher cost on financial performance overpowered the incentive to control costs.

Once consumption was separated from payment, insurers were faced with the vexing question of what to pay for and how to regulate moral hazard. To minimize the risk of overutilization, insurers limited payment to necessary services. Necessary services were defined as treatments that alleviated a pressing medical issue. Insurers did not want to pay for preventive care or routine checkups because the risk of overutilization was too great. Insurers would cover applying a cast or performing a surgery, but they did not pay for services that provided little therapeutic value. Early insurance plans often would not pay for an x-ray if there was no fracture; patients seeking an x-ray for an injury would be responsible for payment if the x-ray revealed no break. Payment systems discouraged evaluation and management visits for which the duration and outcome were often indeterminate and encouraged overutilization of procedures.

Besides encouraging the use of procedures and discouraging preventive care, these systems compensated specialists better than generalists. The resource-based relative value scale (RBRVS) was an attempt to correct the inequitable reimbursement that grew out of this system in which surgeons received disproportionately larger payments for procedures than family practitioners and internal medicine physicians received for visits. The effect of this payment system can be seen in the shift of physician training away from lower-compensated general medicine toward specialization. Under RBRVS, physicians are paid according to practice expense, liability insurance, and the time and effort required to provide a service. Similar to DRG hospital reimbursement, RBRVS was an attempt to rebalance incentives by reducing payment for procedures and encouraging evaluation and management services.

Examining the potential effect of reimbursement systems on quality is a complicated task. Quality must be paid for, but, as will be shown, the quality incentives of reimbursement systems simultaneously encourage and discourage specific types of services. As stated earlier, health care demand was restrained by patient willingness and ability to pay when the patient was responsible for a large percentage of health care costs. Providers may have wished to expand their services, but they had to convince patients that the service was a good use of their money.

The advent of third-party insurance, which reimbursed providers on the basis of charge, encouraged the overuse of curative services but typically did not pay for preventive care or experimental treatment. The reduction in patient copayments, the institution of Medicare and Medicaid, and the growth in defensive medicine led to a rapid expansion in health care expenditures but also raised issues of "unmanaged" care, overuse of unnecessary services, underuse of preventive care, and lack of access for the uninsured.

If we confine the discussion to hospital care, DRG (per case) reimbursement was an attempt to impose external control over medical decisions. Under cost- and charge-reimbursement systems there are incentives to admit too many patients, keep them hospitalized for too long, and overuse tests and procedures. One of the first reforms was to deny payment for unnecessary admissions. This, combined with the fixed payment per case, which discourages early admissions, lengthy hospitalizations, and overuse of services, can improve quality of care *if* overuse is the problem. Reducing admissions and LOS reduces the risk to patients from possible hospital-acquired infections and pressure ulcers; reducing the use of low-value tests and procedures similarly eliminates the accompanying risks that arise from use of medical services.

If overuse is not the problem, DRG reimbursement can exacerbate underuse. Given the financial incentive to keep patients out of the hospital, DRG payment can encourage "quicker and sicker" discharges. This possibility was considered and reduced by denying payment for any readmission for the same condition within 30 days, the point being that providers should not be able to gain an additional case payment because of their failure to adequately treat a patient during his first stay.

managed care
the use of payment policies and personnel to control utilization of health care treatment and lower costs

With the rise of **managed care**, the redefinition of incentives started by Medicare began to be extended into private health insurance. Private payers had seen their outlays rapidly increase when public programs reduced reimbursements, and the payers wanted to prevent providers from raising their prices to increase their revenue. The adoption of per case or per diem reimbursement by private insurers was intended to put additional pressure on providers to limit their use of services and increase efficiency. Per case and per diem reimbursement provide similar incentives, except that per diem reverses the per case incentive to reduce LOS. Under per diem reimbursement providers can increase their income by extending LOS (as long as the insurer deems these days as medically necessary), while under **per case reimbursement** additional days typically represent an expenditure of resources without commensurate reimbursement.

per case reimbursement
a reimbursement system that pays hospitals a flat fee per admission; in the Medicare DRG system this fee is based on type of care provided and the severity of the patient's condition

As seen under per case reimbursement, per diem payment can improve quality if the problem is premature discharge. Concurrent review, in which hospital or insurance personnel assess whether continued hospitalization is medically necessary, was designed to prevent overuse. Some providers have argued that while per diem reimbursement provides an incentive to retain patients, utilization review pushes providers toward underuse by encouraging early discharge. Managed care plans introduced in the 1980s and 1990s also attempted to address the underuse of preventive care by paying for annual wellness visits for their subscribers.

Managed care organizations had initial success containing their medical outlays; often their medical outlays were 10% to 15% less than those of indemnity insurers. Part of their success was accomplished by reducing utilization, including ER visits (only true emergencies were reimbursed) and obstetric care (one-day OB stays). Public outcry over restricted access resulted in legislation reducing managed care plans' ability to limit coverage. Rules requiring payment for ER visits deemed necessary by the patient and two-day minimum OB stays were mandated. Although these reforms addressed issues of underuse, they also encourage overuse. At the same time that legislation was undercutting managed care insurers' ability to manage utilization, insurers and third-party payers began to roll back their coverage of well visits. The companies instituted and raised copayments, which moved the system back toward encouraging the overuse of procedures and discouraging preventive care.

The most radical approach to paying for health care services is capitation, but once again the effect of the payment system on quality cannot be definitively determined. Although most would say that a payment system that pays a flat fee per member for a defined time period is aimed at restricting care, this can be positive if overuse is the concern. However, many accuse capitation systems of cherry picking (selecting only healthy enrollees who will need little or no care) and limiting necessary services since no additional revenue will result. On the other hand, capitation encourages preventive care when it is cheaper to provide preventive services than curative care; providers reap financial benefits by keeping patients healthy rather than treating them after they become ill. The incentive toward preventive care is weakened by the movement of patients across insurance plans; that is, preventive care delivered and paid for in 2012 may not yield lower health care costs until 2022, and by that time the patient may be insured by another insurer.

The difficulty for a hospital in developing an operating plan incorporating these different reimbursement systems is that they are financially contradictory. Optimizing treatment under one reimbursement system may reduce revenue for treating patients who are covered by other mechanisms. Assume a hospital optimizes care for Medicare patients (50% of its patients) by streamlining treatment and reducing LOS, which improves quality and the hospital's income from Medicare. For patients covered under charge or per diem systems, the reduction in LOS is accompanied by a reduction in reimbursement. Since the majority of hospitals' costs are incurred in the early part of the stay, the reduction in LOS under a per diem system may reduce reimbursement more than cost. Similarly, expansions of care, like Medicare's requirement for a predischarge pneumococcal vaccine, will improve quality and increase cost but will not increase a provider's DRG payment. Under per case, per diem, or capitated reimbursement, the expenditure of resources for vaccination will not increase revenue. The dilemma for providers is that efforts to improve quality may have an adverse effect on an organization's bottom line and possibly on their viability.

Dealing with the problem of misuse of services is more straightforward than dealing with the issues of overuse and underuse. The difficulty with misuse is that it is costly to detect and hard to determine, but once detected, the solution is clear. Under charge- and cost-reimbursement systems, providers can redo incorrect work and submit additional bills for their services. Per case, per diem, and capitation systems provide a solution because they curtail misuse by providing incentives to do things right the first time; under these systems hospital reimbursement will not increase regardless of how many times a test or procedure is redone.

As we have seen, depending on the reimbursement system, improving quality will not always have an entirely positive impact on financial performance. When we look at quality, we see that each reimbursement system can lead to overuse and underuse. But when we look at net income, we see that reimbursement, the amount paid to a provider, is definitively determined by changes in treatment. Attempting to achieve a specific treatment goal or optimal care by manipulating reimbursement systems would require knowing the specific problem faced by every organization and instituting individually designed payment systems. There is no way to institute a one-size-fits-all payment system that can adequately address the quality issues of individual providers. The inability of regulatory, legal, and economic forces to ensure quality requires that other tools be used to identify specific problems and their possible solutions.

Return on Investment on Delivering High-Quality Care

Reimbursement has had a significant effect on how health care has evolved in the United States, yet economic incentives may be insufficient to tackle the problems of overuse, underuse, and misuse. Although a one-size-fits-all solution is not possible, economic factors will still determine how seriously institutions pursue quality improvements. This section introduces a formula to calculate the **return on investment** (ROI) on actions aimed at improving health care quality. In the following formula, Q=quantity, P=price, QI=quality improvement, and Δ is change, or the difference

return on investment
the net income created per dollar invested in an activity, calculated as total additional income divided by the total investment

between the baseline amount and the amount after improvements have been undertaken.

$$\Delta \text{Profit} = \Delta \text{Revenue} - \Delta \text{Cost} \qquad\qquad 3.1$$

$$\Delta \text{Profit} = (\Delta Q \times \Delta P) - \Delta \text{Cost of Treatment} \qquad 3.2$$
$$- \Delta \text{Cost of QI (Grote et al. 2007)}$$

$$\Delta \text{Profit} = (\Delta Q \times \Delta P) - (\Delta Q \times \Delta \text{Outputs} \qquad 3.3$$
$$\times \Delta \text{Inputs per output} \times \Delta \text{Cost per input}) - \Delta \text{Cost of QI}$$

$$(\text{Volume} \times \text{Intensity} \times \text{Efficiency} \times \text{Input Price})$$

The accounting equation 3.1 holds that profit is the difference between revenues and costs, and that profit will increase if quality-improving actions increase revenue, decrease costs, increase revenue more than they increase cost, or decrease revenue but decrease costs by a larger amount. Quality improvement initiatives will have a greater chance of being pursued and institutionalized if they increase profits, that is, if the change in net income is positive.

Revenue is straightforward: the number of units sold multiplied by price (reimbursement). Cost, on the other hand, is multifaceted. When the formula is broken down, it is clear that implementing quality improvement adds new costs. Implementing quality improvement systems requires manpower, supplies, and equipment; monitoring performance, reporting results, and implementing correction (when required) will also impose new costs on an organization (ΔCost of QI). The key question is: What will be the impact of quality improvement on revenue (ΔRevenue) and on the cost of treatment (ΔCost of Treatment)?

Equation 3.3 demonstrates that the impact of quality improvement on the profitability of an organization will depend on how it affects revenues and treatment costs and the cost of QI. Like revenue, a prime driver of treatment costs is volume, ΔQ = volume. The second driver is intensity, ΔOutputs = Intensity, which measures the number of services provided to treat a patient. Intensity could be measured as the number of days hospitalized for an inpatient, the number of tests or procedures performed, and so on. The third component of production costs is the how these services are produced. Efficiency, Δ inputs per output, examines the number of labor hours needed to produce a service, the amount of supplies consumed to produce an output, and so on. The final driver is the price paid to acquire resources, Δ cost per input = input price. Input prices track the cost an organization pays to acquire labor, supplies, and other resources. The following sections focus on how quality improvement may increase or decrease revenues and treatment costs and thus its impact on profitability.

Revenue

Efforts to improve quality can affect revenue in only three possible ways: an increase, a decrease, or no change. Higher quality can affect revenue in sometimes surprising ways given its impact on volume and reimbursement. Organizations often see quality enhancement as a means of attracting more customers, and they work continuously to add features, increase reliability, improve service, and lower prices to increase their customer base, and thus revenue. At the extreme, organizations that do not deliver the expected level of quality go out of business. There appears to be a distinct possibility that improved quality will increase the volume of care delivered; patients as well as payers may want to patronize providers with superior outcomes. However, if every provider increases quality by the same amount, there may be no change in volume.

A potential problem for health care providers noted earlier is whether higher quality will lead to lower volume. One possibility is that doing things right will reduce the total number of admissions, tests, and procedures performed. This will reduce revenue (under cost- and charge-reimbursement systems). If higher quality reduces patient volume then the impact on revenues will hinge on whether payers are willing to pay more for better care.

The third possible result of improved quality is no change in volume; that is, consumers do not recognize the improved quality or they do not care. As stated above, if all producers improve simultaneously, there may be no change in the relative competitiveness and market share of any organization.

The same outcomes are possible for changes in price (reimbursement).

pay for performance
a reimbursement system that seeks improved quality by tying provider payments to process and outcome targets

A program that is receiving wide attention is **pay for performance**, tying reimbursement to quality goals. Three programs, Hawaii, Michigan Blue Cross, and CMS (Centers for Medicare and Medicaid Services), have instituted bonuses, $500,000 lump sum, 4% of payments, and 2% of payments, respectively, based on achieving defined quality thresholds. High-quality producers may also be able to raise their prices if the marketplace recognizes their products and services are superior to competitors.

Although it seems counterintuitive that reimbursement may decrease as quality increases, it is very likely. Third-party payers monitor the care they pay for, and if an insurer notes declining lengths of stay (due to improved quality) delivered to their enrollees, they may expect reimbursement concessions (lower per case, per diem, or PMPM rates) in their next negotiation. The final possibility is that an improvement in quality may have no effect on reimbursement. Table 3.6 summarizes the possibilities and their effect on revenue.

Table 3.6 Potential Changes in Revenue Quality

	Increase in Quantity	No Change in Quantity	Decrease in Quantity
Increase in Reimbursement	Higher Revenue $\uparrow Q^* \uparrow P = \uparrow$Revenue	Higher Revenue $\leftrightarrow Q^* \uparrow P = \uparrow$Revenue	Indeterminate $\downarrow Q^* \uparrow P = ?$Revenue
No Change in Reimbursement	Higher Revenue $\uparrow Q^* \leftrightarrow P = \uparrow$Revenue	No Change in Revenue $\leftrightarrow Q^* \leftrightarrow P = \leftrightarrow$Revenue	Lower Revenue $\downarrow Q^* \leftrightarrow P = \downarrow$Revenue
Decrease in Reimbursement	Indeterminate $\uparrow Q^* \downarrow P = ?$Revenue	Lower Revenue $\leftrightarrow Q^* \downarrow P = \downarrow$Revenue	Lower Revenue $\downarrow Q^* \downarrow P = \downarrow$Revenue

Table 3.6 demonstrates that providers should strive to implement quality improvements that will increase revenue and that they may be less than enthusiastic about initiatives that lower revenue. Typically when organizations produce higher-quality products, they attract a larger number of customers and the value-adding inputs can be passed on as higher prices (cell 1). Organizations research product enhancements to determine if the cost of improvement is valued enough by customers that they will be willing to pay more for the product. Under a charge- or cost-based system, health care providers could determine what constitutes an improvement and pass these costs on to consumers. The advent of fixed-price reimbursement (per diem, per case, and capitation) has dramatically reduced providers' ability to pass on higher costs. To date, there is little evidence to suggest that referral patterns are affected by quality rankings or that revenue will increase appreciably with improvements in quality.

Cost of Treatment

The second financial reason to pursue quality improvement is reducing treatment costs. The cost of treatment is a function of volume of patients treated (Q), the outputs produced for each patient (intensity of care), the inputs consumed to produce each output (efficiency), and the cost per input (input prices). Quality initiatives may increase, decrease, or have no impact on each of these four items. Since the quantity of patients was addressed in the revenue section, this factor will not be reviewed again.

If we start with the number of outputs required to complete a patient encounter, it is easy to conceptualize the effect of quality improvement. If an organization is hampered by overuse and misuse, quality management will lead to a reduction in costs. The elimination of unnecessary tests and procedures (overuse) and poorly performed services (misuse) will reduce the number of outputs produced. It is up to management to translate the reduction of outputs into maximum cost savings. Although the cost of supplies and equipment not used will produce savings, if the employees running these tests are left idle and not switched to other work, there will be zero labor savings. A side benefit of a reduction in outputs is the elimination of all expenses relating to adverse effects.

On the other hand, if patients are currently not receiving all the care they should (underuse), quality improvement will increase the number of services delivered and thus also the cost of treatment. The increase may arise from the necessity of performing more tests and procedures and increasing the amount of resources consumed. The third result is no change in costs; that is, quality improvement will require increases in some outputs and reductions in others.

In terms of efficiency, quality improvement by instituting improved processes could lead to greater efficiency, less time per service delivered. Quality initiatives that are bureaucratic and impede work can easily lead to inefficiency. A quality assurance system built on documenting or double-checking every step in a treatment process will reduce employee productivity. The third possibility is no change; better processes and higher efficiency in one area may be offset by lower efficiency and documentation requirements in other areas.

The fourth variable that determines treatment cost is the price of input. Will improvements in quality require hiring more capable and higher-paid employees or using higher-cost supplies and equipment? Will improvement in processes reduce cost by reallocating lower-skilled tasks to lower-paid employees? Will higher quality affect the cost of inputs?

We'll look at the potential effect of quality improvement on treatment cost by assuming no change in patient volume or input prices to isolate the effect of changes in intensity and efficiency on treatment costs.

Table 3.7 makes it clear that quality initiatives that lower intensity (the volume of services produced) and increase efficiency are most desirable (cell 3). A quality initiative that addresses overuse (lowers intensity) may be financially advantageous even if it lowers efficiency (cell 4) as long as Δintensity ($) is larger than Δefficiency ($). Similarly, if improvements in efficiency exceed the increase in cost due to producing more services (higher intensity), the change will be financially advantageous (cell 1). However, if quality improvement leads to higher costs through increase in intensity and lower efficiency, it will have a devastating effect on a provider (cell 2).

The challenge for organizations is to incorporate quality improvement into operations. As the accounting equation makes clear, it is possible to increase outputs without incurring costs if efficiency can be increased (cell 1) or if inputs can be purchased more economically. On the other hand, reductions in output may not create any savings if previously employed resources are left idle (cell 4). Any estimate of savings in treatment costs and how they will be accomplished must be explicitly defined.

Table 3.7 Potential Changes in Treatment Costs Due to Quality Improvement

	Higher Efficiency	Lower Efficiency
Higher Intensity	Indeterminate	Higher Cost
	ΔOutputs↑ × ΔInputs per output↓ = ?Treatment Costs	ΔOutputs↑ × ΔInputs per output↑ = ↑Treatment Costs
Lower Intensity	Lower Cost	Indeterminate
	ΔOutputs↓ × ΔInputs per output↓ = ↓Treatment Costs	ΔOutputs↓ × ΔInputs per output↑ = ?Treatment Costs

Cost of Quality Improvement

The cost of quality improvement is most likely to add costs to the organization. Establishing quality improvement programs requires the establishment of administrative structures and the redirection of employee efforts from revenue-generating activities to assessment (data collection, reporting, and reviewing). While these activities when properly directed may reduce treatment costs, it is essential that institutions recognize quality improvement costs as adding to the total operating expense of the organization.

Impact on Net Income

An effective quality improvement program, one that can demonstrate better outcomes and lower adverse events, may produce cost savings, including potential reductions in malpractice premiums and settlements. The cost of running a quality improvement (QI) program always adds cost, so providers need to determine whether these costs will be offset by increases in revenue or reductions in cost of treatment to improve the organization's financial performance.

A positive return on investment in quality improvement appears to be driven primarily by the second factor, changes in the cost of treatment (see Table 3.8). Assuming no change in revenue (Q or P), the cost of QI must be more than offset by reductions in cost of treatment to be financially viable (cell 6). Assuming no change in patient volume but an increase in reimbursement (pay for performance), there are three possible paths to financial viability (cells 1 through 3). The first is the change in revenue combined with a decrease in treatment cost may be likely to more than offset QI costs (cell 3). The second case requires the increase in revenue to offset QI costs while treatment costs remain constant. Least likely is that the change in revenue must more than compensate for the increase in treatment and QI costs (cell 1).

If quality improvement leads to higher total costs, the question will not be what the "right" reimbursement mechanism is but rather whether society is willing to pay for higher health care quality. If quality improvement leads to lower total costs, that is, if reductions in the cost of treatment exceed the increase in QI costs, then quality improvement can be pursued at an organizational level. The problem for providers is that care is typically delivered in a consistent manner across patients (different treatment is not delivered based on how the patient's services will be reimbursed), so a treatment plan that meets both quality and financial objectives for one group of patients may have a negative impact on the organization's overall financial performance.

Table 3.8 Potential Impact of Quality Improvement on Net Income

	Increase in Treatment Cost	No Change in Treatment Cost	Decrease in Treatment Cost
Increase in Revenue	Increase in net income, if $\Delta Rev > \Delta TC + \Delta QI$	Increase in net income, if $\Delta Rev > \Delta QI$	Increase in net income, if $\Delta Rev + \Delta TC > \Delta QI$
No Change in Revenue	Decrease in net income	Decrease in net income	Increase in net income, if $\Delta TC > \Delta QI$
Decrease in Revenue	Decrease in net income	Decrease in net income	Decrease in net income

Pay for Performance and the CMS Quality Initiative

Pay for performance is an explicit attempt to increase provider revenues for organizations that deliver high-quality care and to decrease payments for poor-quality care. Pay for performance systems must navigate four major issues: what to reward; the size of reward; whether to reward high performers, those achieving the greatest improvement, or both; and whether rewards will be given to individuals, teams, organizations, or all of the above (Petersen et al. 2006).

The first issue is what to reward. Donabedian's framework is a good place to start: Should incentives be given for having resources in place (structure), doing the right things (process), or achieving results (outcomes)? If employing higher-skilled and higher-paid workers or the latest technology improves outcomes, then reimbursement systems should provide the funds to hire the best workers and rapidly update their equipment and facilities. The rationale for process incentives is that medical outcomes are not solely the result of medical care, so incentives should be provided to providers who practice evidence-based medicine. The argument in favor of outcomes rests on the fact that outcomes are why people seek care; they are what is important to patients and society. A fourth element, satisfaction, requires additional discussion even though it is included as an outcome in both Donabedian's and Nash's systems. Should rewards be given for achieving a medical outcome and restoration of health, or should rewards be based on keeping patients happy? Medical results can be achieved and patient satisfaction can be increased by a higher expenditure of resources, so there is also a need to encourage efficiency as a way of providing more resources without raising the cost.

The second question is size of the reward. How much incentive is required to get people to change their behavior? Small incentives, such as 1% to 2% of a provider's payments, may not catch their attention. Large incentives, 20% to 25% of a provider's payments, may produce the desired behavior, but the issue that then arises is where the funds will come from to pay for these incentives. As seen in health care and education, attempts to fund rewards to higher-performing institutions by reducing funds to low performers presents a dilemma. Low-performing institutions may be the least capable of sustaining revenue reductions, and any reduction to their funding may exacerbate quality problems.

The third issue is what types of performance should be rewarded. The first choice is rewarding high performers, those who have consistently outperformed others. In this situation, the reward may not encourage further improvement; in an extreme case, an institution at the top of its field may not be capable of improving its results. Another option is to reward those showing the greatest improvement. Although improvement is the goal of quality management, rewarding improvement creates inequity. Assume hospital A has 45% compliance with a recognized medical protocol and hospital B has 90%. If A and B increase compliance by 2%, A will have a 4.4% improvement (2% ÷ 45%) while B will only improve by 2.2% (2% ÷ 90%). Payments based on improvement may disadvantage higher performers. Obviously, incentive programs should reward consistently superior performance as well as encourage improvement among low-performing institutions. To achieve equity, incentive programs may have to sacrifice simplicity and develop multiple reward plans.

Giving people a personal stake in improvement encourages them to change. The last issue is whether to reward individuals or groups. Health care is a team endeavor; caring for a patient requires input from multiple individuals. Rewarding individuals is the surest path to improvement, but similar to rewarding process or outcome, encouraging better care requires moving the entire system. Placing incentives at the group level, or above, could discourage individuals if they believe the rest of the system will not be changed and could reward free riders who believe they can do nothing and reap the rewards of others' activities.

In 2003 Medicare established a demonstration project to reward high-quality hospitals, and the program ran through 2009 (CMS 2011). A key element in the project was the top 20% of performers would receive a financial bonus, while the bottom 20% could see reductions in their Medicare payments of 1% or 2%. Medicare used a mix of process and outcome measures; for example, acute myocardial infarction (AMI) has eight process variables and one outcome variable (mortality). Table 3.9 details the medical conditions included, the number of measures assessed, and the change in performance between 2003 and 2009. (CABG is coronary artery bypass surgery, and SCIP is Surgical Care Improvement Project.)

Table 3.9 Hospital Quality Initiative Demonstration: Clinical Conditions

Condition	Process	Outcome	Total	2003	2009
AMI	8	1	9	87.5%	98.1%
CABG	7	1	8	84.8%	97.6%
Heart Failure	4	0	4	64.5%	95.5%
Pneumonia	7	0	7	69.3%	94.8%
Hip and Knee Replacement	5	1	6	84.6%	98.0%
SCIP (year 6)	5	0	5	85.8%	96.2%

Source: CMS (Centers for Medicare and Medicaid Services), 2011, Premier Hospital Quality Incentive Demonstration, http://www.cms.gov/Medicare/Quality-Initiatives-Patient-Assessment-Instruments/HospitalQualityInits/Downloads/HospitalPremierPressRelease-FactSheet.pdf, 2.

Table 3.9 documents substantial improvement in provider adherence to care standards. Incentive payments were made to the top performers as discussed earlier, but additional awards were made for attaining or exceeding median performance and achieving the greatest improvement. In the sixth year of the program, 216 hospitals completed the demonstration and 211 received awards totaling $12 million.

Lindenauer et al. (2010) examined differences in hospital 30-day mortality and readmission rates between 2006 and 2009 based on CMS's National Pneumonia Project. They found that 30-day mortality rates, adjusted for CMI (case mix index) averaged 11.6% and ranged from 6.7% to 20.9%. Similarly, CMI-adjusted readmission rates averaged 18.2% and ranged between 13.6% and 26.7%. The authors did not attempt to determine why rates varied substantially, but their work provides insight into the potential improvement that can be achieved in pneumonia care.

Glickman et al. (2007) examined differences in the use of the process of care measures that define CMS's pay for performance project for acute myocardial infarction. They studied 54 hospitals that participated in the quality incentive program and 446 control hospitals to determine if processes or outcomes were different between the two groups. The difference between the two groups on the CMS measures was minimal; there was no difference between the two groups on the six variable composite measures; and only aspirin at discharge and smoking cessation were better in the participating hospitals.

A concern in quality management is that concentration on one set of measures, in this case the six CMS variables, could lead to lower performance on another set of measures. Glickman et al. evaluated performance on a set of uncompensated measures and found no significant difference between the participating and control hospitals on the composite measure and seven of eight individual measures. Only lipid-lowering medication had significantly higher rates of delivery in the participating hospitals. Mortality, the outcome measure, was not different between the two groups. The authors conclude that financial incentives had "limited incremental impact" on AMI processes and outcomes.

Summary

For better or worse, medical purchases are made in markets that depart significantly from markets for other goods and services. These departures were designed to alleviate patients' informational disadvantage and inability to afford expensive medical care. The remedies for these problems encouraged overutilization of medical services and raised the question of whether society is receiving sufficient return on its investment in health care.

Ensuring the quality of health care was initially reserved to the medical profession, but over time oversight has shifted to government and nongovernmental organizations. Regulatory approaches, including licensing, accreditation, and credentialing have not proved to be entirely satisfactory, as evidenced by the continuing calls for action regarding quality. The failure of regulation to ensure quality has led patients to seek relief in the legal system. While the legal system has produced significant financial settlements for injured patients, there are serious questions of whether it effectively compensates negligently treated patients and levies judgments on nonnegligent providers.

Quality issues combined with the rapid increase in health care spending led to a search for an economic solution to both issues. Economics provides two insights; the first is that more health care reduces the amount of other goods and services a person or society can consume. The second insight is that the benefit of health care declines as more health services are consumed. Opportunity costs and diminishing marginal returns require that we analyze health care purchases not only from a medical perspective but also allow ourselves to ask whether a different set of outputs would produce better health for patients and society.

Solutions to overuse, underuse, and misuse will require identifying specific problems, their causes, and potential solutions and implementing effective solutions where each problem arises. Health care problems can arise from personnel, supplies, equipment, facilities, and processes and often are location-specific. Improvement will require understanding how specific systems operate and implementing solutions that consider how the parts of the system interact. Regulation, law, and economics can support these solutions, but they cannot solve health care quality issues.

KEY TERMS

Accreditation	Law of diminishing marginal utility
Budget constraint	Licensure
Capitation	Law of demand
Capture theory of regulation	Managed care
Charge reimbursement	Marginal benefit
Consumer surplus	Medium of exchange
Copayments	Moral hazard
Cost reimbursement	Need-based decision making
Credentialing	Opportunity cost
Deadweight loss	Pay for reimbursement
Demand	Per case reimbursement
Demand curve	Per diem reimbursement
Diagnosis-related groups	Premiums
Elasticity Supply	Principal-agent relationship
Equilibrium price	Public interest theory of regulation
Externality	Return on investment
First dollar coverage	Supply
Hippocratic oath	Supply curve
Information asymmetry	
Insurance	

REVIEW QUESTIONS

1. Contrast medical and economic decision making.

2. What are the strengths and weaknesses of licensing, accreditation, and credentialing? How effective have these systems been?

3. What are the two purposes of malpractice actions?

4. Explain moral hazard and how a deadweight loss comes into existence.

5. Compare and contrast the incentives that arise under different reimbursement systems.

6. Describe the conditions that must be present for a provider to receive a positive return on investment in quality improvement.

PROBLEMS

1. The following table shows the quantity demanded and supplied of physician office visits at various prices. Draw the demand and supply curves. What is equilibrium price and quantity?

Price (P)	Quantity Demanded	Quantity Supplied
$50	9	1
$70	7	3
$90	5	5
$110	3	7
$130	1	9

2. The following table shows the quantity demanded and supplied of physician office visits at various prices. Draw the demand and supply curves. What is the equilibrium price and quantity? Assume the patient gets a job and has employer-provided health insurance that reimburses 50% of the cost of physician visits. What is the new equilibrium price and quantity?

Price (P)	Quantity Demanded	Quantity Supplied
$40	12	2
$60	10	4
$80	8	6
$100	6	8
$120	4	10
$140	2	12
$160	0	14

3. A surgeon currently earns $250,000 a year performing 100 surgeries on Medicare patients. On order to contain costs, Medicare institutes a reimbursement reduction of 20%, reducing the per surgery payment from $2,500 per case to $2,000. How many surgeries will the physician have to perform to maintain his income of $250,000 after the reimbursement reductions are put into place?

4. Assume a quality improvement program will increase a hospital's revenue by 1%, increase treatment costs by 0.5%, and add $500,000 in administrative costs. What will be the impact on the organization's net income if its revenues, total treatment costs, and administrative expenses are currently $100,000,000, $70,000,000 and $25,000,000?

References

Cardarelli R and Licciardone JC, 2006, Factors Associated with High Severity Disciplinary Action by a State Medical Board: A Texas Study of Medical License Revocation, *Journal of the American Osteopathic Association* 106 (3): 153–156.

CMS (Centers for Medicare and Medicaid Services), 2011, Premier Hospital Quality Incentive Demonstration, http://www.cms.gov/Medicare/Quality-Initiatives-Patient-Assessment-Instruments/HospitalQualityInits/HospitalPremier.html, accessed June 14, 2012.

Chen J, Rathore SS, Radford MJ, and Krumholz HM, 2003, JCAHO Accreditation and the Quality of Care for Acute Myocardial Infarction, *Health Affairs* 22 (3): 243–254.

Glickman SW, Ou FS, DeLong ER, Roe MT, Lytle BL, Mulgund J, Rumsfeld JS, Gibler WB, Ohman EM, Schulman KA, Peterson ED, 2007, Pay for Performance, Quality of Care, and Outcomes in Acute Myocardial Infarction, *JAMA* 297 (21): 2373–2380.

Grote K, Fleming E, Levine E, Richmond R, Sutaria S, Wiest FC, and Daley J, 2007, The "New Economics" of Clinical Quality Improvement: The Case of Community-Acquired Pneumonia, *Journal of Healthcare Management* 52 (4): 246–258.

Joint Commission, 2009, http://www.jointcommission.org/AboutUs/Fact_Sheets/overview_qa.htm, accessed September 2, 2009.

Joint Commission, 2012, Facts about Scoring and Accreditation Decisions for 2012, http://www.jointcommission.org/assets/1/18/Scoring_and_Accreditation_Decisions_for_2012_4_3_12.pdf, accessed June 12, 2012.

Kohatsu ND, Gould D, Ross LK, and Fox PJ, 2004, Characteristics Associated with Physician Discipline, *Archives of Internal Medicine* 164 (6): 653–658.

Kohl HK, Berwick DM, Clancy CM, Baur C, Brach C, Harris LM, and Zerhusen EG, 2012, New Federal Policy Initiatives to Boost Health Literacy Can Help the Nation Move Beyond the Cycle of Costly "Crisis Care," *Health Affairs* 31 (2): 434–443.

Lindenauer PK, Bernheim SM, Grady JN, Lin Z, Wang Y, Wang Y, Merrill AR, Han LF, Rapp MT, Drye EE, Normand SL, and Krumholz HM, 2010, The Performance of US Hospitals as Reflected in Risk-Standardized 30-day Mortality and Readmission Rates for Medicare Beneficiaries with Pneumonia, *Journal of Hospital Medicine* 5 (6): E12–18.

Localio AR, Lawthers AG, Brennan TA, Laird NM, Hebert LE, Peterson LM, Newhouse JP, Weiler PC, and Hiatt HH, 1991, Relation between Malpractice Claims and Adverse Events Due to Negligence: Results of the Harvard Medical Practice Study III, *New England Journal of Medicine* 325 (4): 245–251.

Menger C, 1871, *Principles of Economics*, New York University Press, New York, NY.

Miller MR, Pronovost P, Donithan M, Zeger S, Zhan C, Morlock L, and Meyer GS, 2005, Relationship between Performance Measurement and Accreditation: Implications for Quality of Care and Patient Safety, *American Journal of Medical Quality* 20 (5): 239–252.

Miller RD, 2006, *Problems in Health Care Law*, 9th ed., Jones and Bartlett Publishers, Sudbury MA.

Morrison J and Wickersham P, 1998, Physicians Disciplined by a State Medical Board, *JAMA* 279 (23): 1889–1893.

NCDOC (North Carolina Department of Commerce), Occupations Requiring a License in North Carolina, http://eslmi03.esc.state.nc.us/navigator/jc/licensed/index.htm, accessed May 12, 2013.

NSHD (Nevada State Health Division), 2009, Health Division Reaches Settlement with West Hills Hospital, http://health.nv.gov/PIO/PRs/2009/PR-2009–07–17_WestHillsSettlement.pdf, accessed June 7, 2012.

OECD (Organisation for Economic Co-operation and Development), *OECD Health Data 2009*, Paris, France.

Petersen LA, Woodard LD, Urech T, Daw C, and Sookanan S, 2006, Does Pay for Performance Improve the Quality of Health Care?, *Annals of Internal Medicine* 145 (4): 265–272.

Pozgar G, 1996, *Legal Aspects of Health Care Administration*, Aspen Publications, Gaithersburg, MD.

Schyve PM, 2000, The Evolution of External Quality Evaluation from the Joint Commission on Accreditation of Healthcare Organizations, *International Journal for Quality in Health Care* 12 (3): 255–258.

Sloan FA, Conover CJ, and Provenzale D, 2000, Hospital Credentialing and Quality of Care, *Social Science and Medicine* 50, 77–88.

Starr P, 1982, *The Social Transformation of American Medicine*, Basic Books, New York, NY.

Statistical Abstract of the United States, 2003, http://www.census.gov/compendia/statab/.

Statistical Abstract of the United States, 2012, http://www.census.gov/compendia/statab/.

Texas DSHS (Department of State Health Services), General Hospitals—Health Facility Program, http://www.dshs.state.tx.us/HFP/hospital.shtm, accessed June 15, 2013.

Thornlow DK and Merwin E, 2009, Managing to Improve Quality: The Relationship between Accreditation Standards, Safety Practices and Patient Outcomes, *Health Care Management Review* 34 (3): 262–272.

U.S. Department of Health and Human Services, 2012, National Practitioner Data Bank 2010 Annual Report, http://www.npdb-hipdb.hrsa.gov/resources/reports/2010NPDBAnnualReport.pdf, accessed May 15, 2012.

Woodwell DA, 1999, National Ambulatory Medical Care Survey: 1997 Summary, National Center for Health Statistics, Hyattsville, MD.

PART 2

QUALITY MANAGEMENT TOOLS

Chapter Four introduces the reader to a variety of tools to document and understand how a system is operating. These tools are designed to take data and organize it into information from which decisions can be made and action taken. Ten tools are introduced to identify problems, identify the potential causes of problems, reduce a list of solutions to one or two to be implemented, and monitor implemented solutions to determine if they produce the desired effects. A correctly defined problem is half solved, so improvement is contingent on the ability to understand a situation. Rigorous data analysis is essential to defining problems and causes, and the chapter demonstrates how the reader can take a large amount of seemingly indecipherable data and highlight the key features of a system through a limited number of charts and diagrams.

Chapters Five and Ten focus on root cause analysis (RCA) and on failure mode and effects analysis (FMEA). Both are techniques for investigating and preventing problems. RCA focuses on problems that have already arisen, generally a single event; FMEA examines the potential for failure and reviews systems and subsystems to identify where problems could appear and their impact on desired outcomes. Both chapters review prevention and recovery techniques to improve outcomes and build safer systems.

Chapters Six through Eight cover statistical process control (SPC). SPC monitors outputs and outcomes to determine when systems should be investigated and possibly corrected. Every system produces outputs and outcomes that vary; the challenge for quality management is to determine when the amount of variation warrants investigation. There are two types of variation: natural variation is a constant within a stable system while special cause variation signals change or instability in a system. Distinguishing the two types of variation is essential; quality management does not seek to impede production by interrupting stable and capable systems. Investigation and action should be limited to unstable systems that fail to meet desired standards; employees should be free to work at their discretion as long as their outputs and outcomes remain within acceptable limits.

Three chapters are needed to demonstrate how SPC is adapted to the desired goal. Health care produces various outputs and outcomes, and they are measured on different scales; continuous variables measure timeliness and response to care, binomial measures indicate success/failure or acceptable/unacceptable performance, and counts record the number of events. All require different analytical techniques. While the analytical technique varies with the phenomenon measured, the analytical process and interpretation are constant. Three chapters provide the reader with the ability to practice and reinforce their skills by examining different data and drawing insights across chapters.

Chapter Nine introduces chi-square, ANOVA, ANOM, and regression, which can be used to identify problems and causes and assess whether improvements have been achieved. While Chapter Four emphasized defining problems and identifying causes, Chapter Nine more formally addresses the question of whether a change has improved outcomes. While run charts document the direction of change, Chapter Nine asks the question: Is the magnitude of change sufficient to conclude improvement? Are the results in a postintervention group significantly better than the preintervention group; that is, are results after a system change significantly better than before? Like SPC, the idea is that there will be period-to-period changes in performance, and true improvement must be sufficiently larger than chance period-to-period movements.

CHAPTER 4

PROCESS ANALYSIS TOOLS

Introduction

Many organizations are **data** rich and **information** poor. Organizations and especially health care providers have tremendous amounts of data but rarely the ability to make optimal use of the data. Think about the amount of physician notes, nursing notes, test results, medications ordered, and other information recorded in the medical record as well as the data captured by the billing system. Each piece of information is collected for a specific purpose, which it fulfills (answer a question about a patient's health status at a particular point in time, submit bill to a payer), but it is seldom used to assess the performance of the system. Health care providers have vast amounts of data, but in many ways they are among the worst organizations for using this data to answer questions of quality and efficiency.

Health care information systems are designed to collect data on individual patients and distribute information to individual care givers, but these systems often fail to provide information on how the system is performing relative to groups of patients. In addition to the problem of the orientation of data systems, health care must also work around the orientation of providers. The Hippocratic oath, to do no harm, is often implemented interpreted as to do everything possible for the patient. Providers, like the data system, are trained to focus on the needs of the individual patient, and the skills required for quality management (taking a population-based perspective or looking at outcomes across groups of patients) are not emphasized in medical education. Health care providers are often ill-prepared to interpret system performance data and address quality management questions.

LEARNING OBJECTIVES

1. Explain the differences among data, information, and knowledge

2. Apply process analysis tools to identify problems

3. Use process analysis tools to identify potential causes of problems

4. Use process analysis tools to reduce a list of potential solutions to a manageable number for implementation

5. Monitor the effectiveness of solutions implemented using process analysis tools

data

symbols, numbers, text, images, sounds, and so forth; data is unorganized information

information

answers questions and provides insight into phenomena; information is organized data

knowledge

the condition of possessing sufficient understanding of information to identify the appropriate action for a particular situation; knowledge is useful information

This chapter introduces the basic tools to move from data collection to action. Providers must learn how to collect, organize, and analyze aggregate data to gauge system performance. Individual failures can justifiably be attributed to a number of causes and may not provide any particular insight into system performance. However, multiple failures arising from one or more causes may highlight systemic weaknesses that should be corrected. This chapter equips the reader to pinpoint systemic problems and their causes, select a potential solution, and monitor the effectiveness of solutions implemented.

The amount of data that is readily available in today's world is astounding, but it is also disturbing that this data is often biased, if not incorrect, and ineffectively used when it is correct. The knowledge hierarchy, Figure 4.1, emphasizes the need to transform data into information and information into **knowledge**. Data is simply numbers, text, images, sounds, and so forth; data are simply symbols that, outside of context, are frequently meaningless. Data is unorganized information; to obtain meaning, the data analyst must put it into context, analyze it, and summarize it to answer questions.

Data → Information → Knowledge

Unorganized → Organized → Useful Information
Information   Data

Data Collection →   Data   → Policy Formulation/
                   Analysis   Decision Making

Figure 4.1 The Knowledge Hierarchy

To create information, the data analyst may calculate sums or averages, place the data into sequence (typically chronological but ascending or descending order also adds insight into performance), and compare the calculated values to known thresholds. Information comprises organized data that answers questions. Information provides the user with insight into the phenomenon from which the data was drawn. Is the patient or system improving, deteriorating, or stable?

Knowledge is the condition of possessing sufficient understanding of information to identify the appropriate action for a particular situation. Knowledge is useful information or the ability to apply information, that is, to do what should be done based on what is known. For example, blood pressure data has been collected over six points in time. To convert this raw data into information, it is plotted chronologically as a line chart (or placed into a data table). Once the data is placed in chronological order, it is easy to determine if blood pressure is rising or if it is stable. In addition to any trend, the blood pressure reading must be compared against known thresholds; stage 1 hypertension is a systolic blood pressure greater than 140 mm Hg or a diastolic reading greater than 80. The next step is to determine what action should be taken; for example, if blood pressure is rising and over 140 mm Hg, should the patient be placed on medications such as diuretics, beta blockers, ACE inhibitors, or calcium channel blockers, or should lifestyle modifications be advised?

The final step is to take action based on knowledge. If the appropriate action is not taken, the value of data collection, data analysis, and developing the appropriate response is lost and the effort is wasted. The goal of process analysis is to improve patient care and system performance. Unfortunately many quality initiatives devolve into meaningless data collection and analysis, often asking the wrong questions, and having no effect on patient outcomes or on how care is delivered.

The goal of quality management is identifying how systems are performing; this requires identifying not individual errors but common errors. Common errors have significant impact on multiple patients and are errors that should be fixed. Employees engaged in quality management must understand what data is available, how to convert the data into information, and formulate the appropriate questions to evaluate performance. Once system performance data is generated, various tools can be used to identify problems, identify the causes of problems, identify potential solutions and select a solution, and determine if the solution remediated the problem, as shown in Table 4.1.

Table 4.1 Uses of Process Analysis Tools

1.	Identify problems.
2.	Identify the potential and primary causes of problems.
3.	Identify potential solutions and select a solution to be implemented.
4.	Monitor implemented solution; did the solution reduce or eliminate the problem?

Tools will be introduced to *expand* the scope of investigations into system performance to ensure that problems and causes are not overlooked and to *narrow* the search for primary causes and effective solutions. The challenge is to take the voluminous data residing in data systems and turn it into useful information that illuminates areas for improvement, guides decision making, and determines if actions undertaken are producing the desired results. These challenges require users to take a broad perspective and consider whether the important factors and relationships between factors have been identified. At other times, thinking must be narrowed to avoid information overload; what are key factors, can they be changed, and what can be done?

Chapter Four departs from prior chapters in that it focuses on building skills. Chapters One through Three discussed the current situation in health care, including the history of quality management, the main challenges to quality management, and the economic and legal factors influencing health care delivery. Chapter Four describes tools to convert data into information and presents the reader with raw data so they can perform the applications for themselves. This chapter aims at providing the reader with both knowledge and skills.

The following discussion of the ten primary quality management tools differentiates between data analysts and users. Data analysts are employees tasked with manipulation of data; that is, they are producers of information. Users are the consumers of information, people who manage operations, determine what issues and problems should be studied, and how data is categorized and manipulated. In many cases the data analyst and user will be the same person. I believe this is the optimal case as problems can arise if the data analyst does not understand the data or how it will be used or if the user does not understand how the data was collected, organized, and analyzed. In either case the underlying data may be unwittingly mishandled and produce useless, if not harmful, information. To guard against this outcome, data analysts and users must understand the process that generated the data and how the data has been handled.

Tools to Identify Problems

Pareto Charts

Pareto chart
a column chart that displays the frequency of events in descending order

Pareto rule
80% of consequences arise from 20% of causes

The **Pareto chart** is designed to separate major issues from minor issues. It is used to illuminate the issues and problems that should receive attention from managers and workers. The **Pareto rule** is related to the Pareto chart. The Pareto rule, a.k.a. the 80-20 rule, states that 80% of consequences arise from 20% of causes. The Pareto rule would conclude that 80% of patient complaints arise from 20% of patients and subsequently corrective action would require identifying this group of patients and determining why they are unhappy. A generalization of the Pareto rule would conclude 80% of the problems are produced by 20% of causes. Effective quality management programs focus on improving this 20%, thereby reducing or eliminating

80% of problems. In quality management all things are not created equal, and focusing on a small group of causes often produces disproportionate improvements in operations.

The problem with data is that unless it can be organized into a useful and easy-to-interpret format, it has little value. The problem can be seen in Table 4.2 of the top ten medications involved in adverse events. A cursory view of the data does not readily yield useful information. The table does not highlight the high-risk medications. Pareto charts convert table data into easily understandable information.

Table 4.2 Top 10 Medications in Adverse Events

Medication	Number of Events
Acetaminophen	14
Amoxicillin	32
Anticoagulants	47
Aspirin	19
Cephalexin	12
Hydrocodone-acetaminophen	17
Ibuprofen	16
Insulin	60
Penicillin	10
Trimethoprim-sulfamethoxazole	17

The problem with Table 4.2 is it does not readily answer the question of what medications should be focused on. By examining the table it is clear the medication with the most adverse events is insulin, but it requires the user to scan the entire list and identify the one with the highest number of events. This type of data display is subject to error and becomes more onerous to handle as the number of items increases. A Pareto chart is an ordered column chart that identifies the cause (medication) associated with the highest number of errors in the first column and displays the remaining causes in descending order. The user does not have to search out the important issues since they are prominently displayed and the relative importance of each issue is visually displayed.

The first step in data analysis is to acquire the data and place it into a form that can be imported into a software package, which often requires manual data entry. The data for Table 4.2 is available online in an Excel worksheet, Ch04Pareto.xls, under the Figure04–03 tab.

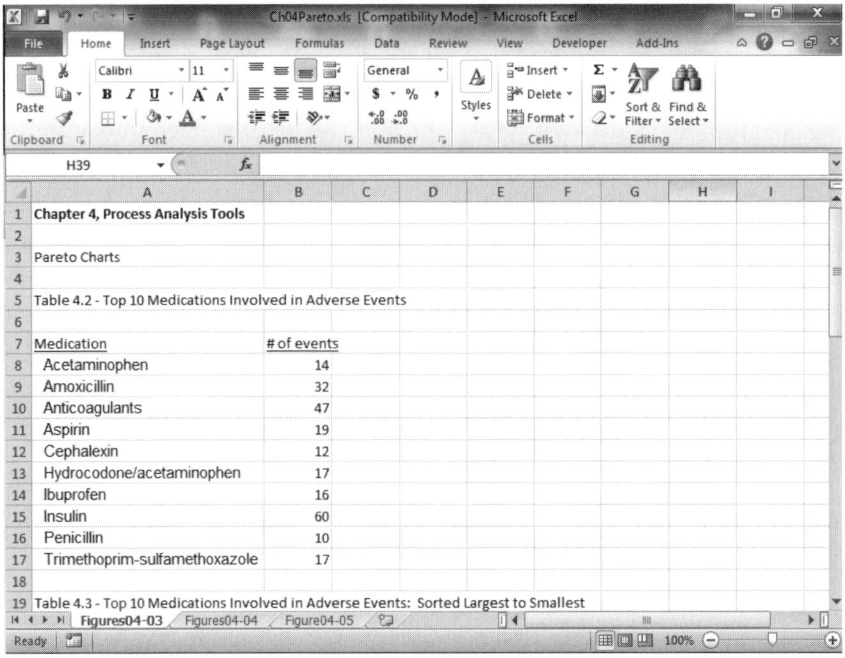

Figure 4.2 Top 10 Medications in Adverse Events

After acquiring the data in a usable form, the first thing the data analyst needs to do is to highlight the relevant range, A8 through B17. After highlighting the range, the data analyst would click on **Data** on the Excel main menu which reveals the following: **Connections, Sort & Filter, Data Tools**, and **Outline**. Clicking on Sort brings up **Column, Sort On**, and **Order**. **Column** allows the data analyst to specify how the data will be sorted. Medications in Table 4.2 are in alphabetical order, but since Pareto charts are ordered column charts that highlight the most frequently occurring events, the data is sorted based on the number of events. So column B is selected. **Sort on** allows the data analyst to specify what to sort on. Typically a data analyst wishes to sort based on the values in each cell; however, Excel also offers the data analyst the ability to sort based on cell color, font color, or cell icon. Table 4.3 will be produced using the default: VALUES OR NUMBER OF EVENTS. Finally **Order** allows the data to be displayed in ascending or descending order. Since the goal is to display the medications involved most frequently with adverse events, descending (largest to smallest) is selected.

Table 4.3 is a major improvement over Table 4.2 since it produces a clear ranking based on the number of events. However, it still requires some effort to evaluate the relative importance of each medication in adverse events. A Pareto chart establishes a visual representation that not only ranks the data but allows a user to easily see the relative difference in adverse events

Table 4.3 Top 10 Medications in Adverse Events: Most Frequent to Least Frequent

Medication	Number of events
Insulin	60
Anticoagulants	47
Amoxicillin	32
Aspirin	19
Hydrocodone-acetaminophen	17
Trimethoprim-sulfamethoxazole	17
Ibuprofen	16
Acetaminophen	14
Cephalexin	12
Penicillin	10

for each drug. To create a Pareto chart from Table 4.3 the data analyst selects **Insert**, which reveals the submenu: **Tables, Illustrations, Charts, Links**, and **Text**. The **Charts** option allows the data analyst to create **Column, Line, Pie, Bar, Scatter**, or **Other Charts**, so Column is selected.

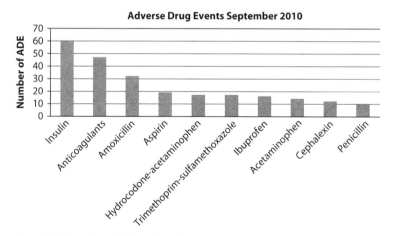

Figure 4.3 Pareto Chart of Adverse Drug Events

The Pareto chart presents information more succinctly than either Tables 4.2 or 4.3. The chart allows the user to see that the top three medications (insulin, anticoagulants, and amoxicillin) account for the lion's share of adverse events and that adverse events involving the remaining seven are rare. This type of presentation is designed to grab people's attention and focus it on the most important issues.

In addition to recording the number of adverse medication events, the Pareto chart should also document the time period covered, location, and source of the data. This information is essential so the user can evaluate the seriousness of the situation, how many events are occurring within what period of time, where are the events occurring, and the reliability of the data source.

We can see how closely the adverse drug events follow the Pareto rule: 20% of causes produce 80% of issues. Table 4.2 includes a total of 244 events; the top 20% of causes would be insulin (60) and anticoagulants (47), which account for 107 of the total events, or 43.9%. While this example does not meet the prediction of the Pareto rule, it demonstrates that focusing attention on a small group of medications (events) can produce disproportionate improvement.

Figure 4.4 presents a slight variation of the Pareto chart by measuring the y-axis as a percentage of total adverse events. Users now see that approximately 25% of adverse events arise from insulin and 20% from anticoagulants. None of the bottom seven medications accounts for more than 8% of the total, and two medications, cephalexin and penicillin, account for less than 5% of the adverse drug events.

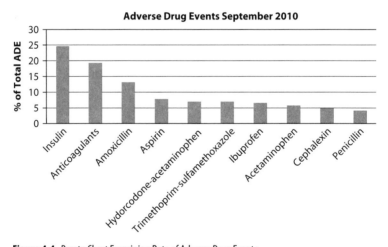

Figure 4.4 Pareto Chart Examining Rate of Adverse Drug Events

To improve health care quality, the Joint Commission collects information from hospitals on sentinel events, unexpected occurrences that could or do produce death or serious injury, and reports the accumulated information back to hospitals so they can assess the risk of these events occurring and institute safeguards to minimize their likelihood of occurrence and their impact if they do occur. Table 4.4 presents the statistics collected from 1995 through 2009.

Table 4.4 Joint Commission Sentinel Event
Statistics: January 1995–March 2009

Event	Cases
Wrong-site surgery	784
Suicide	715
Op/post-op complication	659
Medication error	503
Delay in treatment	472
Patient fall	367
Unintended retention of foreign body	252
Assault/rape/homicide	224
Patient death/injury in restraints	192
Perinatal death/loss of function	181
Transfusion error	135
Infection-related event	118
Medical equipment related	109
Patient elopement	91
Anesthesia-related event	88
Fire	88
Maternal death	78
Ventilator death/injury	56
Abduction	31
Utility system-related event	25
Infant discharged to wrong family	8
Other less frequent types	725

Source: Joint Commission, Summary Data of Sentinel Events
Reviewed by the Joint Commission, www.jointcommission
.org/assets/1/18/2004_4Q_2012_SE_Stats_Summary
.pdf; site currently reports events through 2012.

As stated earlier, tables of numbers are difficult to read. When this data is presented in a Pareto chart, a clearer picture emerges.

The goal of the Pareto chart is to ensure that organizations allocate their limited resources in the most effective manner. Organizations have a limited amount of manpower and other resources and to achieve maximum effectiveness, so they must determine where these resources will have the greatest impact. As the Joint Commission statistics indicate, it may be better to achieve a 50% reduction in wrong-site surgery (392 adverse events eliminated) than total elimination of unintended retention of foreign body (252 events). Pareto charts suggest that improvement should begin with

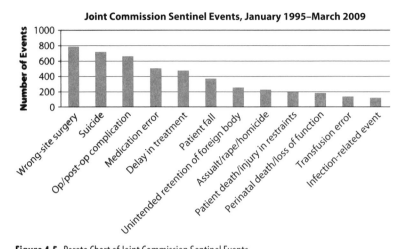

Figure 4.5 Pareto Chart of Joint Commission Sentinel Events

high-frequency events, but it is up to users to determine the seriousness of each type of event and assess how much effort will be required and how much improvement can be achieved when performance improvement projects are undertaken.

Stratification Charts

stratification chart
a chart that displays data in groups to identify commonalities

The purpose of the **stratification chart** is to group things into categories. Stratification charts are similar to Pareto charts in that they identify problems and use column charts. Whereas the Pareto chart reports total events, stratification charts attempt to peer into the data to discover the potential causes of the events. Stratification, the ability to drill down into the data, enables a user to assess more information (if contained in the data set). Typical factors associated with production and errors are the personnel involved (who), equipment and materials used (what), location (where), and day or time (when).

Table 4.5 records patient falls over a three-month period, although the table displays only the first eight days. Assume an organization has initiated a fall prevention program and as part of the program it records the date of each fall, the patient's age and level of medication, the location of fall, the time of day (shift), and the presence of staff at the time of the fall. The raw data does not highlight any particular relationships between the events and possible factors, and it needs to be organized to produce useful information. In terms of risk assessment the first question we might ask is, how does patient age or level of medication impact patient falls?

To determine the effect of age, the data analyst could sort the data, but the output would simply be a listing of patients in ascending or descending order, which would not be particularly useful. What a user wants is the information aggregated into understandable (or logical) subgroups. For age the user may want to know how many of the patients who fell were under 18 years of age, between 18 and 40, between 41 and 64, and over 65. To produce a count of patients in each age category, the Excel **Frequency** function is used.

Table 4.5 Patient Falls

Date	Patient Age	Medication	Location	Shift	Staff Present
Thursday, January 01, 2009	77	Heavy	2N-Med	First	Yes
Thursday, January 01, 2009	59	Heavy	2N-Med	Second	No
Thursday, January 01, 2009	102	Heavy	3S-Surg	Second	No
Friday, January 02, 2009	68	Moderate	3N-Surg	Third	Yes
Friday, January 02, 2009	83	Light	2S-Med	First	No
Saturday, January 03, 2009	20	Heavy	Clinic	First	No
Saturday, January 03, 2009	36	Heavy	3N-Surg	Second	Yes
Sunday, January 04, 2009	24	Moderate	ER	Third	No
Sunday, January 04, 2009	29	Moderate	2N-Med	First	No
Sunday, January 04, 2009	83	Light	Clinic	Second	Yes
Sunday, January 04, 2009	94	Heavy	2N-Med	Second	No
Monday, January 05, 2009	70	Heavy	2N-Med	Third	No
Monday, January 05, 2009	69	Moderate	3S-Surg	First	No
Monday, January 05, 2009	77	Moderate	3N-Surg	Second	Yes
Tuesday, January 06, 2009	71	Light	2S-Med	Second	No
Tuesday, January 06, 2009	88	Heavy	2N-Med	Third	No
Wednesday, January 07, 2009	101	Heavy	2N-Med	First	Yes

The first thing the data analyst must do is determine how the user wants the data organized. Intuitively we group patients as 18 and under (adolescents), 19 to 39 (young adults), 40 to 59 (adults), 60 to 79 (senior citizens), and 80 and older (octogenarians). Other categorization schemes could be used such as 0–9, 10–19, 20–29, and so on. The ultimate scheme will be based on the goals of the analysis and may be influenced by the data. If 90% of events fall into a single category (for example, 90% of patient falls with injury occur in the 60 to 79 population), the user should consider subdividing the groups into smaller divisions. Excel's Frequency function will review the data and count every value that occurs at or below the user-specified value. Excel calls the user-defined ranges "bins." Using the categorization scheme described above, the data analyst enters 19, 39, 59, 79, and the maximum age + 1 to ensure that all values are counted into five empty cells in the worksheet. So, entering "19" results in Excel counting every patient with an age less than 19, that is, patients 18 and under.

After entering the bin values (the desired age ranges), the data analyst must highlight the five cells next to the bin values to be filled with the counts. Highlighting the four cells adjoining the bin values creates a concise table and facilitates the creation of the stratification chart. On the Excel main menu the data analyst selects **Formulas**. Formulas contains the following choices: **Function Library, Defined Names, Formula Auditing**, and **Calculation**. Under Function Library, select **Insert Function**, which allows the data analyst to search for a function or select a category of functions to browse. Selecting **All** provides alphabetical access to every function, and the data analyst can browse until they find **Frequency**. After selecting Frequency, the data analyst must specify a data range in Data_array. This specifies the data to be sorted and a range for Bins_array, the categories to sort the data into or how to sort. At this point it is tempting to hit **OK**, but hitting OK will result in only the first category being counted; that is, only patients under 18 will be counted. To obtain the counts for each category, the data analyst must simultaneously hit **Crtl**, **Shift**, and **Enter** to produce the frequency counts in cells K12–K16.

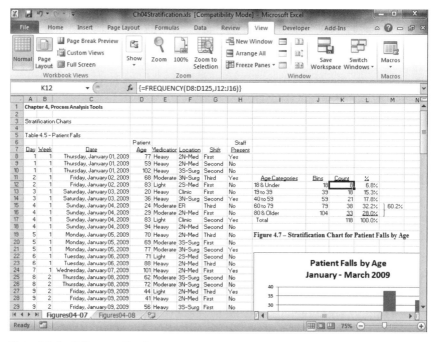

Figure 4.6 Excel's Frequency Function

A common problem in data analysis is lost or uncounted data. The total number of falls should be double-checked in the data set and frequency table to guarantee that all patient falls have been counted; making decisions based on incomplete data may lead to erroneous conclusions. The data analyst should go back to the original data set and count the number of patient falls. This can be done by inserting the function **=COUNT(data range)** and compare the total to the total of the frequency table, **=SUM(data range)**. In this example, **=COUNT(A8:A125)** yields 118 falls and equals the sum of the frequency table, **=SUM(K12:K16)**, so all patient falls have been counted. The last step is to produce a column chart. The data analyst highlights the data range he wants to build the graph from, that is, the column labeled Count, and selects **Insert**, and **Column**. To enter the column titles, the data analyst right-clicks on the produced chart and selects Select Data followed by Horizontal (Categories) Axis Labels.

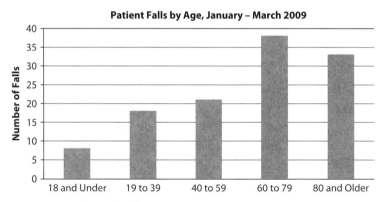

Figure 4.7 Stratification Chart for Patient Falls by Age

The graph is easy to interpret. The over-60 population accounts for 60.2% of all falls, and both the 60 to 79 and 80 and over groups account for more falls than the other three age groupings. The problem with using raw counts is that we would expect the number of patient falls to vary proportionally with the number of admissions in each age group. Introducing the number of admissions would add an important element to assess organizational performance and risk. What an organization wants to know is how its rate of patient falls compares to that of other institutions. A 500-bed hospital will have more falls than a 200-bed institution, so equalization requires a common metric, falls per admission. Falls per admissions allows users to compare outcomes across dissimilar organizations. Internally, falls per admission stratified by age group facilitates risk assessment; for example, examining total falls by patients over 80 divided by total patients over 80 allows the organization to determine which age group has the highest rate of falls.

Does the level of medication have an effect on patient falls? Unlike patient age, which is a numeric value, level of medication is categorized as heavy, moderate, and light. These are labels rather than numbers and neither =FREQUENCY nor =COUNT can analyze nonnumeric data. To determine the relationship between medication and patient falls we use **=COUNTIF(data range, criteria)**, which requires the data analyst to enter a data range to be reviewed and a criterion to be counted. **=COUNTIF(E8:E125,"Heavy")** reviews the specified data range and counts the number of times a label occurs that matches the user-specified value "Heavy" and documents 49 occurrences. Note that the criteria must be entered in double quotation marks to find and count the specified character string.

Data analysts can avoid directly entering labels by specifying a flexible cell reference, **=COUNTIF(E$8:E$125,I14)**, which allows the data analyst to copy this function through a data table without having to type the criteria into each function. Note that the data range is a fixed cell reference due to the inclusion of the "$" in front of the row number. The second argument, I14, is a flexible reference, meaning the row number will be incremented if the function is copied down a spreadsheet, cell I12 is "Light," I13 is "Moderate", and I14 is "Heavy." Copying **=COUNTIF(E$8:E$125,I12)** down two rows directs Excel to count the occurrences between E8 and E125 that meet the desired character strings specified in cells I12 through I14.

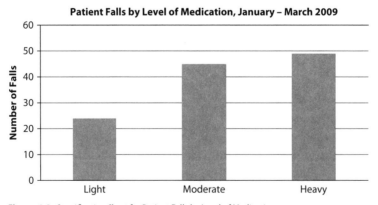

Figure 4.8 Stratification Chart for Patient Falls by Level of Medication

Figure 4.8 demonstrates that there is little difference between the number of falls occurring between the moderately and heavily medicated patients. In terms of risk assessment and instituting precautions, this information should lead providers to pay extra attention to both groups of patients (as opposed to lightly medicated patients). With Figures 4.7

and 4.8 users can begin to develop a profile of patients most likely to fall: patients over 65 who are moderately or heavily medicated. The other data in Table 4.5 could be used to examine the influence of location, time of day, and whether the patient was alone or with an employee at the time of the fall and further define our risk profile by adding organizational characteristics to patient characteristics to focus fall prevention efforts.

The goal of stratification is to subdivide data to identify factors associated with a large percentage of events. The identification of common factors should move the user closer to finding the ultimate causes of a problem by focusing attention on a small number of factors and focusing the development of solutions on specific issues.

Histograms

A **histogram** is another method for visually displaying information. Unlike Pareto and stratification charts which record the number of times a discrete event occurred, histograms analyze events that have an outcome that can be measured on a continuous scale. Histograms are based on the **normal distribution** (bell curve). When data is normally distributed, the majority of events fall close to the average and exceedingly high and low values are rare.

The mean (average) birth weight in the United States is 3175 grams (or seven pounds) and low birth weight is considered to be less than 2500 grams. The second variable that defines a normal distribution, in addition to the mean, is the standard deviation. The standard deviation used for birth weights in Figure 4.9 is 600 grams; if weight ranges are established using this standard deviation, the expected number of babies in each category as shown in Figure 4.9 is produced.

histogram
a column chart that displays the frequency of occurrence

normal distribution
a distribution that approximates the density of many phenomena where 68.3% of events fall within one standard deviation of the mean and 95.5% and 99.7% within two and three standard deviations

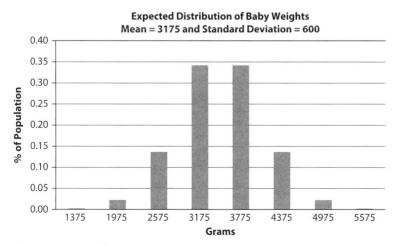

Figure 4.9 Histogram for Baby Weights

Babies weights in this histogram are normally distributed: 68% of the population falls within one standard deviation of the mean. The histogram shows that 34% of babies weigh between 3175 grams (the mean) and 3763 grams (the mean plus one standard deviation), and 34% weigh between 3175 grams and 2587 grams (the mean minus one standard deviation). We expect 95% of babies will weigh between 1999 and 4351 grams, the mean plus or minus two standard deviations. Conversely we expect less than 5% of babies would weigh less than 1999 grams or more than 4361 grams (more than two standard deviations from the mean). To be exact, only 2.27% of babies should fall more than two standard deviations above the mean and 2.27% should fall more than two standard deviations under the mean. Figure 4.9 also displays the occurrences beyond three standard deviations, below 1411 grams and above 5527 grams. At these weights the graph becomes undecipherable, but statistical theory tells us that these extreme values occur at a rate of 0.0013, or 13 births per in 10,000 cases.

Suppose a data analyst wants to examine inpatient length of stay (LOS) for groups of physicians, between hospitals within a state, or between states across the United States. The goal would be to identify physicians, hospitals, or states that have inappropriately high or low LOS. If LOS is too low, patients may be being discharged too quickly and may not be receiving proper care. If LOS is too high, this could indicate a different problem. LOS may be too high because care was not rendered at the appropriate time or inappropriate care injured the patient, necessitating an extended stay. In addition to quality issues, LOS must be examined to ensure that beds are available for future patients and resources are being effectively used. Effective management of quality and capacity dictates that patients who do not require inpatient care not be admitted to or allowed to linger in the hospital.

Table 4.6 LOS by State

State	Number of Hospitals	Staffed Beds	Total Discharges	Patient Days	Gross Patient Revenue ($000)
AK—Alaska	12	998	34,421	219,344	$1,538,741
AL—Alabama	99	15,859	653,176	3,532,253	$24,307,131
AR—Arkansas	57	8,137	325,221	1,736,664	$9,950,236
AZ—Arizona	64	11,394	664,559	2,843,523	$23,717,971
CA—California	351	75,854	3,156,632	18,647,141	$174,565,816
CO—Colorado	45	8,082	375,654	1,930,955	$16,965,279
CT—Connecticut	32	7,966	377,905	2,289,142	$13,733,179
DC—Washington DC	7	2,892	123,307	824,655	$5,163,822
DE—Delaware	6	2,070	96,563	585,331	$2,580,914
FL—Florida	175	52,773	2,267,578	12,215,719	$98,979,587
GA—Georgia	109	23,140	891,250	5,914,639	$32,451,158

Source: American Hospital Association, http://www.ahd.com/state_statistics.html.

Table 4.6 is a partial listing of hospital activity by state. (The full data is available online in the Ch04Problems.xls file, under the States tab.) The data table is less than informative, but by manipulating the data it can be converted into insightful information. Average LOS by state can be calculated by dividing patient days (column 5) by total discharges (column 4). For example, LOS for Alaska is 6.37 days (219,344 ÷ 34,421). The question is, how do Alaskan hospitals' LOS compare to the rest of the country?

After calculating LOS for each state, the next step is to calculate the minimum and maximum LOS across the United States. The minimum is calculated by entering **=MIN(data range)** and the maximum is calculated with **=MAX(data range)**. The minimum and maximum are required to determine the interval length, that is, how the data will be categorized or how many groups will be presented in the histogram. In this data set the minimum, **=MIN(G9:G61)**, is 4.28 (Arizona) and the maximum, **=MAX(G9:G61)**, is 8.50 (New York). LOS was almost twice as long in New York as in Arizona. Why? The difference, the range, between the minimum and maximum is 4.22 days. The interval length will be displayed in a histogram using columns and the desired histogram will have seven columns. A common rule of thumb is that a histogram should have between five and eight columns. Fewer than five columns does not provide sufficient differentiation of activity (too much aggregation) while more than eight results in too much information that may be difficult to interpret because it obscures natural breaks in the data. In this example seven columns were chosen but a user should review the produced histogram to determine if too many observations fall within an interval and, if so, should increase the number of intervals. Conversely, if multiple intervals have a small number of observations, the user may elect to increase the size of the interval and reduce the number of intervals in the chart. Interval length for each column is calculated by subtracting the minimum value from the maximum value and dividing the difference by the desired number of columns. In this example the interval length is 0.604 days, (8.50 − 4.28) ÷ 7.

Excel's **Frequency** function is used to sort LOS into the user-defined categories. The first bin is calculated as the minimum plus the interval length, 4.88 (4.28 days + 0.604 days). =FREQUENCY counts all states with a LOS equal to or less than 4.88 days. The second bin is the first bin plus the interval, 5.49 (4.88 + 0.604). The preceding bin calculated should continue to be incremented (by the interval length) until the maximum is reached. The first column of Table 4.7 shows the top of range LOS (bins) that Excel will use to summarize the data; that is, =FREQUENCY will count every state with a LOS equal to or under 4.88. In the second row Excel counts LOS equal to or under 5.49 and greater than 4.88. The procedure for operating Frequency is the same as discussed in stratification charts: the data analyst highlights the range adjacent to the established bins, selects Insert Function, enters the range to be sorted and bins, and hits Ctrl+Shift+Enter. This procedure will reproduce Table 4.7.

Table 4.7 LOS Frequency

Top of Range	Count
4.88	5
5.49	18
6.09	17
6.69	8
7.30	0
7.90	0
8.50	5
Total	53

After producing the frequency table, the data analyst highlights the counts (the range he or she wants to build the graph from), and selects **Insert** and **Column**. To enter the column titles, the data analyst must right-click on the produced chart and choose Select Data followed by Horizontal (Categories) Axis Labels to enter the LOS categories on the x-axis.

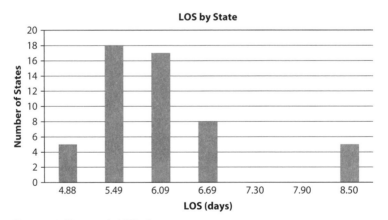

Figure 4.10 Histogram for LOS by State

The frequency table and histogram show that the vast majority of states have an average LOS of less than 6.69 days, but there are five states that have LOS considerably higher than the other states. New York has the highest LOS, and the other four states are Hawaii, North Dakota, South Dakota, and Montana. Except New York these states are all western states and have very few hospitals (group average = 19, U.S. average = 71). A sum is calculated to ensure that all states and territories were counted. The total records

53 occurrences; the data source included Washington DC, Puerto Rico, and Guam, in addition to the 50 states. The histogram in Figure 4.10 is skewed to the right, reflecting the fact that there is no upward limit on LOS.

Figure 4.11 examines common histogram shapes.

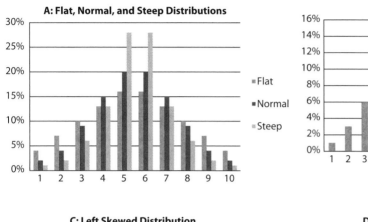

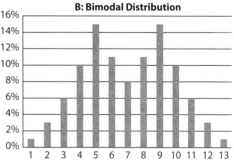

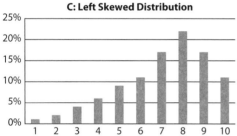

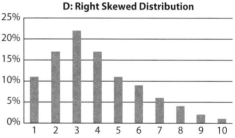

Figure 4.11 Histogram Distributions

The first histogram in Figure 4.11 shows three distributions. The first is the normal distribution (the gray columns). Contrasted against this is a more tightly distributed curve (the dark green columns), which demonstrates more consistent performance or outcomes. The last distribution (the light green columns) demonstrates less consistency, in which performance or outcomes are more evenly spread across the possible continuum. The steepness or flatness of a distribution allows a user to predict performance or outcomes. A user would be quite confident in predicting performance under the steep distribution. Predictions under the normal distribution would follow the standard pattern (68% within one standard deviation and so on), but with the flat distribution almost any outcome is equally likely.

The bimodal distribution suggests the possibility that two different groups with different performance or outcomes are being measured. The "valley" represents the demarcation between the performance of the higher- and lower-performing groups. The histogram skews to the left when performance has an upper limit, for example, 100%, but no significant lower limit exists. A good example is school grades. They cluster between 70% and 100%, but extremely low values do occur. When a distribution is skewed to the right, the phenomenon has a lower limit, typically zero, but no upper limit. Money incomes follow this pattern; the majority of American males cluster around the median income of $33,161 and there is a small number of individuals who earn billions of dollars per year skewing the distribution to the right (*Statistical Abstract of the United States*, 2011).

Histograms can also be produced using the Histogram function located in Excel's Data Analysis ToolPak. If the histogram function is used, the data analyst can specify the bin_array or allow Excel to default. If the default option is used, Excel produces an eight-column chart.

The power of histograms is they provide great insight into how a system is operating when the variable of interest is a continuous variable. In the LOS by State example (Figure 4.10), the data could have been analyzed as attribute data: how many states have LOS over 6.70 days. The output would be five states above and 48 states and territories below. What is lost in the analysis is any indication of what average performance was or the distribution of performance. Figure 4.10 demonstrates that average LOS generally falls between 5.49 and 6.09 days, but five states have LOS substantially above this range, with no states lying between 6.69 and 7.90 days.

Check Sheets

check sheet
a tool to collect data and display how many times an event occurs

The **check sheet** is the fourth tool that can be used to identify problems. Check sheets serve two purposes: they are a tool to collect information and can also be used to analyze performance. There are four major types of check sheets that allow a user to monitor aspects of a production process and move beyond simple identification of a problem to explore its potential causes. Check sheets are designed to require minimal data collection effort; data entry often is limited to making a check mark in the appropriate field. One variant requires the user to note the date of the occurrence rather than a check mark in the appropriate field. Check sheets are also designed to be informational without any data organization or analysis. Unlike the data analysis tools used to create Pareto charts, stratification charts, and histograms, a check sheet can be understood immediately after the data is recorded without manipulation.

The four types of check sheets are process distribution, defective item, defect location, and defect factor, a.k.a. defect concentration diagram

(Goetsch and Davis 2010). Process distribution check sheets are concerned with the variability of a process while defective item, defect location, and defect factor check sheets are concerned with the type of defect, where the defect occurred, and why the defect occurred.

Process Distribution Check Sheet

Like the histogram, the **process distribution check sheet** is designed to monitor the variability of the output from a process. A check sheet could be set up to record times, temperature, weight, height and width, or quantity/dose. Table 4.8 records wait times for ten patients over a week in an ER; however, the data in this format is not insightful.

process distribution check sheet
a tool to record and display the variability of a process

Table 4.8 ER Wait Times (in Minutes)

	PATIENTS									
	1	2	3	4	5	6	7	8	9	10
Day 1	5	29	32	39	46	59	55	63	72	71
Day 2	14	40	46	65	79	82	99	110	145	187
Day 3	7	14	29	32	49	58	52	74	63	88
Day 4	22	36	43	47	57	62	71	89	92	109
Day 5	13	16	19	38	41	59	46	49	73	83
Day 6	2	28	41	43	49	58	57	46	76	92
Day 7	28	22	39	33	48	54	62	72	81	104

To improve the usefulness of the data, we will convert the data from a table into a check sheet. If a check sheet was originally used to capture the data, all that would be needed is a check mark in the appropriate row. After the conversion, Figure 4.12, one can see immediately that the average wait is between 45 and 60 minutes and that there are infrequent occurrences of long waits.

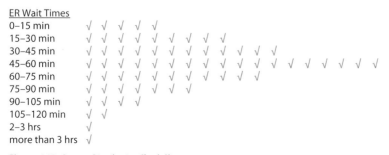

Figure 4.12 Process Distribution Check Sheet

Figure 4.13 uses the same data as Figure 4.12 but uses numbers rather than check marks to record not only how long a patient waited but the date of their visit. In this example, the ER manager randomly sampled ten visits per day for one week, "1" equals the first day of the week, "2" the second, and so on. The addition of the date of occurrence provides more information and allows a user to identify patterns. In this example, the first day of the week had short wait times; there were no patients who waited more than 75 minutes, but patients on day two often waited 90 minutes or more for treatment.

ER Wait Times

Category																	
0–15 min	1	3	3	5	6												
15–30 min	1	2	3	4	5	5	6	7	7								
30–45 min	1	1	2	3	4	4	5	5	6	6	7	7					
45–60 min	1	1	1	2	3	3	3	4	4	5	5	5	6	6	6	6	7	7
60–75 min	1	1	1	2	3	3	4	4	5	7	7						
75–90 min	2	2	3	4	5	6	7										
90–105 min	2	4	6	7													
105–120 min	2	4															
2–3 hrs	2																
more than 3 hrs	2																

Figure 4.13 Process Distribution Check Sheet with Dates

The use of the day of the week instead of a check mark is helpful in identifying deviations from normal operation and diagnosing why wait times are long because it identifies specific days to begin the investigation. In the case of Figure 4.12, the wait time may be deemed acceptable by an observer but with the addition of date of occurrence, Figure 4.13, it becomes clear that while average wait time over the week may be acceptable, there is a problem on day two. Day two had the two highest wait times over the period, and more than half the visits sampled had a wait time greater than 75 minutes. Does this day of the week regularly have high patient volume and subsequently long wait times, or was this particular day adversely affected by an infrequent occurring event such as a major accident or the absence of more than one employee? Improvement demands that users understand the situation before attempting change, and more information is preferred to less when drawing conclusions concerning the performance of a system.

The process distribution check sheet is similar to the previously discussed histogram in that we expect the output of a process to follow a normal distribution, with some high and low occurrences but with the majority of events falling in the middle. The next three check sheets—defective item, defect factor, and defect location—are more closely related to Pareto charts, which examine how often an event occurs, and stratification charts, which examine what the characteristics of an event are.

Defective Item Check Sheet

The **defective item check sheet** is used to identify the type of event occurring. Assume you work in the pharmacy and want to start a program to reduce medication errors. The first question is where to start. Which type of medication error should be focused on? The first step is construction of a check sheet with the major types of errors: prescribing errors, dispensing errors, administration errors, and drug delivery devices, as seen in Figure 4.14. The user must precisely define each type of error to minimize misclassification; definitions must be clear enough that if different people observe the same event it will be consistently recorded. Prescription errors are errors by physicians on the type or dosage of medicine prescribed or the failure to recognize adverse reactions with other prescribed drugs. Dispensing errors would be any deviations from the prescribed orders. For example, an illegible prescription filled incorrectly would be a dispensing error as it would be the pharmacist's responsibility to clarify the prescription before filling it. Administration errors would be any error by the person responsible for delivering the medicine to the patient. Potential administration errors include delivering the medication at the wrong time (too soon, too late, or not at all), wrong route (orally, intravenously, or rectally), or giving it to the wrong patient. Drug delivery device errors include misprogramming, equipment failure, and intravenous (IV) line mix-ups. The second step is recording data over a period of time: week, month, or year.

defective item check sheet
a tool to record and display the type of errors or defects occurring

Medication Error
Prescribing   √ √ √ √ √ √ √ √ √ √ √
Dispensing   √ √ √ √
Administration   √ √ √ √ √ √
Drug Device   √ √

Figure 4.14 Defective Item Check Sheet

Figure 4.14 shows that the most frequent type of error is prescribing. At this point the user may wish to further subdivide prescription error into more distinct categories before initiating corrective action. The defective item check sheet can assist in defining the order of process improvement by focusing attention on the most frequent types of errors. In this example, prescribing errors should be tackled first, followed by administration errors, dispensing errors, and finally drug device errors.

Defect Factor Check Sheet

The **defect factor check sheet** records the factors present when an event occurred and attempts to determine if these factors contributed to the

defect factor check sheet
a tool to record and display the factors present when an error or defect occurs

error. For example, are prescription errors related to a specific physician, patient group, manufacturer, day and time, or level of activity? Besides these factors, errors may also be related to external or physical factors such as temperature, lighting, and weather.

Physician
Physician A	√ √ √
Physician B	√ √ √ √
Physician C	√ √ √
Physician D	√ √ √ √
Physician E	√ √ √ √
Physician F	√ √ √ √ √
Physician G	√ √
Physician H	√ √ √ √
Physician I	√ √ √ √

Day of Week
Monday	√ √ √ √
Tuesday	√ √ √
Wednesday	√ √
Thursday	√ √
Friday	√ √ √
Saturday	√ √ √ √ √ √ √ √ √
Sunday	√ √ √ √ √ √ √ √ √ √

Figure 4.15 Defect Factor Check Sheets

Figure 4.15 provides two examples of defect factor check sheets; the physician factor check sheet is used to record the prescribing doctor. In this example errors appear to be independent of provider. There were 33 prescription errors, and they were evenly distributed across the nine identified physicians. The average number of errors per physician was 3.67, and physician F had the highest number of errors with five while physician G had only two. The other seven doctors had between three and four medication errors.

The day of the week check sheet indicates that the day of the week affects prescription errors. The average daily error is 4.71 errors per day, but Saturday saw nine errors and Sunday had ten. The user can see that the average weekend error rate is 9.5 versus 2.8 during the week. The spike in error rates over the weekend indicates that improvement efforts should first explore what is occurring on the weekend that may contribute to the higher number of errors.

defect location check sheet
a tool to record and display where errors or defects are observed

Defect Location Check Sheet

Similar to the defect factor check sheet, the **defect location check sheet** attempts to pinpoint the cause of problems. The defect location check sheet focuses on where events arise: is one location more error prone and, if so, what operating conditions impact the number of errors made? Figure 4.16 demonstrates that the largest number of medication errors occurs in the ER. One could speculate that the hectic environment and lack of information in that location increase error rates. In the next section we will look at tools that help determine the actual cause of the errors.

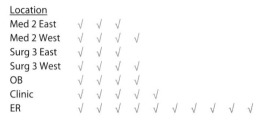

Location
Med 2 East	√	√	√							
Med 2 West	√	√	√	√						
Surg 3 East	√	√	√							
Surg 3 West	√	√	√	√						
OB	√	√	√	√						
Clinic	√	√	√	√	√					
ER	√	√	√	√	√	√	√	√	√	√

Figure 4.16 Defect Location Check Sheet

Check sheets are an easy-to-use tool to collect data on operations. The user can define what parts of the process to monitor, and data recording takes minimal effort. A major advantage of check sheets is that after the data is recorded, they provide an immediate visual representation of system performance.

Tools to Identify Causes

While the initial discussion focused on tools to identify errors, the second section of this chapter begins the task of identifying the cause of problems. The defect factor and location check sheets started the process by shifting the focus from what was happening to examining the factors present when an error occurred and where the error occurred. This section introduces three additional tools to identify the potential causes of problems: cause and effect diagrams, **scatter diagrams**, and **flowcharts**.

Cause and Effect Diagrams

Cause and effect diagrams (also known as fishbone diagrams or Ishikawa diagrams) are designed to provide structure to the search for the causes of a problem, which is often an ad hoc process. When errors are discovered, a natural reaction is to leap to a conclusion to their cause. This tendency, though it facilitates rapid action, is susceptible to error. The cause and effect diagram establishes a framework to guide the process to ensure that multiple parties are involved, the process receives a thorough review, and causes rather than symptoms are identified and corrected.

The problem with ad hoc problem solving is that it may reflect only the views of those involved (other affected parties' concerns may be ignored),

scatter diagrams
a chart used to assess the relationship between two variables

flowcharts
a tool to document the steps a process should or does follow

and it may hang the problem on a single cause (or symptom) when multiple causes are at play. Consequently a solution designed to correct one part of the process may fail to prevent reoccurrence of the error when factors are interrelated.

The cause and effect diagram is designed to focus a team's attention on a single error or problem. The output of the process is a graph that organizes and displays the multiple potential causes of the identified problem. The diagram should provide insight to the users and highlight the relationships among multiple factors that could be related to a problem. After a problem is identified, the search for the cause begins with identifying the potential major causes. Once the major causes are established, users attempt to break down the major issues into particular factors that could have caused or contributed to the problem. If a problem is believed to be due to labor, the particular labor factors that could be responsible for the problem are considered: inadequate staffing, undertrained staff, fatigue, and so on.

The process of developing a cause and effect chart includes:

1.   Assemble the problem-solving team; this should include all involved or affected parties to see the problem from all perspectives. Health care issues should be explored by a team that includes physicians, nurses, other health care providers, quality improvement experts, administration, and patients.

2.   Clearly define the problem; the goal is to eliminate disagreement over what the problem is and ensure that all team members agree on the problem and work toward the same goal. Given the often substantial disagreement that arises among committee members over their task, this step operates on the premise that a well-defined problem is half solved.

3.   After the problem is agreed upon, it is placed in a box on the right side of the page, as shown in Figure 4.17.

4.   A horizontal spine is drawn from the left side of the page to the box containing the problem.

5.   Brainstorm to identify potential major causes of the problem; Table 4.9 shows the most common causes.

6.   Place each major cause in a box with a rib connecting it to the central spine; a common rule of thumb is the number of major causes should be between two and seven.

7.   Identify sub-causes; each identified sub-cause is attached to the appropriate rib (major cause), this process continues until the committee is satisfied that all likely causes have been identified.

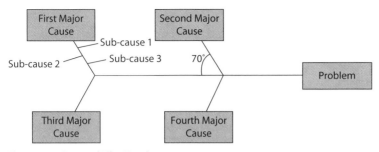

Figure 4.17 Cause and Effect Template

The causes and sub-causes vary according to the problem being explored, but some generalizations can be made. Five major causes are commonly identified: people, supplies, equipment, process, or environment. These can also be remembered as the five Ms: manpower, materials, machines, methods, or mother nature. When problems arise, they can be traced to errors in human performance, a failure in the materials or equipment being used, an error-prone system, or environmental factors (or a combination of these). The extensive use of root cause analysis in health care can be gauged by the multitude of articles that have been published. As of December 5, 2012, PubMed reports 121 articles with "root cause analysis" in the title.

Table 4.9 Five Majors Causes and Frequent Sub-causes

People (workforce or manpower; should be used to reinforce 5Ms): Cause and effect diagrams often divide manpower into two major causes—employees (production or staff) and management (supervision)—to distinguish errors due to poor worker performance from the failure of management to provide necessary support and oversight of the production process. Typical production sub-causes include lack of knowledge (improper or no instruction on how to perform a task), lack of skill (employee knows how to complete a task but is unable to perform at the required level), inconsistency (employee is knowledgeable and skilled but is inconsistent due to absence, inattention, carelessness, willingness to skip steps, or refusal to use safety devices). Managerial sub-causes include assignment (supervisors select individuals who lack knowledge or skills), supervision (insufficient oversight), and lack of incentive (superior or inferior performance is not rewarded or penalized).

Supplies (materials): design (supplies unsuitable for use), inferior (poor-quality materials used, such as purchase of supplies at lowest unit cost versus lowest total cost), defective or damaged (reliable materials impaired before they enter production and impairment is not recognized), and unavailable (supplies not available at time of need).

Equipment (machines): design (appropriateness), assembly (performance hindered by poor construction), age (old or outdated), maintenance (periodic or necessary maintenance not performed), inappropriate use (equipment employed in unintended use), unreliable (performance dependent on environmental factors or continuous recalibration), or unavailable (equipment unavailable when needed).

Table 4.9 *(Continued)*

Process (method): process problems arise from how work is organized independent of labor, materials, and equipment used, and the process is susceptible to error. Typical process problems include procedures (poor or missing descriptions of how work should be performed), fragmentation (noncontinuous processes that increase probability of error), excessive hand-offs (frequent transfer of responsibility disrupts continuity of performance), and unavailability of information (employees do not have timely or accurate information to complete tasks).

Environment (mother nature): environmental problems are defined as organizational culture issues such as low performance expectations among staff, inadequacy of staffing, and internal (employee) versus external (customer) orientation. These types of issues are clearly managerial problems. Environmental issues also include external factors that cannot be controlled but must be recognized and accounted for, such as inadequate space, distractions, interruptions, temperature, light, and moisture.

The final step is to determine which major cause and sub-cause is the most likely to produce the problem. The reader is reminded of Occam's razor, which states: "Entities should not be multiplied unnecessarily." That is, there is little to be gained by making things more complicated than they need to be. Newton provided a more eloquent interpretation: "We are to admit no more causes of natural things than such as are both true and sufficient to explain their appearances." Occam's razor is often interpreted to mean that simple solutions are better than complicated or convoluted theories when searching for the explanation of some phenomenon or problem.

Cause and Effect Example: Medication Error

A hospital wants to analyze medication errors and uses the "five rights" of medication administration—right patient, right medication, right dosage, right time, and right route—as a starting point for their analysis. The five rights of medication administration highlights the five ways medication errors can occur; any of the rights can be done wrong. The hospital has collected data and determined that the most frequent problem is wrong medication. The cause and effect diagram asks: What are the potential causes for the wrong medication being administered to a patient?

Six major categories will be used (and they differ from the five major causes given in Table 4.9): staffing, patient information, drug labeling, prescribing, environment, and process.

More than one sub-cause could be contributing to the problem. For example, unlabeled drugs could result from understaffing in the pharmacy

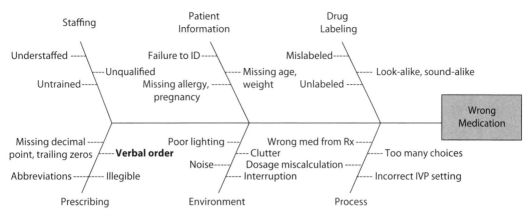

Figure 4.18 Cause and Effect Diagram for Wrong Medication

or from poor quality labels that fall off if they get wet—a purchasing problem. Let's assume the hospital determined that the problem is mistranslation of verbal orders (note this sub-cause is in bold on Figure 4.18). The responses could be to prohibit verbal drug orders (which could not be enforced), or to require mandatory read-backs of all verbal orders, and/or 24-hour physician sign-off on verbal orders. Prohibiting verbal orders fails to recognize that there are times when it is undesirable to delay treatment until a written order can be obtained. Mandatory read-backs and 24-hour sign-offs recognize the necessity of verbal orders but attempt to reduce the susceptibility to error by instituting processes by which errors can be quickly recognized and corrected.

A common mistake that occurs when the problem is not well defined is that people will focus on the types of errors occurring rather than on the reasons that errors occur. For example, when dealing with the five rights, if the wrong route is determined to be the problem, the analysis could focus on what the wrong administration routes are rather than on why the wrong route was used.

Scatter Diagrams

Scatter diagrams (also known as XY charts) are used to determine if there is a relationship between two variables. Does one variable (x) produce or predict changes in another variable (y)? To be statistically precise, scatter diagrams assess correlation—whether two variables move together; they do not assess causation. If a relationship is observed, we cannot assume that x causes y or that y causes x, so all we can say with confidence is that the variables are correlated. The case for causation can be strengthened by relying on theory, time dependency (x always precedes y), or by testing (elimination of x changes y). The reader must remember that causation cannot be determined through graphs or statistical methods.

Scatter diagrams graph points in a two-dimensional space (x on the horizontal axis and y on the vertical axis) to determine if a change in one variable is correlated with a change in the other variable. The x variable is often deemed the independent variable, and y is the dependent variable. The question is: How does y change when x increases? Does y increase, decrease, stay the same, or increase to a point and decrease thereafter?

Figure 4.19 displays four cases. The points in graph A indicate that as x increases, y increases. In this example, average ER wait time and number of patients are graphed. The graph indicates that as the number of patients increases, average wait time increases. This is called a positive or **direct relationship**. The effect of the number of patients on wait time is obvious and expected. We do not expect average wait time to drive the number of patients, so the direction of causation is clear—an increase in patients should result in longer waiting times.

Graph B demonstrates a negative or **inverse relationship**. The y variable remains average wait time, but the independent variable is number of ER staff. The direction of correlation is obvious: the greater the level of staffing, the faster patients should be seen, all other things constant. Graph B demonstrates that our thinking is correct: as staffing increases, wait time decreases. If graphs A and B reflect the situation in the ER, the actions that can be taken to reduce patient wait times are clear: the hospital could reduce the number of patients seeking treatment in the ER by redirecting less serious cases to other sites or increase the size of the staff.

Graph C demonstrates **no relationship**; that is, wait time does not change with time of day. If wait time were changing systematically with time of day, the solution would again be obvious: add staff or divert patients during that time. Graph D demonstrates a **nonlinear relationship**. In this case, there is a positive relationship—y increases with increases in x over a certain range—but after the inflexion point is reached there is an inverse relationship. This case may represent the relationship between patient well-being and the dosage of pain medication. There is an optimal range of medication to reduce pain. Where the graph changes direction and beyond this point, the patient will experience reduced well-being and potential drug dependency or overdosing.

The first scatter diagram in Figure 4.19 displays a positive or direct relationship; as x, the number of patient arrivals, increases, y, wait time, increases. The second diagram shows a negative or inverse relationship; as

direct relationship

an increase (or decrease) in the independent variable predicts or causes an increase (or decrease) in the dependent variable; variables move in same direction

inverse relationship

an increase (or decrease) in the independent variable predicts or causes a decrease (increase) in the dependent variable; variables move in opposite directions

no relationship

a change in the independent variable has no effect on the dependent variable

nonlinear relationship

a relationship between two variables that cannot be described by a straight line; the dependent variable may increase or decrease with increases in the independent variable

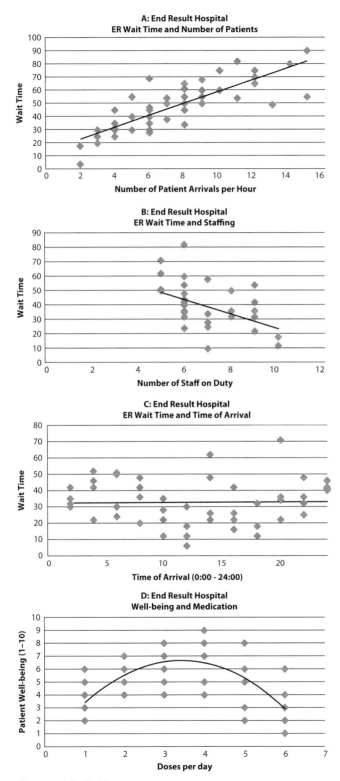

Figure 4.19 Scatter Diagrams

x increases, y decreases—more staffing leads to lower wait times. The third diagram shows no relationship; that is, y is unaffected by changes in x—wait time cannot be predicted based on time of arrival. The fourth diagram shows a nonlinear relationship; y increases with increases in x to a point and then decreases. In this case patient well-being improves as medication is increased, but past the inflection point further doses reduce well-being.

Assume that a hospital wants to determine if the number of cases it admits is correlated with LOS. One possibility is that hospitals with higher case volumes will develop more efficient processes and move patients through their hospital stay more expeditiously. On the other hand, greater volume could complicate patient scheduling and prolong a visit. A third option is that volume may have no impact on LOS. The data in Table 4.10 was collected by the Pennsylvania Cost Containment Council for patients in DRG 143.

Table 4.10 DRG 143 Length of Stay, 2005

Hospital Name	Cases	Length of Stay	Average Charge
Abington Memorial	1293	1.5	$23,308
Albert Einstein	845	1.5	$20,960
Aliquippa Community	31	1.9	$7,700
Allegheny General	237	1.6	$11,481
Alle-Kiski	242	1.7	$10,276
Altoona Regional	147	1.7	$8,943
Armstrong County Memorial	42	1.7	$3,967
Ashland Regional	23	1.4	$5,369

Source: Pennsylvania Cost Containment Council, http://www.phc4.org/.

To produce a scatter diagram, the data analyst highlights the data range (Cases and Length of Stay), clicks on **Insert**, and selects **Scatter**. Excel produces a scatter diagram, but the user can see from examining the data points that there is no clear trend. To obtain greater insight, the data analyst should right-click on one of the data points and add a trend line. In most cases a linear trend line will be appropriate, but the data analyst should examine the scatter plot to determine if a nonlinear trend line would do a better job fitting the data. The trend line shows a slight decline in LOS as number of cases decreases. The complete data shows that hospitals performing 50 to 100 cases have an average LOS of approximately 1.7 days while those performing more than 1,000 have an LOS of about 1.6 days. The last task is to format the graph so it is easy for a reader to interpret by adding a title and labels on the x- and y-axes.

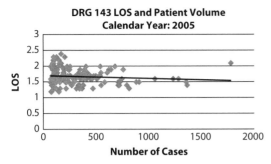

DRG 143 LOS and Patient Volume
Calendar Year: 2005

Figure 4.20 Scatter Diagram of LOS and Patient Volume

The goal of assessing scatter diagrams is to determine if changing one variable (the independent variable) is likely to have an impact on another variable (the dependent variable). Unlike the cause and effect diagram, in which the correct cause is determined by group consensus, the scatter diagram is based on data and evidence. Readers should be cautious in attempting to pinpoint causation based on a scatter diagram; the correlation of two variables does not determine causation and can obscure the fact that a third, unknown variable may be affecting both variables. In Figure 4.20 a lower LOS is correlated with a higher number of cases, but both may be the result of the skills and reputation of the medical team. A highly skilled medical team may attract patients and capture more cases and may deliver care more expeditiously.

Flowcharts

Flowcharts are tools to increase comprehension of how a system operates or should operate. A flowchart, which visually represents a process using a standardized set of symbols, attempts to trace the major steps of a process, noting the entry of inputs into the system, functions performed, decisions made, and outputs produced.

Flowcharts outline relationships and document or record what is happening in a system, including the start and finish of a process and what functions should occur. Elaborate flowcharts may expand on the basic steps by identifying who is responsible for the completion of each function, how long each function should take, or how performance will be assessed. Flowcharts are communication devices; they communicate how a system should operate and can be used to inform all participants (workers and customers) of what is expected.

While a detailed flowchart may seem unnecessary, one must remember the multiple actors in a process. Sinanan et al. (2000) found in a study of patient scheduling that there were six departments "and a cadre of patient care coordinators" involved in planning patient visits *before* any clinical activities were undertaken. A flowchart, by explicit recognition of the people and elements involved in patient scheduling, provided the first step toward simplifying and improving the process.

When a problem arises, it is useful to study a flowchart that documents the expected process in order to identify the source of the problem if one exists. Did the process begin in the expected way, were all the steps completed, were the steps completed in the proper sequence, were the steps completed properly, and did they generate the expected outputs? The first step in exploring a problem is to determine what should have been done and what was done.

Unfortunately flowcharts are often created *after* a problem arises. Rather than being prescriptive, describing how the process *should* operate, flowcharts frequently document how a process *is* operated and serve as a launching point for contemplating what was missing or what was done wrong. The second step in many error investigations, after a team is assembled, is to develop a flowchart. Figure 4.21 reviews the major symbols used in flowcharting, describes how to produce a flowchart in Word, and presents an example of a flowchart.

Microsoft Word provides an easy-to-use feature to create flowcharts. On the main Word tool bar, a data analyst would select **Insert**, which offers the data analyst the choice to create Pages, Tables, Illustrations, Links, Header & Footer, Text, and Symbols. In the **Illustrations** group the data analyst can select Picture, Clip Art, **Shapes**, SmartArt and Chart. The Shapes menu includes **Flowchart**.

Flowchart provides the data analyst with a wide variety of flowcharting symbols. The data analyst simply right-clicks the desired shape and left-clicks to position it on her flowchart. The data analyst can enter text in the symbol by right-clicking within the inserted symbol and selecting Add Text. The data analyst can size the symbol by right-clicking on the symbol and dragging it to the desired size.

Tools to Identify Solutions

Once a potential cause has been identified, a means of correction must be selected. Since there are many ways to solve a problem, users are faced with multiple choices, some more popular than others, and a team is unlikely to immediately agree on one approach. The committee must devise a process for reducing a list of options to one or two items to implement. The quality improvement team should not attempt to introduce multiple changes to a process at the same time because it is then

1. Event (inverted triangle): start of a process, such as patient arrives, triggering a set of operations.

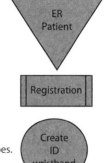

2. Procedure (rectangle with vertical lines on each side): a process that requires multiple steps.

3. Operation (circle or rectangle): a single-step function, a task that an employee does.

4. Operation with inspection (circle in a square): a single-step function plus subsequent inspection; one person performs task, second person checks or verifies.

5. Decision (diamond): a decision that often requires a yes-or-no answer. Yes meets the condition, and no does not meet the condition. The answer to the question determines the future path; such as triage or true emergency?

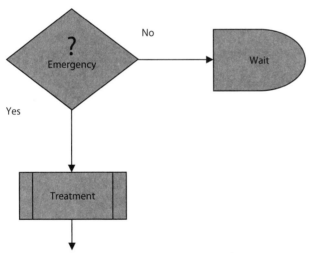

6. Document (rectangle with scalloped bottom): production of a report, receipt

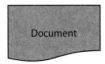

Figure 4.21 Common Flowchart Symbols

impossible to determine which changes were effective and which may have had no impact. The quality improvement team should also consider workers within the process and not overwhelm them with multiple changes within a short time. If multiple changes are required, their

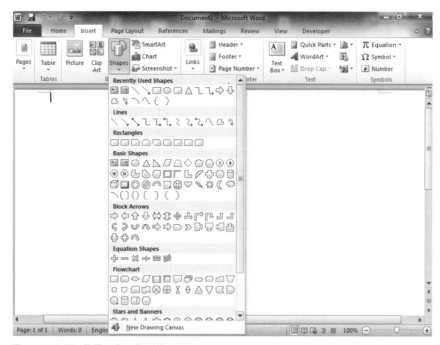

Figure 4.22 Word's Flowchart Capability

implementation should be staggered to give employees time to adjust to new processes.

Peter Drucker suggests four criteria that should be considered when selecting a solution: risk, economy of effort, timing, and resources (Drucker [1954] 1982, 362–363). Risk is concerned with the ratio of the expected benefit and cost of an action. Economy of action aims at achieving the maximum result with the least effort. Timing speaks to how quickly a problem must be resolved, and resources demands that any action be within the abilities of those who must carry it into action.

Multivoting and **Q-sort** are forced ranking techniques. The problem is that all proposed solutions have merit in that they were deemed worthy of consideration. But not all solutions are created equal; some are more likely to be effective and more likely to succeed than others. The challenge is to reduce a list of potential solutions to a manageable and implementable number.

Multivoting
an iterative technique for narrowing choices when faced with a wide range of alternatives by limiting the number of alternatives an individual may choose and selecting the most supported options in the voting group

Q-sort
a technique for ranking choices along a continuum when there are small differences among alternatives

Multivoting

The first technique provides each team member with a limited number of votes and forces each individual to select his or her top choices. A series of votes are held until a single solution or set of solutions is determined. Table 4.11 lists the steps involved.

Table 4.11 The Multivoting Process

1.	Label a set of potential solutions with letters or numbers. Post the list.
2.	Determine the desired outcome and how many solutions are sought; in the following example the goal is a single solution.
3.	Determine how many potential solutions each group member will be allowed to vote on; for example, the group may determine that all members can vote their top two choices.
4.	After the number of votes is established, the votes are weighted and a member's first choice is given the highest weight and the less preferred choices are given lower weights. If only two votes are allowed, the top vote typically is allocated two points and the second vote one point.
5.	Tally votes.
6.	Determine minimum vote total for list reduction; that is, what is the minimum vote (or cut-off) required for a potential solution to remain in consideration?
7.	If the vote concludes with strong support for one solution, the voting process ends. If no clear winners emerge, drop the least supported solutions and revote; again, if one clear solution emerges, stop. If more than one solution continues to receive strong support, drop the least supported solutions and revote. Continue revoting and dropping until only one solution remains.

Assume that a three-person team (Kerry, Jerry, and Terry) has developed six potential solutions (labeled A – F) to institute to reduce the number of late OR starts. The group has decided that initiatives will be implemented one at a time until an acceptable rate of late starts is achieved. Table 4.12 lists the preference of each team member.

Table 4.12 Multivoting Table of Preferences

Member	First Choice	Second Choice	Third Choice	Fourth Choice	Fifth Choice	Sixth Choice
Jerry	A	C	E	F	B	D
Kerry	B	F	E	D	A	C
Terry	D	B	C	E	A	F

If each team member votes for his or her top choice, the team will be deadlocked in a three-way tie between initiatives A, B, and D. The group decides they will use multivoting to determine the first initiative to implement. Each member will vote for his or her top two choices, with first choice worth two points and second choice worth one point. After votes are tallied, they will drop low-tallying initiatives and revote until only two choices remain. Once the initiatives are reduced to two, each member will receive one vote for their top choice. Table 4.13 shows the tallies for the first round of voting.

Table 4.13 First Vote Results

Initiative	Top Vote	Second Choice	Total
A	Jerry 2		2
B	Kerry 2	Terry 1	3
C		Jerry 1	1
D	Terry 2		2
E			0
F		Kerry 1	1

The group decides to eliminate the low-supported initiatives, those with vote totals under 2, so initiatives C, E, and F are dropped, and the group will revote on A, B, and D. Table 4.14 shows the tallies for the second vote.

Table 4.14 Second Vote Results

Initiative	Top Vote	Second Choice	Total
A	Jerry 2		2
B	Kerry 2	Jerry 1, Terry 1	4
D	Terry 2	Kerry 1	3

The second vote reveals the strongest support for initiatives B and D, so the final vote pair these two solutions. At this stage, each vote is worth only one point.

Table 4.15 Final Vote Results

Initiative	Top Vote	Total
B	Kerry, Jerry	2
D	Terry	1

The final vote concludes that there is higher support for B than D. This vote came down to Jerry's preference for initiative B over D. While these were Jerry's fifth and sixth preferences, his support was vital to breaking the deadlock between Kerry and Terry, whose top picks were B and D. Kerry is satisfied with the result as B was her top pick, and Terry is content as B was his second choice.

Q-sort

Multivoting does not allow each member of the team to express a preference for each alternative. To remedy this drawback, a team could use Q-sort. Q-sort is a technique in which each committee member gets to evaluate every solution from highest to lowest preference in a single voting process. Table 4.16 presents two different Q-sort processes: the standard process and the forced normal distribution process. The standard process should be used when team members see distinct differences in alternatives; the forced normal distribution should be used otherwise. The forced normal distribution is based on the bell curve and recognizes that in the middle of the distribution there may be little difference among alternatives.

Table 4.16 The Q-sort Process

Standard Process
1. Team members rank all potential solutions from highest to lowest.
2. Assign highest weight to most preferred solution; given ten solutions, the most preferred alternative typically receives 10 points, the second highest alternative receives a lower weight, in this example 9 points (10 – 1), and lesser preferred solutions continue to have their weights reduced by 1 point until the least preferred alternative receives a single point.
3. Tally rankings.
4. Rank alternatives from highest vote total (most favored by the group) to lowest (least favored).

Forced Normal Distribution Process
1. Determine number of categories; for example, seven categories, from most promising (first tier, 7) to least promising (seventh tier, 1).
2. Each committee member receives one most-promising, first-tier vote (worth 7 points), two second-tier votes (6), four third-tier votes (5), six fourth-tier votes (4), four fifth-tier votes (3), two sixth-tier votes (2), and one least-promising, seventh-tier vote (1).
3. Vote.
4. Tally votes.
5. Solutions are ranked in declining order from the highest vote total to the lowest.

Table 4.17 displays the rankings of the three team members for ten possible interventions using the standard process, Table 14.18 translates the rankings into a numeric vote tally, and Table 14.19 sorts the vote tallies from the most preferred to the least preferred intervention.

Table 4.17 Q-sort Table of Preferences

	PREFERENCE									
	1st	**2nd**	**3rd**	**4th**	**5th**	**6th**	**7th**	**8th**	**9th**	**10th**
					Weight					
Member	**10**	**9**	**8**	**7**	**6**	**5**	**4**	**3**	**2**	**1**
Jerry	B	D	J	A	C	I	E	G	F	H
Kerry	H	F	E	B	I	C	G	J	A	D
Terry	D	E	G	B	J	H	A	I	C	F

Table 4.18 Weighted Preferences

Initiative	Jerry	Kerry	Terry	Total
A	7	2	4	13
B	10	7	7	24
C	6	5	2	13
D	9	1	10	20
E	4	8	9	21
F	2	9	1	12
G	3	4	8	15
H	1	10	5	16
I	5	6	3	14
J	8	3	6	17

Table 4.19 Ranked Interventions

Initiative	Total
B	24
E	21
D	20
J	17
H	16
G	15
I	14
A	13
C	13
F	12

The ranking shows that initiative B is strongly preferred by the group and that initiatives E and D are ranked second and third. The remaining seven alternatives are clustered between 12 and 17 and demonstrate little consensus on the usefulness of the initiatives.

Tool to Monitor Progress

Run Chart

Run charts

charts that record events in chronological order of occurrence

Run charts record performance over time. They are often used to understand a process and identify problems, yet they can also be used as a tool to monitor progress, answering the question: Does a system demonstrate better performance in the periods after quality improvements are implemented? A run chart records a performance measure on the y-axis and time on the x-axis. Its construction makes it easy for analysts to judge the effectiveness of an improvement initiative because performance before and after the change can be contrasted.

In Excel, the first step that must be taken (after data is collected) to create a run chart is calculating the number of events per time period. This example will use the patient fall data recorded in Table 4.5. The =FREQUENCY function is used to sort the events into time periods, so the data analyst must establish the bins to use and highlight the data range to fill. (For instructions, see the section on stratification charts earlier in this chapter.) After the range is highlighted, the data analyst inserts **=FREQUENCY** and specifies the data range and bin range and hits **Crtl+Shift+Enter**. The data analyst has decided to group patient falls by week to minimize the vagaries that may arise on a day-to-day basis. After falls per week are calculated, the data analyst selects **Insert, Chart**, and **Line Chart**. After the chart is produced, the data analyst formats as desired with a title, x- and y-axis labels, and data legends.

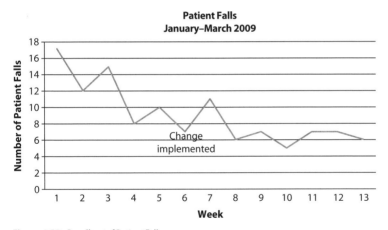

Figure 4.23 Run Chart of Patient Falls

Referents are often useful to understand change over time, and one way to increase the usefulness of a run chart is to add average performance to the graph. The average allows the user to quickly see how the process moves around its average. To add the average, calculate the average for the 13 periods, **=AVERAGE(K10:K22)**, copy average into a new column, highlight count and the new average column, select **Insert, Line**, and select a chart style.

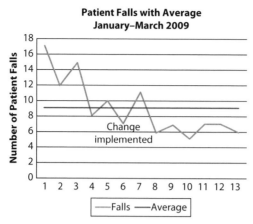

Figure 4.24 Run Chart of Patient Falls with Average

While it is easy to see in Figures 4.23 and 4.24 that patient falls have decreased during the period of observation, sometimes trends are not perceptible. A second variation of the run chart adds a trendline to determine if the process is improving, stable, or deteriorating. To add a trendline, right-click on one of the data points and select Add Trendline. There are six trendline options, and in most cases the use of the Linear option will accurately portray any trend in the data.

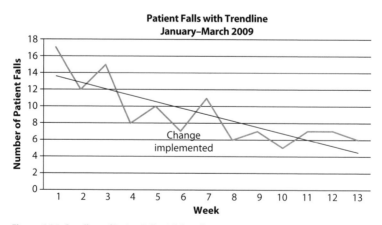

Figure 4.25 Run Chart of Patient Falls with Trendline

The three charts display the same basic information, that patient falls are decreasing over this three-month period. The addition of the average in Figure 4.24 highlights three distinct periods: weeks 1–3 are above average, weeks 4–7 cycle around the average, and weeks 8–13 fall below average, suggesting that performance in the later periods was significantly different than the early periods. The addition of the trendline in Figure 4.25 highlights the downward trend and leads the audience to believe the trend may continue. When trendlines are used, analysts and others must be alert not to extrapolate trends beyond the data. Figure 4.24 demonstrates that the downward trend seen in weeks 1 through 6 has ended; patient falls in weeks 8 through 13 have leveled off and are running parallel to the average.

Run charts are one of the easiest tools to master and one of the most important to use to ensure that quality improvement produces long-lasting change in an organization. One of the biggest problems faced by organizations is that after a quality improvement initiative has been made and success is achieved, attention moves elsewhere and employees revert to their previous habits and the improvement is lost. Continuous monitoring is required to ensure that the organization and workers are aware of their performance so that any slippages can be remediated.

Summary

This chapter highlights the need for medical providers to make better use of the vast amounts of data they collect to move from focusing on individual patients to understanding performance and outcomes across groups of patients. The tools introduced in this chapter facilitate the collection of data, organizing the data into information, and analyzing the information to build knowledge from which action can be taken.

The ten primary tools of quality management were broken into four primary uses. The first four tools, Pareto charts, stratification charts, histograms, and check sheets, are used to collect and analyze data to identify problems. Once a problem is identified, the next step is to identify the potential cause of the problem. Cause and effect diagrams, flowcharts, and scatter diagrams allow users to expand the search for potential causes of problems and then reduce this list to one or more primary causes.

After identifying a primary cause and a list of potential solutions, multivoting and Q-sort were introduced as means to reduce a list of potential solutions to one or more solutions to be implemented. To achieve quality improvement, it is essential to determine whether the implemented solution produced the expected results and, if successful, to ensure that it is maintained over time. The simple tracking of performance over time using a run chart documents results and produces a visual display that quickly and effectively communicates performance to all involved parties.

KEY TERMS

Check sheet	Multivoting
Data	No relationship
Defect factor check sheet	Nonlinear relationship
Defective item check sheet	Normal distribution
Defect location check sheet	Pareto chart
Direct relationship	Pareto rule
Flowchart	Process distribution check sheet
Histogram	Q-sort
Information	Run chart
Inverse relationship	Scatter diagram
Knowledge	Stratification chart

REVIEW QUESTIONS

1. Explain the differences among data, information, and knowledge.

2. Identify which process analysis tools are best for identifying the potential causes of a problem and briefly explain how each identifies causes.

3. What is the purpose of each of the four types of check sheets discussed in the chapter?

4. What are the five most commonly cited major causes of problems? Include at least two sub-causes for each major cause.

5. Describe the major types of relationship between the x and y variables that an analyst may observe using a scatter diagram.

6. Prepare a cause and effect diagram to explain why a patient may fall and sustain injury.

PROBLEMS

1. Using the Ch04Problems.xls file and the States tab, create a Pareto chart showing the top 10 states with the longest lengths of stay and the average length of stay for the remaining 40 states. Your chart should contain eleven columns. Is there any commonality among the states with long lengths of stay?

2. Using the Ch04Problems.xls file and the DRG143 tab, create a histogram of length of stay. Your histogram should contain seven columns. What is the mean and the standard deviation for length of stay? Assume that we suspect there may be quality issues in hospitals with extremely high or low lengths of stay, and we decide to examine institutions that have a length of stay more than or less than two standard deviations from the mean. Which hospitals should be reviewed?

3. Using the Ch04Problems.xls file and the States tab, create a scatter chart examining the relationship between total discharges and total patient days. Describe the relationship between these two variables.

4. Using the Ch04Problems.xls file and the DRG143 tab, create a scatter chart examining the relationship between number of cases and length of stay. Describe the relationship between these two variables.

5. Using the Ch04Problems.xls file and the Patient Falls tab, create two stratification charts examining: (a) the relationship between patient falls and shift, and (b) between patient falls and patient age. If you were in charge of reducing patient falls, where should your efforts be concentrated for maximum effectiveness?

6. You are the manager of the patient transport department at a hospital, and recently the radiology department has voiced a concern over the late arrival of patients for their radiology tests. You have pulled the transport log for the last week to investigate (Ch04Problems.xls file, Transport Log tab). Prepare two check sheets: (a) prepare a process distribution check sheet to document how late arrivals have been and (b) prepare a defect factor check sheet to determine if late arrivals are due to any particular transport employee. Discuss your findings.

Process Distribution Check Sheet

Minutes Late	Number of Occurrences	Total
1–5 min		
6–10 min		
11–15 min		
16–20 min		
21–25 min		
26+ min		

Defect Factor Check Sheet

Transporter	Number of Occurrences	Total
A		
B		

....

C

....

D

....

E

_____

7. Ten projects are being considered by the QM team. Based on team member preferences (below), if a single vote is held, project D will be selected. The chair wants to consider team member preferences beyond simply their first choice. Use a multivoting process and assign three points to each member's first choice, two points to the second, and one point to the third. After the first vote, options that receive fewer than three points should be eliminated and the remaining options revoted. In subsequent rounds, two points will be given to the first choice and one point to the second. Continue to eliminate low vote tallying options until all but two options have been eliminated. On the final vote each team member will get a single vote worth one point. Which option will be selected?

QM Team Preferences

Jacob	D, I, B, C, A, F, E, J, H, G
Isabella	A, C, E, F, G, J, D, H, I, B
Ethan	H, G, E, D, B, I, J, A, C, F
Emma	D, I, F, A, E, G, B, C, H, J
Olivia	B, G, A, J, H, C, F, E, I, D

8. Given the preferences of the four team members below, tally the rankings of projects A through H using a Q-sort process and prepare a list of projects from the most favored to the least favored project. Which two projects should be pursued?

Choice	Deion	Malcolm	Charity	Sue
First	G	A	C	F
Second	F	D	B	D
Third	D	H	G	A
Fourth	E	G	F	E
Fifth	A	C	H	G
Sixth	C	B	A	H
Seventh	B	F	E	B
Eighth	H	E	D	C

9. Using the Ch04Problems.xls file and the Patient Falls tab, create a run chart examining falls per week. Have patient falls been reduced over this 13-week period?

References

American Hospital Association, http://www.ahd.com/state_statistics.html.

Drucker P, (1954) 1982, *The Practice of Management*, Harper Business, New York, NY.

Goetsch D and Davis S, 2010, *Quality Management for Organizational Excellence*, 6th ed., Pearson Prentice Hall, Upper Saddle River, NJ.

Joint Commission, http://www.jointcommission.org/.

Pennsylvania Health Care Cost Containment Council, http://www.phc4.org/.

Sinanan M, Wicks K, Peccoud M, Canfield J, Poser L, Sailer L, Stephens K, and Edwards D, 2000, Formula for Surgical Practice Resuscitation in an Academic Medical Center, *The American Journal of Surgery* 179 (5): 417–421.

Statistical Abstract of the United States, 2011, http://www.census.gov/compendia/statab/.

CHAPTER 5

ROOT CAUSE ANALYSIS

Introduction

In 2000, Ford Motor Company was in the midst of a large problem. Their popular Explorer was rolling over at high rates and causing multiple fatalities. The first question I ask my students is: How does a manufacturer know a vehicle is unsafe? On the surface this appears to be a trivial question, but it is complex. In 2000, the *Statistical Abstract of the United States* reported that 43,354 Americans died in motor vehicle accidents. These accidents included every type of driver and every type of vehicle. Identifying a problem based on the data was like looking for a needle in a haystack.

One of the problems with SUVs compared to passenger cars is their design increases the probability of rollover; they are heavy vehicles with high centers of gravity. The first step was to recognize that Explorers were rolling over at higher rates than other SUVs. Data revealed that Explorers were 13% more likely to roll over than other SUVs, and when coupled with equipment failure they were 53% more likely to roll. After identifying the problem, Ford's next step was to identify the cause.

Identifying causes was discussed in Chapter Four; cause and effect diagrams are a great tool to explore the potential causes of a problem. If we had worked at Ford, we may have identified the SUV design, drivers, equipment, and environment as the potential major causes. Drivers could be the cause of the rollover problems if Ford drivers were younger or engaged in more risky driving behaviors. Similarly, the environment influences vehicle crashes by changing traction and stopping distances; that is, rain, snow, and ice increase the probability that accidents will occur. The impact of drivers and the environment are only

LEARNING OBJECTIVES

1. Understand the relationship between unsafe practices and major problems

2. Distinguish among slips, lapses, mistakes, and violations

3. Understand the causes of error

4. Understand the root cause process

5. Apply investigative techniques

6. Apply data techniques to identify commonalities in aggregate root cause analysis

7. Explain prevention and recovery techniques

important if there are differences between the drivers and driving conditions of Ford and other SUV manufacturers. There was no evidence that Ford drivers or driving conditions differed substantially from those of other auto makers, so the cause must lie elsewhere.

The design of SUVs makes them more likely to roll over than standard passenger cars, but again the differences are minimal between manufacturers of SUVs, so this cause can be discounted as well. The fourth major cause is equipment. Auto makers use different suppliers for parts, and in the end it was equipment that explained the higher Explorer rollover rate. The equipment that produced the higher rollovers was the tires. The tires were losing their tread and the tread loss produced rollover.

After the tires were pinpointed, the problem was traced to a change in the tire manufacturing process at a single plant in Illinois. Ford and the tire manufacturer, Firestone, had had a 100-year history, but the problem and its handling terminated the relationship.

Root cause analysis

a technique for identifying the primary causes of an undesirable event or a poor outcome

Root cause analysis (RCA) is a technique for identifying the primary causes of an undesirable event or a poor outcome. RCA uses a systems perspective to analyze inputs, processes, outputs, outcomes, and feedback and control mechanisms. RCA assumes that undesirable events or poor outcomes are seldom due to a dysfunction at a single point but are the result of a systemic breakdown. In systems there are many points at which problems can start but many more opportunities to monitor quality and correct deficiencies. Undesirable events may arise at one point in a process, but controls can be created at any preceding or succeeding steps to prevent these events from occurring or from impairing outcomes.

RCA is concerned with determining why undesirable events arise and how future outcomes can be improved. RCA in health care is designed to build understanding of care processes, identify the causes of undesirable outcomes, determine if and how these causes can be monitored and prevented, and ultimately assist in implementing changes to improve patient outcomes. RCA is *not* an attempt to quickly get answers or place blame to put an undesirable event to rest—it is a knowledge-building device. Efforts to short-circuit or fast-track the process will increase the probability that underlying problems will arise again and produce similar undesirable outcomes. Attempts to introduce superficial corrective actions (for example, changing the responsibility for a function or requiring additional paperwork) without a firm understanding of the entire process are destined to fail.

Root Cause Analysis

Efforts to minimize the impact of quality problems can be made at three distinct points. First, systems can be designed and built to minimize problems. Second, monitors and controls can be implemented at various production points to identify variations as they occur. Finally, postproduction problems can be explored after negative outcomes have occurred and changes can be implemented to prevent reoccurrence. RCA is a process for examining problems *after* poor outcomes have been identified and is an appropriate tool for addressing existing quality problems in health care.

Health care has a long history, with many current practices rooted in the 19th century. The health care system cannot be torn down and rebuilt to minimize problems. Changes must be made within the existing structure. In an industry with more than 5,000 hospitals, 600,000 physicians, and 33,600,000 admissions that consumes more than 16% of U.S. economic output, attempts to implement controls are hampered by the question of where to start. RCA provides one answer: the health care industry should address major issues that produce substantial patient harm first and after resolving these issues move to less pressing problems. The goal of zero defects is as commendable as it is impractical—the best designed and monitored system will produce undesired outcomes. These occurrences underscore the fact that the ability to identify root causes is a desirable skill for workers to possess.

RCA requires two sets of knowledge and skills. The first is to understand the process to be studied, and the second is to understand how to investigate and place the process into context for problem solving. One of the problems with RCA is that seldom does a single person possess both sets of knowledge and skills. Medical personnel have vast understanding of health care processes but generally little training in RCA. Management engineers understand RCA but are often unfamiliar with health care systems, including organizational structure, decision-making processes, and culture. Differences in perspectives bedevil RCA teams and reduce the likelihood that RCA will produce substantial improvement to health care processes. Those invested in a process may find it difficult to critique the process, while those trained in problem solving may arrive at simplistic, out-of-context solutions.

Medical personnel need to recognize that there is no single procedure for RCA. Authors describe different processes, and organizations rely on different systems. The user must focus on the goal of RCA rather than on its steps. Vincent et al. (1999) note that RCA is not an end in itself but a means to accomplish three ends. The first is to obtain the greatest possible benefit from medical knowledge and clinical experience. The goal is to improve patient care by understanding outcomes, what produced the outcome, and what can be changed to improve outcomes. The second end is to create a climate of openness and learning in which lower-than-desired outcomes are recorded and are analyzed to understand the role of systems and individuals. The third goal is to structure the analysis process to ensure comprehensiveness, consistency, and ease of use.

One of the problems hampering process and quality improvement in health care, and in other industries, is the defensive reaction of workers when confronted by an error or poor outcome. Defensiveness is a natural human response to a threatening situation, and RCA signals to workers that a problem is severe enough to warrant the attention of their superiors. One of the dysfunctional side effects of defensiveness is an unwillingness to disclose the problem or the solution to allow others to learn from errors (Gosbee and Anderson 2003). A known and structured approach to RCA should demonstrate to employees that the process is neither ad hoc nor arbitrary and is aimed at improvement rather than placing blame and punishing those who make errors (Vincent et al. 1999).

A problem corrected in one area cannot benefit others if the event remains undisclosed. The lack of awareness of vulnerabilities and shared learning result in unnecessary reoccurrence of problems and the need to reinvent the wheel each time a problem arises. Employees who understand the parameters of RCA should be less threatened by the process, more capable, and more willing to contribute to outcome and performance improvement initiatives. In the long run, it is hoped that workers will internalize the goals of RCA and systematically study the systems they work in when they see the potential for improvements. RCA will only reach its potential when it is undertaken due to internal awareness of opportunities rather than external recognition of problems.

The Goal of RCA and Types of Error

sentinel event
an unexpected occurrence involving death or serious physical or psychological injury, or the risk thereof

RCA has grown in stature within the health care industry with the Joint Commission's requirement that health care organizations must produce thorough and credible reports on the causes of **sentinel events** (Joint Commission 2010, SE-10). Institute of Medicine (IOM) reports have trumpeted the use of RCA to improve quality and patient safety in health care (IOM 2004). The Joint Commission requirement touches just the surface of RCA potential, requiring its use only for the most serious events, whereas the IOM recommends a broader application, to include errors that produce no harm or minimal harm. The IOM philosophy is that attention to **no-harm events** could transform medicine by elevating health care workers' awareness of quality and safety issues.

no-harm event
an event that does not meet generally accepted performance standards but does not produce injury or death

adverse event
an event that results in death or injury

The Joint Commission categorizes undesirable events and outcomes as **adverse events** or sentinel events. A sentinel event is "an unexpected occurrence involving death or serious physical or psychological injury, or the risk thereof" (Joint Commission 2010, SE-1). The IOM defines an adverse event as an event that results in unintended harm to the patient by an

error of commission or an **error of omission** rather than by the underlying disease or condition of the patient (IOM 2004). No-harm and **near-miss events** are also important; a no-harm event describes a deviation from accepted medical practice where the patient is not injured. The fact that an inappropriate treatment is rendered but no harm arises can provide insight into resiliency of patients and into remediation practices to counteract harm. Near misses indicate an almost event, an error that was detected and corrected before treatment was rendered. Near misses provide insight into self-correction.

> **error of commission**
> an error arising from performing an action incorrectly

> **error of omission**
> an error arising from the failure to perform an action

> **near-miss event**
> an action that could produce harm that is caught before injury arises

The goal of RCA is to reduce the probability that undesirable harm-causing and no-harm events will occur. Avoidable events should be reduced, and the negative consequences of unavoidable events must be minimized. RCA exists to improve the health care delivery system and patient outcomes by identifying undesirable events and outcomes and tracing them to their causes.

Broad application of RCA is currently impossible to implement given the limited number of health care personnel trained in RCA and the large number of events that could be analyzed. The IOM reports that near misses occur 7 to 100 times as often as adverse events (IOM 2004, 226). Although adverse events, near misses, and no-harm events are widespread, documenting and studying these events is often limited to the medical staff or a full-time quality improvement manager with an ad hoc group of employees assembled to investigate particular incidents.

Kaoru Ishikawa was one of the first quality improvement experts to advance the idea that quality improvement was too important to be left in the hands of specialists (Beckford 1998). Obtaining the greatest possible benefit from RCA requires that all members of an organization understand the process. Workers throughout an organization should be familiar with RCA tools, general causes of failure, and potential remedies. In addition to these topics, this chapter reviews case studies to demonstrate how these components fit together to produce useful information to prevent errors. These studies provide frameworks to follow when analyzing processes or contributing to a RCA.

The relationship between sentinel events and near misses becomes clearer using the **Heinrich triangle**. Heinrich analyzed 5,000 industrial accidents and found that for every major injury there were 29 minor injuries, and 300 no-injury accidents. In addition, he posited that for each major injury there were thousands of unsafe practices and conditions that could produce an accident or injury (Heinrich 1959). Health care faces a similar situation: for every incident that results in a patient fatality, there are numerous injuries and hundreds of no-harm or near-miss events.

> **Heinrich triangle**
> a hierarchical model examining the relationship between major, minor, and no injury events and unsafe practices and conditions

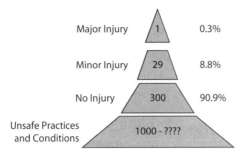

Major Injury	1	0.3%
Minor Injury	29	8.8%
No Injury	300	90.9%
Unsafe Practices and Conditions	1000 - ????	

Figure 5.1 Heinrich Triangle

The problem in health care is that our knowledge of these incidents is an inverted triangle. We produce a large amount of information on the small number of events at the top of the triangle and overlook the knowledge that could be gained by understanding more commonly occurring events. Generally, the unexpected death of a patient results in a large investigation to discover the cause. Patient injury, in many cases, is the result of a large number of low-probability events that aligned to produce the error—the **Swiss cheese model** of error occurrence. Figure 5.2 shows that the potential error can be caught at four points. Only if the failures of the system's safeguards align, similar to the holes in the Swiss cheese in the model, will an error actually occur.

Swiss cheese model
an error prevention model demonstrating that the possibility of a realized error is reduced by building more safeguards in to a system

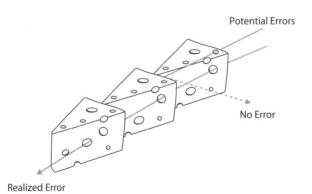

Potential Errors

No Error

Realized Error

Figure 5.2 The Swiss Cheese Model of Error Occurrence

Prevention efforts follow knowledge. The majority of prevention effort is spent on the least frequent but most harmful events. The focus on severity is understandable, but attention should also be paid to whether sufficient effort is allocated to reducing unsafe practices and conditions. Would quality of care be improved by increasing our attention to and understanding of no-harm incidents? Would a reduction in no-harm events do more to reduce major patient injuries than continuing our current level of emphasis on serious but infrequent events?

Why Do Errors Occur?

Medical errors arise due to deficiencies in human performance, equipment failure, insufficient management, poor communication, and lack of information, to name but a few causes. James Reason identifies the three major elements that contribute to the production of an error as being the nature of the task and environmental circumstances, the mechanisms governing performance, and the individual (1990, 4). The Joint Commission's classification scheme of human, equipment, and controllable and noncontrollable environmental factors parallels Reason's categories. Reason sought to build a theory to account for the conditions that produce error and the types of error that arise.

Reason focuses on why humans err rather than on environmental or mechanical factors since humans may be the single most important factor in producing error. Understanding why human performance fails to meet expectations requires the observer to determine if the action was intentional or unintentional (1990, 195). Unsafe and undesirable actions are divided into two different spheres, depending on the intent of the actor. One sphere requires understanding why undesirable activities occur unintentionally, and the other sphere, why people knowingly engage in undesirable acts.

Intentional undesirable acts must be further divided into acts that were intentional but mistaken and those undertaken with full knowledge that the action was suboptimal, inappropriate, or wrong. Reason labels the latter group **violations**. Safeguards implemented to improve processes are radically different for violations. The often-used remedy of training is more effective in dealing with unintended actions, where ability is lacking or where intended but ill-chosen actions are taken, than in cases where individuals know what should be done but choose other actions.

Reason draws heavily on Rasmussen's skill-rule-knowledge framework, which divides error into skill, decision-making, and knowledge problems. **Skill-based errors** arise when individuals cannot properly execute actions. A skill-based error occurs when a proper treatment plan is in place but individuals do not follow it or make errors while carrying out the plan. Errors resulting from failure to follow plans are classified as **lapses**; that is, someone overlooks a step or is interrupted and does not recommence the procedure at the point of interruption. Execution errors are categorized as **slips**. Slips are errors in performance where an individual does not complete a task appropriately. Slips include procedures performed on the wrong patient or site, pushing the wrong buttons, and incorrect recording of data.

violation
an undesirable action that is undertaken with full knowledge that it was suboptimal, inappropriate, or wrong

lapse
the failure to complete one or more steps in a process

slip
the failure to complete a task according to generally accepted performance standards

Rule-based errors occur when an incorrect plan is followed. A rule-based error occurs when a patient's condition is properly assessed, but the plan of treatment is inappropriate, for example, when medical personnel are unable to identify the proper treatment (rule) to apply to the patient's condition. *Knowledge-based errors* arise when individuals do not comprehend the situation (misdiagnosis) and consequently do not develop an appropriate action plan. Rule- and knowledge-based errors are classified as **mistakes**. The primary difference between skill-based errors and rule- and knowledge-based errors is that in the former, a plan is not executed while in the later, an inappropriate plan is chosen when the situation has been correctly assessed (resulting in a rule-based error) or due to a failure to understand the situation (resulting in a knowledge-based error) (Reason 1990, 43).

Rasmussen's framework does not cover violations, that is, inappropriate actions intentionally undertaken with full knowledge that the action is inappropriate or will not produce the desired end. Reason notes three types of violations: **routine violations**, **exceptional violations**, and **sabotage**. Routine violations occur when there is a prescribed way of doing things but individuals regularly or always deviate from the correct procedure. An example of a routine violation is a provider checking one patient identifier before administering a drug or treatment when organizational policy requires that two IDs be checked. Other examples of routine violations include failure to use safeguards because they get in the way, failure to log off computers, and failure to return floor medicines to centralized storage. Routine violations are not intended to cause harm, but the circumvention of defined procedures weakens systems and increases the probability of harm occurring.

The second type of violation is exceptional; that is, a policy, rule, or procedure is not followed due to extraordinary circumstances or an emergency in which adverse consequences may occur if standard practice is followed. Exceptional violations, even more so than routine violations, are not intended to cause injury but to reduce patient harm. Exceptional violations involve a conscious decision to bypass established ways of doing things because the increased probability of harm resulting from deviation from standard practice is considered less than the potential harm that may occur if standard practice is followed.

The third type of violation is sabotage. Sabotage is a deliberate contravention of mandated or safe practice undertaken to advance the private interests of the actor. These interests can range from malice and vengeance to contrariness, monetary gain, or delusion. Saboteurs not only recognize the harm they may cause but often engage in this behavior specifically to cause harm.

mistakes
errors arising from the failure of an actor to correctly assess a situation or select an appropriate action

routine violations
a generally accepted circumvention of generally accepted performance standards

exceptional violations
infrequent circumventions of generally accepted performance standards undertaken to minimize harm

sabotage
intentional circumvention of generally accepted performance standards often undertaken to cause harm

Classifying Error

The preceding discussion examined how and why individuals err. But what exactly is an error? Error is commonly classified in two categories: active and latent. An **active error** defines the most immediate or direct cause of an adverse outcome, what produced or triggered the error. Patient injury may arise from the action of a health care worker, an error of commission: the provider did something he should not have done, or he performed a necessary function poorly—a slip, mistake, or violation. Injuries also arise from failure to act, an error of omission: a function was required to prevent harm, but the action was not performed—a lapse. Active error may pinpoint an incorrect action or nonaction, but it may fail to illuminate why an action was inappropriate or why it was not performed.

active error
the immediate or direct cause of an adverse event

Latent error focuses on the context surrounding the active error. Latent error recognizes that error is unavoidable and that systems increase or decrease the probability of undesirable events occurring. Latent error attempts to explain how the opportunity for error arose. It looks at whether there are systemic or organizational weaknesses that increase the potential for error, such as inadequate training, poor communication, inappropriate delegation of tasks or decision making, poor supervision, and so on. In addition to organizational issues, latent error may include external, or environmental, issues, process design flaws, and problems with the facilities, equipment, or materials used to deliver care.

latent error
weaknesses in a system that increase the possibility of adverse events

Medication errors illustrate the difference between active and latent error. An example of active error is when an employee administers an incorrect medication or dose to a patient. Was the employee the primary cause of the problem? Was the medication error due to lack of necessary diligence on the part of the employee or was it due to weaknesses in the system? Is it possible that another employee would have made the same mistake?

The search for latent errors may reveal systemic causes that place responsibility for the error on other parts of the system. Was the wrong drug provided by the pharmacy, was it mislabeled, was the wrong drug prescribed, were patients transferred during shift change? The search for latent errors is designed to identify system issues that increase the probability that anybody working in the system would be likely to make the same error. Latent causes include overwork, look-alike or sound-alike drugs, and a history of poor communication between employees. Latent causes have less to do with the slips, mistakes, or lapses of individuals and more to do with the existence of systemic causes that make slips, mistakes, and lapses more probable.

Table 5.1 demonstrates one of the difficulties health care workers encounter when they enter the quality improvement field: language is not consistent. Table 5.1 shows how 11 terms are commonly used by authors to describe active and latent errors.

Table 5.1 Classifying Error

Author(s)	Active Error	Latent Error
Reason	Active	Latent
Garnerin et al.	Specific	General
Massachusetts Medical Society	Proximate	Contributing
Joint Commission	Proximate or Special	Systems and Processes or Common
Batty, Holland-Elliot, & Rosenfeld	Immediate	Underlying

Taken as a whole, the various terms illustrate the underlying difference among the types of error and may extend a person's understanding of what each represents. However, if someone does not know the jargon, a Tower of Babel situation arises in which one person speaks of active causes while another of proximate causes, and a meeting of minds does not occur.

The Causes of Error

There are three sources of error: humans; facilities, equipment, and materials; and the environment. Some attribute all error to humans. System failures are the result of design problems—a human failure. When facilities, equipment, and materials fail due to maintenance or design issues, these are human-caused problems. When facilities are not adapted to the demands and threats of their environment, these errors may also be caused by humans. While it is debatable whether all error can be attributed to human failings, the key point is to understand the causes of error and reduce it to a minimum.

Human

As we have seen, human errors can be either intentional or unintentional. Unintentional errors arise from four sources. The first is lack of knowledge, for example, the selection of a treatment based on failure to understand that it is inappropriate, or not selecting an appropriate treatment due to unawareness of its existence. The second is assessment or perception problems, an inability to assess the situation or need. The provider understands the available treatments but has incorrectly assessed the patient and selected an inappropriate treatment. The third source is decision problems: the provider correctly assesses the patient's situation and is knowledgeable of treatments but fails to select the best treatment. The final source of error is skill-based errors; the provider understands treatments and the patient's situation and has arrived at a correct decision but does not or cannot carry out the selected treatment plan. Failure to deliver effective treatment may arise from lack of skill or from carelessness, fatigue, or other factors.

Errors arising from knowledge, assessment, or decision making are all **cognitive errors**. The last type of error is an execution error. Improving outcomes when cognitive or execution errors arise may simply require training, additional information, or defined procedures. Defining the source of the error is vital as it should dictate the type of training or remediation required to prevent reoccurrence. Remediation must be appropriate to the type of error. For example, providing skill-based training is not going to improve outcomes for workers making cognitive errors, nor will cognitive training be beneficial for employees who lack the dexterity to execute treatment.

Intentional error arises because of a different type of judgment; it is not a lack of understanding of treatments or patient need but rather a decision not to follow standard procedure. As we have seen, circumvention of an established procedure may be undertaken to better serve the patient, as in the case of exceptional violation. However, the other two types of intentional error, routine violation and sabotage, arise when an employee deliberately circumvents a defined or accepted method of performance to satisfy an internal goal rather than serving the patient. Employees intentionally engaging in potentially harmful actions may be motivated by maliciousness, delusion, profit, unwillingness to accept direction, or a conscious attempt to reduce the amount of work they must perform, among other reasons. When intentional errors are being made, training, information, and procedures may not correct the situation. Intentional error is not undertaken due to cognitive errors or inability to execute a plan of action but rather a willingness to continue action knowing it is inappropriate. In these situations, monitoring and inspection are the minimum requirement to prevent this behavior. Continued violations may require disciplinary action against the violator.

cognitive errors
errors arising from insufficient knowledge and assessment or poor decision making

Facilities, Equipment, and Materials

Medical error can be the result of problems with the facilities where care is rendered or with the equipment and materials used to provide care. Facility, equipment, and material problems can be divided into controllable and noncontrollable categories.

Controllable failures include errors that arise from using a resource for an application it is ill-suited for, operating conditions, poor maintenance, storage and deterioration, or distribution of the resources. Machines or facilities that will not function or that operate erratically because they have not been properly used or maintained are clearly controllable; procedures should be developed to document proper use and maintenance, and checks should be routinely made to ensure compliance. As for materials and supplies, mislabeling or improper storage can produce problems including improper distribution and spoilage.

Controllable equipment errors hark back to human failures. However, when equipment failure occurs, we know that the person delivering care in the facility or using the equipment or materials may not be the primary cause of the error. The active error (who was providing care) may not be the main focus of prevention. Instead, the latent errors that allowed the facility, equipment, or materials failure to arise should be examined. This may require establishing regular maintenance programs, increasing purchases to ensure the availability of resources, and inspections to ensure that resources are used for their intended purposes.

Facilities, equipment, and materials can fail without noticeable signs. Design and structural problems, manufacturing errors, programming errors, and metal fatigue can produce failure and not be easily observed by employees. In these cases, the best that can be hoped for is early identification of problems and termination of use until reoccurrence can be prevented. Metal fatigue on aircraft is a notable example of a problem that is not apparent on visual inspection; aircraft are often grounded when a crash occurs so fleets can be tested for similar defects. Battery problems that have caused laptop computers to ignite present an example of an undiscoverable problem. The probability of catching fire was estimated to be 1 in 1,000,000, so a user would be unlikely to perceive a problem until his laptop was on fire.

Environment

Error and harm also arise due to environmental factors. For this discussion we will limit our focus to four issues—weather, construction, power, and demand—and examine the interaction between the organization and its environment, and the extent to which external forces can be controlled. Similar to materials and equipment, environmental factors can be viewed as either controllable or noncontrollable. One could say, "Everything is controllable," but the cost and benefit of control must be taken into consideration.

Hurricane Katrina in 2005 exemplifies the environmental issues. Was the magnitude of the catastrophe controllable? Yes, but at what cost? The Army Corps of Engineers designed a 500-year levy system, so New Orleans was protected to withstand all but the most severe storms. Was the impact of Katrina controllable? Yes, more money could have been invested in the levy system, but a conscious decision was made to accept some risk. Controlling environmental hazards always involves comparing the cost of control against the probability of an event and the harm it may produce.

New Orleans's health care institutions could have constructed better buildings to withstand flooding since executives knew that parts of the city were located below sea level. Their choice of building design and location may have been prudent. Only with hindsight knowledge of the storm's magnitude we can now question their degree of preparedness.

The power failure that accompanied Katrina provides another example of controllability. Hospitals anticipate external power failures and build their own generating systems. The question is, how much back-up capacity should an institution have; should it prepare for short-term interruption or long-term interruption?

The last environmental issue is demand for services; hospitals build excess capacity to deal with surges in demand. The question is, how much excess capacity should be available to deal with infrequent spikes in demand? Given reimbursement reductions, health care organizations must balance the ability to handle high and irregular increases in patient volume against the cost of excess capacity. The cost of a hospital bed in 2003 was reported by Loudown Hospital to range from $530,000 to $1,070,000, so hospitals' wanting to minimize excess beds is understandable.

Organizations should take all prudent steps to minimize the risk of harm to their patients and employees. In this chapter, environmental issues have not been specifically divided into controllable and noncontrollable categories, because most environmental risk can be controlled. But the difficulty arises from the fact that safeguards may come at an unaffordable price. The reader should view environmental risks along a continuum rather than attempting to classify them as controllable or noncontrollable. Along the continuum, it is up to the institution to decide what level of risk is acceptable and how many resources to invest in controlling environmental factors.

The Root Causes of Medical Events

The error classification system defines the conceptual level of error and possible remedies, a foundation on which specific errors and common causes can be explored. In "Sentinel Event Data: Root Causes by Event Type, 2004–2012," the Joint Commission (2013) lists human factors (such as staffing levels, staff supervision, rushing, fatigue) as the number-one root cause in 68.1% of all sentinel events in 2012. Leadership and communication followed closely, arising in 61.8% and 59.0% of events, respectively. Typical of RCA, the Joint Commission list of root causes demonstrates that most events are the result of a system in which poor outcomes arise from multiple causes, thus results do not add up to 100%. The Joint Commission notes this data is voluntarily reported and no conclusion should be drawn concerning the true frequency of occurrence of any particular cause. Figure 5.3 shows the number of occurrences for the top ten root causes in 2012.

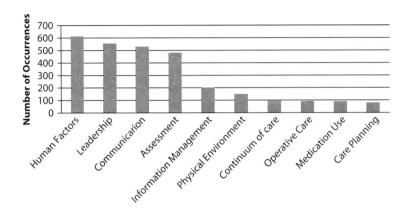

Figure 5.3   Root Causes of Sentinel Events, 2012

Source: Joint Commission Office of Quality Monitoring, Sentinel Event Data: Root Causes by Event Type 2004–2012, 8.

The drawback of the Joint Commission list is the difficulty of moving from the identified causes to correction. Identifying communication as a cause of error is logically and intuitively appealing. Unfortunately finding a remedy for poor or absent communication is infinitely more difficult. Chassin and Becher (2002) note: "We have found no proven, effective interventions to improve communication and teamwork in health care delivery."

Others have attempted to provide more insightful categories that transition easily from actions that could produce an undesirable outcome to action that can be taken to prevent its reoccurrence. The categorization described next is the synthesis of other root cause categorization systems and emphasizes understanding how errors arise (Decision Systems Inc. 2005; NHS 2013b; MMS 2001; Grenier-Sennelier et al. 2002; van Vuuren, Shea, and van der Schaaf 1997).

According to van Vuuren, Shea, and van der Schaaf (1997), "technical" includes design, construction, and materials; "human" comprises knowledge-based, qualifications, coordination, verification, intervention, monitoring, slips (failure of fine motor skills), and tripping (failure in whole-body movements); "organizational" involves knowledge transfer, protocols, management priorities, and culture; "patient-related" involves patient characteristics beyond the control of staff or treatment; and "unclassifiable" encompasses anything outside the other categories.

Some of the categorization systems in Table 5.2 provide more detail than others, and while there is no silver bullet, these five systems provide

Table 5.2 Typologies of Root Causes

Decision Systems Inc.	UK National Health System	Massachusetts Medical Society	Grenier-Sennelier et al.	van Vuuren, Shea, & van der Schaaf
Design and Engineering				
Equipment and Materials	Equipment		Equipment	Technical
Human Performance	Staff/Team	Human Resources		Human Behavior
Management	Organizational	Leadership		Organizational
Communication	Communication	Communication	Coordination	
Training	Education and Training			
External Phenomena	Work Environment	Environment		
Barriers				
Technical Information		Information Management	Perception of Risk	
Inspection				
			Lack of Assistance	
	Patient		Individual	Patient-related
			Hospital Structure	
	Task			
				Unclassifiable

guidance to investigate and resolve system issues. The ultimate success of root cause identification is determined by the skills of the analyst. The reviewed causes and categories can individually or in combination be "the cause" of an adverse event. An individual may be ultimately responsible for an action (an active error), but the system in which she works can increase (or decrease) the probability of error occurring (latent errors). Safeguards can be built or procedures can be specified to reduce the probability of error, but if they are not enforced, the staff will be green-lighted to improvise at their discretion, thus increasing the possibility of error.

Although a straightforward event such as wrong-side surgery could be attributed to a single person (surgeon error) or process (failure to check patient chart before surgery, lack of a consistent marking system), errors should be viewed as the final link in a long chain of events. The Joint Commission does not consider an RCA acceptable if it focuses on individual performance rather than on systems and process (Joint Commission 2010, SE-9).

The point is that one can attribute an error to a single point or person, or one can ask how a process can be restructured to prevent reoccurrence. Placing responsibility on a single person or point in the process overlooks the greater opportunities that could be undertaken to prevent reoccurrence and guarantees a defensive reaction among employees. Instead of placing responsibility and control at a single point or on an individual (for example, the surgeon must be more careful in the future), systemic safeguards should ensure multiple checks and focus the efforts of all involved parties on achieving better outcomes.

Types of Root Cause Analyses

There are two types of root cause analyses. The most common is an analysis of a single event: a patient falls, a wrong pharmaceutical is administered, a nosocomial infection occurs. Single-event RCA is best typified by the Joint Commission's sentinel event policy, which encourages an RCA for any event that results in unanticipated death or permanent loss of function. The Joint Commission encourages analysis for other events even if death or disability does not occur (Joint Commission 2010, SE-6).

aggregate root cause analysis
an RCA that seeks the causes of undesirable outcomes by identifying common attributes across a number of events

The second and more powerful analysis is an **aggregate root cause analysis**, which studies multiple events. While it is important to understand individual cases, multiple-event analysis allows an organization to understand risk: What is occurring in a series of falls, incorrect medications, or infections? Where are processes regularly producing undesirable events, and where should improvement efforts be focused? Staff may minimize the importance of isolated failures or those resulting from a series of factors that are unlikely to reoccur ("the perfect storm"). Staff often feel that time spent analyzing a problem or developing safeguards and remediation plans for events that are unlikely to reoccur draw resources away from more pressing and valuable activities. When failure with or without harm is a regularly documented event, employees may more readily recognize the need for prevention and become more invested in changing the process for the benefit of patients.

The Joint Commission has embraced the concept of shared learning, and its requirement that RCA be performed for sentinel events is used to build a database and issue alerts when they determine that member organizations can learn from the experiences of others. The problem with this approach is the rarity of sentinel events at the organizational level. One need only contrast total sentinel events reported from January 1995 through December 2006—4,074, or roughly 340 per year—against the IOM estimate of 44,000 to 98,000 preventable deaths annually to understand the chasm between what is reported and what is not reported. An additional problem is the inability of organizations to comprehend the commonalities when sentinel events from various institutions are combined. Health care organizations are known for considering themselves to be unique. Health care workers commonly believe that their field is different from other industries and their organization is different from other health care institutions. The result of these beliefs is that quality improvement methods proven effective in other places are often dismissed as being inapplicable to the special circumstances of their organization.

The focus on sentinel events is obviously limited; widespread improvement requires organizations to analyze a broader class of adverse and potentially adverse events for which the Joint Commission does not require an RCA. Building a quality culture will occur only if individual departments record and analyze events to recognize similarities and implement safeguards to address frequently occurring issues. A quality culture will not develop from a centralized, top-down approach driven by sentinel events.

The first steps toward a quality culture begin with instilling a drive to improve among employees and introducing data collection at a department level. Studies report that neither the rate of adverse events nor their impact is definitively known. Ricci et al. (2004) relate that two different reporting systems in a pediatric ICU produced 112 incident reports in one system and 143 reports in the second. Remarkably, only 44 incidents were reported in both systems, a concurrence rate of only 20.9%. Among the incident reporters, there was wide disagreement over the seriousness of events. One system reported that 25.5% were major or life-threatening incidents; the other system reported 40.5%. Similarly, Grenier-Sennelier et al. (2002) report that an administrative incident reporting system documented a fracture rate of 5.0% for patient falls, but a review of medical records found a 10.0% fracture rate.

One of the major questions that arises when quality improvement is suggested is: Will the effort of recording and analyzing events, especially no harm or near misses, be worth the cost? Bates et al. (1995) estimated that the additional cost created by a patient fall is $4,233 while a later study, Bates et al. (1997), reported additional costs incurred after an adverse drug event as $4,685. The cost-effectiveness of quality improvement revolves around how efficient an organization is in collecting and analyzing data and its ability to implement change that reduces the probability of an event, the damage produced, and the costs of remediation. These studies suggest that a substantial opportunity exists to lower health care costs if institutions can identify the causes of undesirable outcomes *and* implement controls that reduce adverse events at a reasonable cost.

Single-Event Analysis

There are three primary components of an RCA: data collection, data analysis, and corrective or preventive action. RCA has an obligation to identify corrective action and follow-up to ensure that change is undertaken and to determine the impact of the recommended changes. The difference between an analysis of an individual case and one analyzing multiple events is primarily focus. Single-case analysis relies more on data collection while multiple-event analysis is driven by data analysis. For an individual case, the analyst may need to talk to all or the majority of individuals who participated in a patient's treatment. On the other hand, the analyst who has access to a database of information from multiple events may elect to mine the data to identify the most at-risk parts of a process.

Individual case analysis requires knowledge of the appropriate questions to ask and the interpersonal skill to effectively ask questions. The interviewer must be able to elicit trust and gain the cooperation of her subjects while exploring potentially sensitive issues dealing with job performance, teamwork, and other issues. For multiple-event analysis, data analysis skills are required to identify commonalities. Creating Pareto charts and histograms is an effective way to produce information to focus quality improvement efforts. Data analysis, including the creation of frequency tables, will be demonstrated when multiple-event analysis is discussed. Both types of analysis require the analyst to understand the RCA process and its goals.

It makes intuitive sense to explore how a single event is examined before expanding into the analysis of multiple events, since individual cases provide the raw data for multiple-event analysis. Table 5.3 summarizes the three basic steps in RCA: data collection, data analysis, and initiation of corrective action.

Table 5.3 Single Case Root Cause Analysis Processes

Data Collection	
1.	Identify event or improvement opportunity
2.	Assemble team based on knowledge and authority
3.	Build timeline of activities
Data Analysis	
4.	Analyze process and identify potential causes
5.	Identify root cause(s)
Corrective or Preventive Action	
6.	Identify potential corrective or preventive changes
7.	Select and implement change
8.	Follow-up: Was change implemented, continued, and effective?

Table 5.3 synthesizes the root cause process recommended by four different authors (Knudsen et al. 2007; Mills et al. 2005; Perkins et al. 2005; Rooney and Vanden Heuvel 2004). These authors propose processes ranging from four to eleven steps. Table 5.3 highlights the transitions from data collection to data analysis to corrective or preventive action. The authors using more steps to describe the process provide the reader with a greater understanding of what is required while the four-step version defines the fundamentals. The reader may again benefit from recognizing the different terminology: data collection is variously described as flowcharting the current process, describing the event, collecting information, or collecting data. The point is that no matter which process is selected, they all cover the same ground. Comparing and contrasting these approaches will give the reader greater understanding of RCA.

The first task in RCA is to understand what has occurred. This requires describing the outcome and the process leading up to an event in sufficient detail to identify the reasons why the outcome occurred. This is a complex task in treatment processes in which a patient presents with multiple conditions, is seen by several care givers, and receives dozens of tests and procedures. Establishing the timeline of activities is an essential first step when analyzing a process. The timeline should cover what was done, where it occurred, who made decisions, who provided care, and who was present during the activity. Timelines are valuable because they place each event in the context of what came before and after, emphasizing that medical care is a process rather than a series of discrete steps.

Flowcharting is a tool that increases comprehension of a process, illuminates discrepant views of the process and serves as a tool to resolve any divergent views, and records the present state of the system. A primary benefit of documentation is to identify different treatment protocols that may not be recognized by those working in the system. Flowcharts should identify all the significant actions and care givers in a process, where actions or decisions were made, the entry of inputs into the system, the outputs produced, and the results achieved.

After documenting the process, the essential task is to disaggregate the care episode into its constituent steps to identify where the error arose, the potential causes of the problem, and the points at which the error could have been prevented (before), detected (concurrent), or corrected (after). Unlike timeline construction, where we were concerned with what was taking place, discovery of root causes requires the delicate process of documenting every event including who was present when the error arose, when and where it occurred, and why it occurred. After identifying an active cause, the analyst should explore the latent causes that could have contributed to the failure.

RCA can be viewed as asking a structured series of questions to determine why an event or outcome occurred and to trace it back to its root causes. Various methodologies have been advanced to direct the search for root causes. Three techniques are described next, beginning with the simplest and most intuitive approach and progressing to a more structured method.

Data Collection Techniques

The Five Whys

The National Health Service (NHS) in England suggests asking *why* five times when an undesirable event occurs. For example, if a patient receives an incorrect medicine, the sequence of questions could be:

Question 1: Why did the patient receive the wrong medicine? (an obvious question)

> Response 1: The prescription was wrong. (one of dozens of possible answers)

Question 2: Why was the prescription wrong? (an obvious follow-up question in response to the first answer)

> Response 2: Physician made incorrect pharmaceutical decision.

Question 3: Why did the physician make the wrong decision?

> Response 3: Incomplete patient chart.

Question 4: Why was the patient chart incomplete?

> Response 4: Physician assistant did not record test results.

Question 5: Why didn't the physician assistant record the test results?

> Response 5: Tests results were phoned to secretary and secretary did not tell physician assistant (NHS 2013a).

The first *why* defines the problem, and the first response establishes the overall direction of the inquiry. Successive *whys* flow naturally from the received responses. Successive responses limit the potential cause and suggest the follow-up question that should be asked. Analysts must recognize that the initial response, and perhaps even the initial question, may not be appropriate and that multiple attempts using the **Five Whys** may be required.

Five questions may or may not uncover the root cause. One may be able to discern a cause using fewer than five questions, and at other times more than five questions will be needed (especially when more than one cause is at work). The general rule holds that an analyst will be reasonably close to

Five Whys
a technique for identifying the root cause of an undesirable event or outcome by asking five questions, starting with a broad question of what occurred and ending with why it arose and how it can be prevented

identifying a root cause after framing five *why* questions. More important than the general rule is the recognition that identifying a root cause need not be an overwhelming and time-consuming process but rather is based on a straightforward and effective questioning technique. Information-gathering techniques are the first skill an analyst must develop.

In the preceding scenario, a narrow interpretation could be that the secretary made an error in failing to inform the physician assistant—the active error. In many cases, the identified cause may be both an active and a latent error. Is illegible handwriting an active error? Yes. Is an organizational culture that tolerates illegibility a latent error? Yes.

A narrow interpretation could lead to the conclusion that the secretary must be more careful. A broader view would ask: Why does a patient care system depend on such a tenuous transmission of information, a sixth *why*. Should the telephone be used for relaying clinical information? If so, should a secretary relay clinical information? If so, should there be a defined procedure for recording the call, recording the relayed data in the patient chart, and notifying care givers? These questions attempt to uncover latent errors that may contribute to medical error.

System weaknesses are often difficult to identify because people have grown accustomed to doing things in a particular way, and these processes often work. The problem for root cause identification is that accepted practices work the majority of the time but can fail when a confluence of events, issues, or pressures arise. The analyst's job is to identify unsafe practices, recognize the conditions under which practices may fail, and design and implement safeguards to handle these conditions.

The Why-Why Diagram

A variation of the Five Why technique is the **Why-Why diagram**. The problem with the Five Whys is that it is linear; a problem is identified and subsequent exploration follows a single path. The administration of the wrong medication can arise from a multitude of causes, so a wrong prescription is only one of several explanations. The patient may have forgotten to inform staff of a previous allergic reaction, the prescription could have been misread, an unprescribed drug could have been administered, or there may be some other cause.

The primary difference between the Five Whys and the Why-Why diagram is the former asks why an event occurred; the latter takes a broader view by exploring how an event could arise. The Why-Why diagram, rather than seeking a single cause, attempts to expand understanding of the many potential causes that could lead to an undesirable event. To construct a Why-Why diagram, the analyst should first ask why an event occurred

Why-Why diagram
a technique for identifying the root causes of an undesirable event or outcome by exploring multiple ways the event or outcome could have arisen

(identical to the Five Why approach) but instead of being satisfied with a single answer would continue to inquire into other possible explanations: What else could have caused the event? One can think of this as pursuing the most likely causes for an event instead of a one-track, five-question exercise. An analyst could find himself with dozens, if not hundreds, of potential causes. The potential causes are best viewed as branches in a tree diagram where a single event could result from one or more causes.

The Why-Why diagram, Figure 5.4, demonstrates how a wrong medication could arise from various causes. For display purposes, the example has been limited to two responses to each question. Accordingly, the two main causes of a wrong medication are: the prescription was wrong (a rule or knowledge error) and the wrong medication was administered (a skill error or violation). This diagram shows that when only two responses are allowed per question, five levels of questioning produces 32 potential causes. Each question doubles the number of causes; $2 \rightarrow 4 \rightarrow 8 \rightarrow 16 \rightarrow 32$. If each question produces three answers, five levels of questioning produces 243 potential causes. The general rule is that the number of potential causes will equal the number of responses raised to the fifth power (potential causes = number of responses^5). The Why-Why diagram is more difficult to manage than the Five Whys but does more justice to clinical situations where more than one cause can produce an undesired outcome.

The procedure for the Five Whys and Why-Why diagram is question and response: an analyst follows each response to one or more possible causes to pursue the root cause. The Why-Why diagram is more time consuming given its broader focus (what could have occurred versus what did occur); however, the greater upfront investment can lead to higher benefits later. By recognizing multiple potential causes, corrective or preventive action can be developed to address more than one weakness at a single point in time (rather than waiting for each to occur before action is taken). A second advantage is that if the analysis arrives at a wrong conclusion (X was caused by Y when X was actually the result of Z), the team does not have to restart the data collection process but can return to the Why-Why diagram to assess why the event reoccurred. Did the event result from one of the previously recognized potential causes that was not pursued?

The Why-Why diagram demonstrates that a single event may be the result of multiple causes. The next technique begins with the premise that undesired outcomes are generally the result of a combination of factors and that one factor is insufficient to explain an adverse event. Normally reliable processes may fail when they are placed under extreme pressure. The goal of the third technique is to identify why normally reliable processes fail, to discover what change or changes produced the failure.

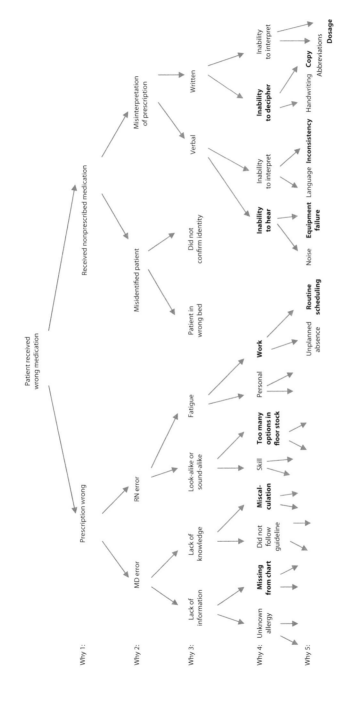

Figure 5.4 Why-Why Diagram

The Is–Is Not Matrix

Kepner and Tregoe (1965) developed a more structured and general system of searching for root causes that is not dependent upon the responses offered to prior questions. The **Is–Is Not matrix** approach to problem specification is based on the assumption that a process has a known standard of performance and that a deviation from the standard has been observed. Deviation provides the impetus for a precise defining of the problem: who or what is affected, where did it occur, when did it occur, and how extensive is the deviation?

Is–Is Not matrix
a technique for identifying the root causes of an undesirable event or outcome that focuses on identifying differences between situations when an error did and did not arise

The process begins by answering the following series of questions:

- What is the deviation: who or what was affected?
- Where was the deviation observed?
- When did the deviation appear?
- How big is the deviation or how many deviations are observed?

These questions provide half the information required to identify the cause of a deviation. The second step is to ask the opposite questions: Who is not affected, and where and when does the deviation not arise? The analyst must identify where deviations are not observed. This could be the same process operating at a different point in time or an identical or similar process operating at a different location. The assumption is that there are identifiable characteristics which distinguish deviations from the outcomes of processes that meet performance standards. The Kepner-Tregoe system requires analysts to define the problem (what *is* the error, where *is* the error) and contrast it with situations in which the same result could arise but did not.

The two sets of data specifying what is a problem and what is not a problem facilitate data analysis. Can an error be traced to readily identifiable differences between situations in which the problem arose and those in which it is not observed? These factors examine differences in what is occurring (process), who is affected (the patient), the individuals providing care, the location of care, and the time or day of care. The Is–Is Not matrix is a balanced approach to the discovery of active and latent errors as it documents the error and the context in which it arose. Kepner and Tregoe's approach to cause discovery is more systematic than the Five Whys or the Why-Why diagram in that it studies the specific event, where deviations from expectations occur, and situations in which similar errors could arise but did not. Rather than an ad hoc, follow-the-data-where-it-leads approach, the Is–Is Not Matrix recommends a review of specific factors that could contribute to variation in performance.

Step one in the Is–Is Not procedure is to clearly state the problem so everyone on the analysis team understands what they are attempting to resolve. **Step two** divides the problem into five parts. A review of the literature shows that specific applications add and subtract elements from the basic five-part framework. The framework is shown in Figure 5.5; column 2 records the basic information on the problem. Similar to newspaper writing, where reporters are supposed to answer who, what, where, when, why, and how, the goal of the Is–Is Not matrix is to assemble the relevant facts on what has occurred (Is).

		Data Collection	Analysis
Step 1 Problem Statement:	Step 2 Is	Step 3 Is Not	Step 4 Difference
Who (what) is affected? What is occurring?	Customers, materials, equipment…		
How important is the problem or what is the extent of the problem?	Frequency, seriousness		
Who is part of the process?	By whom, near whom?		
Where does the problem occur?	Location		
When does the problem occur?	Date, day of week, time of day, proximity to other events		

Figure 5.5 Is–Is Not Template

Unlike with a newspaper article, the analyst also reports nonoccurrences (Is Not). **Step three** requires analysts to explore situations in which the problem is not observed (column 3, the Is Not column). Undesirable outcomes can result from differences in patients as well as differences in care provided. Severely ill patients of advanced age with multiple comorbidities should have lower outcomes than younger or less ill patients. So the question arises, is the problem a medical error or a predictable outcome given the patient's condition? Outcomes also depend on treatment. We must recognize differences in the use of equipment (catheters, ventilators, etc.) and the duration of their use. Step three documents cases in which an undesirable outcome could have arisen but did not.

Step four, which uses the Difference column (column 4), encourages the analyst to contemplate whether the characteristics—who is and is not affected, who was and was not part of care process, where the problem did and did not arise, and when the problem did and did not occur—point to the underlying causes of the event. Are differences between occurrences and nonoccurrences trivial, or are they causal?

The analyst must ask, if the factor were changed—if a different patient, provider, time, or location was involved—would the result be the same? An affirmative answer suggests a system problem (the failure would occur independent of who was involved) or suggests an earlier failure (anyone working with the information would reach the same conclusion). If failure can be traced to a particular person (others would not have performed this way) or time (it was due to the fact that this occurred on the overnight shift or on the weekend), then the solution is somewhat easier: correct the broken component.

control group

the group in a study that receives no intervention and serves as the baseline to evaluate changes in the experimental group

experimental group

the group in a study that receives an intervention

The Is–Is Not Matrix functions similarly to **control groups** and **experimental groups** in random clinical trials, where researchers attempt to hold a number of factors constant, allowing them to attribute any difference in outcomes to one factor that is different between the two groups. For example, we may be able to attribute a reduction in nosocomial infections to the prophylactic use of antibiotics (a *what* factor) when the *who*, *when*, and *where* factors are similar. The strength of the Is–Is Not technique is that it provides a format to explore problems. Asking who (or what) is affected, who is part of the production process, where the problem arises, and when the problem occurs provides the elemental questions to begin exploring a problem. Kepner and Tregoe note that in many cases it will not be a single factor that explains a deviation but a set of circumstances. For example, the fact that patients are over 65 years of age does not satisfactorily explain a patient falling since many patients over 65 do not fall (and some under 65 fall). Root cause identification requires additional information to define why a particular patient over 65 fell and sustained injury when others did not. Was it due to that patient's medical situation or other elements (or both)? Additional information—where, when, and who—is needed to explain the adverse result. Does the combination of patient age, other patient-specific factors, time of day, and location provide the critical elements to identify why a particular patient fell and sustained injury? Unlike the Five Whys, which is geared toward identifying a single cause, the Is–Is Not matrix examines a confluence of issues encompassing active and latent causes. Figure 5.6 explores the problem of patient falls with injury.

The Is–Is Not matrix bridges the transition from data collection to data analysis since the Is and Is Not columns record data, and the Difference column provides a head-to-head comparison that challenges analysts to consider what factors could contribute to the problem and what factors could provide appropriate safeguards to prevent the problem from arising. Specifying all the circumstances in which events are not occurring

Problem Statement: Patient Fall with Injury	Is	Is Not	Difference
Who is affected (or who is primarily affected if looking at a series of falls)?	Patient older than 65 years of age (greater probability of falling)	Patients younger than 65 years of age	Does age explain this fall? A large number of falls?
How important is the problem or what is the extent of injury?	Patients older than 65 are more likely to sustain serious harm		
Who is interacting with the patient or what is the patient interacting with?	Nurses, aides, housekeeping, transport (who), furniture (what)…		Does involvement (or lack of) of personnel explain the fall? Does furniture explain this fall?
Where does the problem occur?	Patient room (or nursing unit x)	Ancillary areas (or nursing units y, z…)	Are some locations more prone? Does department (or level of staffing) explain this fall?
When does the problem occur?	Night/evening (or weekends)	Day (or weekdays)	Does time of day (or day of the week) explain? Is it related to other activities?

Figure 5.6 An Is–Is Not Example

or being observed could be an extremely time-consuming and unproductive task. If we were examining a single patient fall, we could attempt to compare this fall with all the other patients hospitalized that day who did not fall but obviously some comparisons would yield little information, for example, comparing elderly patients to pediatric or ICU patients. Similarly, it would be possible to identify similar patients (similar age and condition treated by the same personnel in the same location at the same time) who did not fall, thus making it impossible to identify differences. The Is–Is Not matrix requires the analyst's judgment to direct it toward productive comparisons.

Besides bridging the gap between data collection and analysis and casting a wider net encompassing active and latent error, the Is–Is Not matrix is a useful tool for comparing multiple instances of an event and identifying commonly appearing elements in the Is and Is Not columns. As stated earlier, because these questioning processes will often identify multiple potential reasons for an event, using the Is-Is Not Matrix to examine multiple events may allow the analyst to focus on substantial differences—those occurring in a majority of cases—and sift out the trivial differences.

Data Analysis and Identifying a Cause

After the data has been collected, it must be studied to identify the root cause. Determining the root cause is a matter of judgment. Particularly in medicine a course of treatment can be second-guessed given differences in practice style, but analysts need to inoculate themselves against **hindsight bias**. Hindsight bias is the tendency, after an adverse outcome has occurred, to attribute predictability to its causes. The question is, without prior knowledge of the adverse outcome would one have been able to find fault with the circumstances that preceded it?

Expert judgment is a method for identifying root causes and reaching decisions based on the insight of recognized knowledgeable individuals. Expert judgment can be solicited through literature review: who has published on a topic and what did it say? Expert judgment is often obtained by assembling a panel of leaders in the field; these individuals may have published in the area, performed a high volume of procedures, or may hold office in professional societies. After the group has been assembled, the members are polled to identify root causes.

Consensus is a decision reached by a group as whole. Unlike expert judgment, no external opinions are solicited and the group relies upon itself to reach a decision. Chapter Four covered two techniques, multivoting and Q-sort, to identify solutions, but these two techniques can also be employed to identify a root cause when more than one factor may be the cause of a problem.

Statistical analysis attempts to quantify the relationship between two variables. Typically, statistics establishes statistical significance at 5%: is there less than a 5% chance that we would observe the change in one variable given a change in another variable? If the probability of observing the relationship is more than 5%, we say the observed relationship may be due to chance. Chapter Nine examines common statistical tools to determine if variables are related.

hindsight bias
the tendency, after an adverse outcome has occurred, to attribute predictability to its causes

consensus
a judgment reached by most, if not all, of a group

statistical analysis
a body of methods applied to quantitative data to summary and explore phenomenon

Implementing Corrective or Preventive Action

The final step is modifying the delivery system to design a new process (with corrective action), document the change, communicate the change to affected parties, and provide the opportunity for feedback. This modification may include altering clinical practice guidelines, changing policies and procedures, and issuing alerts. The point that Shojania et al. (2001) made is worth repeating: "researchers now believe that most medical errors cannot be prevented by perfecting the technical work of individual doctors, nurses, or pharmacists. Improving patient safety often involves the coordinated efforts of multiple members of the health care team, who may adopt strategies from outside health care." A multilevel approach that recognizes why humans err is needed to develop systems and technology to make medical errors less likely to occur and more likely to be identified when they do arise.

Multiple-Event Analysis

There is strength in numbers. The problem with an analysis of a single event is that it is often downplayed. People are quick to dismiss an error as a confluence of events unlikely to reoccur or as aberrant behavior by an individual and thus invest little energy in analyzing, redesigning, and rebuilding the process. While it is widely recognized that changing a system can create more problems than it resolves, single-event analysis provides little insight into whether a system should be changed. Single-event analysis by its nature cannot provide insight into how often adverse events occur nor identify common factors that are present in similar events.

The primary goal of RCA is to prevent the reoccurrence of errors and improve outcomes. To prioritize improvement efforts, organizations need to understand what is happening, how often it occurs, and how serious the issue is. Single-event analysis provides information on what is happening, why it happened, and how serious it is for an individual patient, but it does not provide sufficient insight into other potential causes that might produce the outcome. How many times have similar problems occurred and how serious are these events for the organization? Small errors or near misses occurring on a daily basis may be a greater problem to the organization than a large problem that occurs once. Unfortunately, large problems are more likely to attract the attention of the public, administrators, and accrediting bodies.

The goal of multiple-event RCA is to identify common elements that contribute to undesirable outcomes. Often a sufficient sample size cannot be obtained to perform multiple-event analysis on sentinel events. Joint Commission statistics demonstrate, for example, that the number of occurrences of infant abduction and homicide is low, and many organizations may never experience one of these events. Nevertheless, assessing whether an organization is efficiently allocating its scarce resources to large and small problems can be determined only by looking at the totality of undesirable events, including the total impact of small problems. Large numbers of less serious events occur frequently in hospitals, such as patient falls and medication errors, and these events offer organizations a substantial opportunity to improve patient care. Medication errors are estimated to arise 5.3 times per 100 orders (Bates et al. 1995), while the rate of patient falls in hospitals has been estimated at 8.9 per 1,000 patient days (Schwendimann et al. 2006).

The goal of multiple-event analysis is not to identify a single cause or group of causes to explain an event but to understand common causes for a type of event. What factors are commonly present when humans err? Can common factors be identified in slips, lapses, mistakes, and violations? Can common factors be identified in particular types of events such as patient falls, or medication errors? Multiple-event analysis, being unconcerned with a particular case, shifts focus from individual behavior to system performance. Multiple-event analysis places greater emphasis on examining the qualifications of the people most commonly involved (rather than those of an individual), the equipment and supplies commonly involved in errors, and the clinical situation.

The goal of multiple-event analysis is to combine information collected on individual cases and identify common factors to improve patient care by modifying these factors to reduce the likelihood of problems reoccurring. Multiple-event analysis differs from single-case analysis in that data collection has already occurred; thus multiple-event analysis emphasizes analysis—getting the maximum amount of information from previously collected data. This may require inputting previously collected data from incident reports into a software application so employees can mine the data. For many organizations getting employees to regularly recognize, report, and systematically record data on potentially harmful events is the most difficult part of the improvement process.

Quality reporting systems to date have been driven by external parties, such as the Joint Commission. Kaplan and Fastman (2003) note that the ability to use data distinguishes organizations performing RCA to fulfill external reporting requirements from those seeking to improve their operations. External reports are not generally user-friendly or easily accessible, and they focus on events deemed important by outsiders. Reporting systems designed to fulfill external reporting requirements are generally less-than-optimal tools for employees seeking to improve performance.

An internally oriented event-reporting system should include more information and be more candid than external systems. External systems may focus on sentinel events, while internal systems should include the type of event and the amount of injury (major, minor, no harm, or near miss) as part of the information recorded. Recording no-harm and near-miss events will differentiate institutions striving for quality improvement from those developing minimal systems to meet external requirements. No-harm events and near misses provide data on frequency of events and recovery actions and are targeted toward generating information that employees can use to understand what is occurring and to improve processes. Near misses provide insight into avoidance systems—based on how an error was eluded—while no-harm events provide clues into resiliency or recovery systems—based on examining what amount of error can occur without harm or what remedial actions can be taken to prevent harm.

Data Collection

To demonstrate how data can be analyzed, assume an organization has collected the following information on adverse events—patient identifier, type of event, date of event, patient age, med/surg staff, days after registration (admittance) that the event occurred, shift that the event occurred on, extent of medication, location of the event, and level of injury—and has recorded this data in Excel (see Figure 5.7). The full data is available online in the Chapter05.xls file under the Figure05–07 tab. Raw data does not provide insight; it has the potential to be information, but in its raw form it generally is not very useful. Analysis transforms data into information that may pinpoint where and why problems arise. The starting point for this transformation is to identify a type of event to examine. The obvious choices are the most frequently occurring events or the events producing the greatest injury.

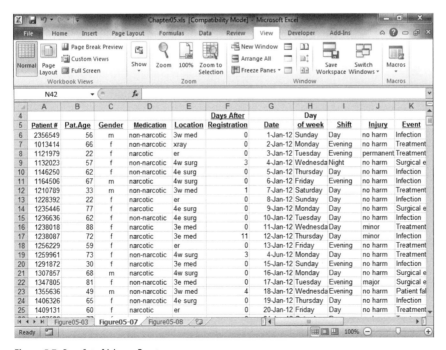

Figure 5.7 Data Set of Adverse Events

Although the Joint Commission focuses on the most severe events, this example will focus on the most frequently occurring event, patient falls. The first task is to sort the data. Using Excel this is performed using **=COUNTIF(range,criteria)**. Entering **=COUNTIF(K6:K465,"Patient Fall")** returns 141 patient falls. To create Table 5.4, the user must specify the other types of adverse events within quotation marks in the =COUNTIF function.

Table 5.4 Frequency of Adverse Events

Type	Number	Percent
Patient fall	141	30.7
Infection	52	11.3
Treatment error	71	15.4
Surgical error	34	7.4
Medication error	132	28.7
Lab/x-ray error	30	6.5
Totals	460	100.0

Reviewing Table 5.4 does not reveal anything more than that patient falls were the most frequent adverse event in 2012. What needs to be established is whether there are there any relationships between the event—the patient fall—and other pieces of data. The easiest way to gain understanding of the data is to construct frequency tables and column charts. Frequency tables divide the total number of cases into user-defined categories; for example, how many falls occurred in a defined time period and what nursing units had the most falls. A column chart presents a visual display of the information in the frequency table.

Frequency tables and column charts are easily created with Excel. The first step is to define the number of groups to be created; typically five to eight groups are used. Suppose we believe that there is a connection between patient falls and how long the patient has been in the hospital. Reviewing column F (days after registration that the fall occurred) we notice that zero is the predominant value; that is, a high number of falls appear to occur on the day of registration. To determine the longest interval between registration and a patient fall, we could again review the data, or we could use Excel to identify the upper limit. Two methods are possible. The first uses the =Max function. Excel will identify the maximum value and minimum values by inserting the **=MAX(data_range) (or =MIN(data_range)** function. The second method is a multilevel sort: the user selects Data, Sort, and **Sort by** (type of event) but then enters a second variable of interest in the **Then by** field. If the second field is days from registration, Excel will sort patient falls based on time lapse from registration, 0 (lowest) to ? (highest) if an ascending sort is selected, or from highest to lowest if descending order is desired.

Either approach identifies 0 as the minimum and 9 as the maximum number of days after registration before a patient fell. A cursory review indicates that values over 4 are rare. When the data is sorted by days after registration, we see that only 15 (out of 141) falls occurred after the fourth day of hospitalization. Using the rule of thumb of five to eight categories of data, a frequency table is built using the listed categories.

Falls occurring:
Day of registration (0)
Day after registration (1)
Two days after registration (2)
Three days after registration (3)
4 to 6 days after registration (6)
7 to 9 days after registration (9)
10 or more days after registration (99)

Excel provides a statistical function, **=FREQUENCY(data_ range,bins)**, that allows the user to count events meeting a user-defined criterion. To count all falls occurring on the day of registration one would enter: **=FREQUENCY(F7:F147,N7:N13)**. This function examines the values in the specified range (F7 through F147) and counts the number of zeros in the specified range; in this case 71 patients fell on the day of registration. =FREQUENCY then counts the number of items matching 1, 2, 3, between 4 and 6, between 7 and 9, and greater than 9 but less than 99 as specified in the bins. Table 5.5 is the resulting frequency table.

Table 5.5 Time between Registration and Patient Fall

Falls Occurring	Count	Percent
Day of registration	71	50.4
Day after registration	31	22.0
Two days after registration	15	10.6
Three days after registration	9	6.4
4 to 6 days after registration	13	9.2
7 to 9 days after registration	2	1.4
10 or more days after registration	0	0.0
	141	100.0

The total number of cases is determined by entering **=SUM(P7:P13)**. The percentage in each category is calculated by dividing each count by the total number of cases. For the day of registration this is **=P7/P$14**. The denominator (total cases) is anchored by the $ preceding the cell row. This formula can be copied to other rows (count categories) without editing. When copied, the numerator is incremented for each row (P8, P9. . .) while the denominator continues to reference cell P$109.

A column chart provides a visual representation of the frequency table and is constructed on the frequency table data. To create a column chart, the user selects the Excel **Insert** function, **Chart**, **Column** and enters the count range, P7:P13. The graph is completed by using the formatting options and specifying the chart location. Compared to the frequency table, a column chart is easier to interpret. Figure 5.8 shows that the majority of patients fall on the day of registration and that the probability of falling declines as patients move farther away from their registration dates.

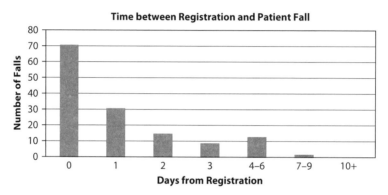

Figure 5.8 Time between Registration and Patient Fall

The column chart shows that the first area of concern should be falls on the day of registration and that falls decline rapidly as the time from registration increases. The number of patient falls should decline with time from admission since outpatients are usually in-house only on the day of registration and only a small percentage of inpatients remain in-house for extended time periods.

Data analysis is designed to transform data into information that provides insight into adverse events to target investigative and corrective efforts. An analyst studying patient falls would want to begin his improvement efforts by analyzing what occurs on the day of registration and determine what changes can be introduced to reduce the number of falls occurring on the day of registration, since it accounts for more than half of all falls. Unlike single-case analysis, which focuses on establishing a time-line of events for a particular patient, an analyst may want to flowchart the treatment process for a typical patient on the day of registration: What is the standard process? Are there vulnerabilities in the process that increase the probability of a patient falling?

Data Analysis

After an adverse event is identified and the standard process has been documented, the analyst should focus on identifying weaknesses in the process that could produce undesirable outcomes. When studying a group of cases, it is likely that multiple causes for an undesirable outcome will exist.

Weaknesses can be identified using a **deductive approach**, an **inductive approach**, or both. The deductive approach relies on gathering a group of people familiar with the type of adverse event being studied and encouraging them to brainstorm over the possible causes of the event. Conclusions will be based on reasoning. Providing more information to the group will facilitate this process. The column chart in Figure 5.8 would allow the assembled group to address the question of why falls are more likely to occur on the day of registration than on other days. Connecting patient falls to other variables, such as patient age, level/type of medication, time of day, and so on would further spur the exploration. The strength of the deductive approach is that a team can be assembled and polled quickly and inexpensively. The prime weakness of this approach is that the brainstormed causes may or may not be valid. The identified causes may represent nothing more than the preconceived biases of one or more of the assembled group members.

deductive approach
the deriving of a conclusion through reasoning

inductive approach
the deriving of a conclusion by assuming that which holds for a part is also true for the whole

The inductive approach, arriving at conclusions by observing part of a population and reasoning that the same conclusion applies to the whole, would pull charts and attempt to identify commonalities through chart reviews. This approach will lead to more fact-based explanations, but it is more time consuming and is dependent on the skills of the chart reviewer.

Returning to the example, assume the analysis group has determined that the probable reasons for the high number of falls on day of registration include:

1. Highest level of impairment
2. More frequent transport
3. Patient unfamiliarity with environment
4. Staff unfamiliarity with patient

The goal of process analysis is to identify fall commonalities; in this situation, the group would determine what common characteristics were present in a significant number of the falls. After completing the analysis and identifying common factors, the analysis group should inform employees of their findings.

Implementing Preventative Action

The utility of the data collection and analysis will be determined by how successful an organization is in reducing the occurrence of adverse events and minimizing the injury resulting from the events that cannot be prevented; that is, the data is only useful if the organization puts it to use. The final step in the improvement process is to create an action plan that can be and is implemented with preventative measures and controls addressing the identified causes. The following questions should be asked: Are the recommended interventions logically related to the identified problem? Can the interventions be implemented (will they be followed, what is the cost of implementation and adherence, etc.)? Can the effectiveness of the intervention be tested?

The success of the action plan will be determined by the validity of the RCA. Were the primary causes of the event identified? Can the recommended interventions reduce the occurrence of an adverse event or the time to recognize and respond to an adverse event? Will the recommended safeguards, alerts, and recovery mechanisms be incorporated into standard operating practice? An effective action plan must specify precisely the actions expected, include resources to support training and equipment purchases to carry out the plan, define responsible parties, set dates for implementation, measure effectiveness, and incorporate performance improvement into the personnel evaluation process. To satisfy Joint Commission requirements, an acceptable action plan for a sentinel event must identify changes that reduce risk, responsible parties, implementation dates, and the effectiveness of the assessment plan (Joint Commission 2010, SE-9–SE10).

Most of the root causes identified by the Joint Commission, Figure 5.3, involve human performance. The Joint Commission's definition of "human factors" includes training, staffing levels, qualifications/competency requirements, and supervision. Other categories shown in Figure 5.3, such as leadership (management), communication (including teamwork), and establishing procedures for assessing patient risk, also reflect human involvement. Two causes, information management and physical environment [name of category], address equipment issues: Are changes to information technology required to improve information availability? Is new equipment required or are controls or guards required for existing equipment? The last cause, physical environment, can be seen as addressing the larger environment in which health care operates: What if anything can be done, to address external factors such as patient condition before arrival at the institution, labor shortages, financial pressures, weather, and so on?

To provide closure to the patient fall example, the analysis team, having collected data and identified causes, has arrived at the following recommendations to reduce patient falls and their severity:

1. Improve patient assessment. Rationale: certain patient characteristics (age, disability, medication) make patients more susceptible to falling and sustaining injury. Staff should be trained to identify high-risk patients, and this information must be communicated among members of the patient care team.

2. Portable testing equipment should be acquired to reduce the need to move high-risk patients. Rationale: reducing the number of high-risk patients that must be transported for tests or procedures will reduce the number of falls that occur. This may be most important during the initial days of a patient stay, when the patient may be most unsteady, staff is less familiar with the patient, and the patient is not fully oriented to his or her surroundings.

3. Increased use of patient protection equipment for high-risk patients, for example, hip protectors, footwear. Rationale: nonslip footwear will reduce the probability of falling, and hip protectors will reduce the probability of injury when a patient falls.

Follow-up is required to determine whether the recommended changes are having the desired impact. Run charts, described in Chapter Four, can be used for follow-up. Effectiveness should be measured as a reduction in the rate of occurrence because superior measures adjust for volume. For example, the percentage of patient falls is the best measure, since the number of falls should change proportionately with the number of patients served; high admission months are expected to have more falls than lower admission months. The number of patient falls divided by number of registrations provides the percentage. The simple number of patient falls over time, however, has the advantage of easy comparison between time periods and is easy to calculate and monitor (did the number of falls per week, month, or quarter decline?). A third measure is patient falls divided by patient days, which recognizes that increases or decreases in average length of stay should have a proportional effect on falls. Falls per 1,000 patient days is the common metric used to compare the frequency of falls across institutions.

If intervention to reduce the number of falls occurring on the day of registration is proven successful (or if it is determined that no improvement can be made), the quality improvement team may want to expand their efforts to the day after registration, when the second highest rate of falls (22%) occurs. Many of the interventions introduced to reduce falls on the day of registration will perform equally well for subsequent days, so the challenge for the analysis team is to identify others factors that may arise after the day of registration. Are there new issues that may affect the rate of patient falls? For example, do attempts to get the patient back on their feet and active after surgery introduce new hazards? Are different controls required to handle these new hazards?

If improvement efforts are not successful, the team may want to reexamine their root causes and the implementation of the recommended remediation efforts. With or without a reduction in adverse events or their severity, the analysis team and care givers should see this as the first step in a never-ending PDCA cycle. Employees should continually review operations to identify opportunities for improvement. After improvement opportunities are identified, interventions should be designed and tested. Those proven successful should be operationalized, and those that do not achieve their goal discarded. Either outcome leads employees back to the beginning—how can outcomes be improved?—thus starting the cycle again.

Adding Cases to the Adverse Event Data Base

Recording of data should be a routine component of every employee's job, and data entry should be made as simple as possible. Excel was chosen for this text because it is widely available and routinely used by many health care workers. Excel provides a platform to extend reporting and analysis to the departmental level.

In the example above, adding cases will not require updating any formulas as long as cases are entered in the prespecified range. For example, add the latest fall, a 65-year-old, heavily medicated male surgical patient who fell the day after registration on 4 North, to the data set of adverse events (Figure 5.7). If a new line is added (**Insert**, **Row**) within the existing data set, after line 6 or before line 465, the formulas are automatically incremented for the new case, and the frequency table (Table 5.4) and column chart (Figure 5.8) are automatically updated with the new case.

The Joint Commission requires an RCA conducted in response to a sentinel event to be acceptable, thorough, and credible. An acceptable RCA must focus on systems and processes, progress from special (active) causes to common (latent) causes, be penetrating (that is, the analysis does not end with the identification of a superficial or obvious cause), and identify potential changes that reduce probability of reoccurrence. Thoroughness requires identification of direct causes, a penetrating analysis that meets minimum Joint Commission requirements (2010, SE-10), identification of risk points, and recommended improvements. Credibility requires the participation and support of upper management and other involved parties, an action plan that is internally consistent, explanation of any "not applicable" findings, and a review of relevant literature (2010, SE-10).

Prevention and Recovery

Undesirable events can be dealt with in two primary ways. The first is to prevent their occurrence, and the second is to mitigate harm after they arise. Action plans should aim for elimination while recognizing that undesirable events occur in the best-designed systems. Prevention and recovery systems must be designed based on the type of error that one wishes to prevent or mitigate.

There is considerable debate over what will improve health care. One side is represented by the medical community, which emphasizes good medicine through professionalism and is skeptical of organizational improvement. On the other side is the recognition that humans cannot be perfected, so systems must be designed to integrate all members of the health care delivery process into early detection and mitigation of errors. The skepticism of the medical community is the result of prior ineffective quality management schemes and emphasizes that regardless of what position one holds, quality management will be judged based on its ability to produce quantifiable evidence of its effectiveness.

One way to prevent errors is safeguards. Safeguards are commonly divided into administrative, physical, and technical categories. **Administrative safeguards** typically deal with the establishment of policies and procedures to guide action, providing education and training to ensure that employees are familiar with the established policies and procedures, and providing oversight to ensure policy and procedures are followed. **Physical safeguards** provide barriers or obstacles to prevent undesired activity from occurring. A simple example is a lock on a door or cabinet that prevents access to unauthorized users. Finally, technical safeguards are the intangible equivalents to locks. **Technical safeguards** include passwords that prevent unauthorized use of equipment or encryption methods that prevent unauthorized access to information. Not all safeguards are equal. Some are highly reliable and require a great deal of effort to circumvent; others depend on whether or not people are willing or able to follow rules.

We can better understand safeguards and recovery systems by examining their effectiveness (ability to produce the intended result by stopping error) and reliability (ability to consistently produce the same result) (see Table 5.6). These two goals will be used to demonstrate the hierarchy of safeguards.

administrative safeguards include policies and procedures to guide action, education and training, and oversight

physical safeguards tangible barriers and obstacles that prevent or impede undesirable action

technical safeguards intangible barriers and obstacles that prevent access to equipment and information

Table 5.6 Reliability and Effectiveness of Safeguards

	Effective (works)	Ineffective (does not work)
Reliable (consistent)	Consistently prevents errors	Produces a consistent result but does not prevent errors
Unreliable (inconsistent)	When followed prevents errors	Not followed and would not prevent errors if followed

Suppose we are concerned about inappropriate and unauthorized use of patient information. Training might provide an effective but unreliable solution. If training is internalized, innocent transgressions will be avoided, but training will not stop deliberate attempts (for example, selling celebrity information to the press). Policies, procedures, and training cannot be expected to prevent willful transgressions. The ease of circumvention of policy and procedures reduces the probability that they will keep patient information from being used inappropriately. On the other hand, information access restrictions, including audit trails and tiered access to data, encumber access and increase the probability that inappropriate use will be discovered, thus providing more effective and reliable deterrence.

The difference between a reliable and effective system and one that produces regular errors is a matter of defining and monitoring processes. The first step is to understand what works and make employees aware of these safeguards. Once effective procedures are defined, measures must be established to ensure they are incorporated into care processes, and management must regularly monitor their use. The job of management is to ensure effectiveness and reliability; that is, management must recognize when actual performance deviates from desired performance and undertake timely corrective action to ensure that care processes proceed as expected.

Systems may rely on single-level error prevention and recovery systems, or they can operate with multiple layered safeguards—the defense-in-depth approach, or Swiss cheese model. Professionalism is a single-level system in which the professional is responsible for defining and ensuring quality. The multiple-layer approach requires more than one error before an undesired outcome occurs. One safeguard may be circumvented, but this is not sufficient to produce a problem since other safeguards will prevent injury. A simple example is a physician ordering a drug that may have an interaction with another medication, a growing concern given the number of medications patients receive. No error will occur if the physician orders the medication through a computerized physician order entry (CPOE) system, which flags potential interactions. If a CPOE is not in place or does not flag the potential interaction, a pharmacist might notice it, providing another line of defense. If the order survives pharmaceutical review, the nursing staff may identify the risk of interaction and provide a final line of defense. Multiple levels of review provide defense in depth: errors must survive repeated review before harm arises.

Although the administrative, physical, and technical approach is commonly used, Dew (2003) provides a more insightful approach that divides safeguards and controls into six categories (see Table 5.7).

Table 5.7 Types of Safeguards

Weak, Passive Safeguards
Knowledge: training and education
Administrative: policies and procedures
Strong, Active Safeguards
Measurement and inspection: human guards, electronic monitoring, two-person rules, audit trails, and so on.
Information: labels, signs, and alarms
Very Strong, Passive Safeguards
Physical: barriers to access or inappropriate use
Natural: introduction of time or distance into an activity

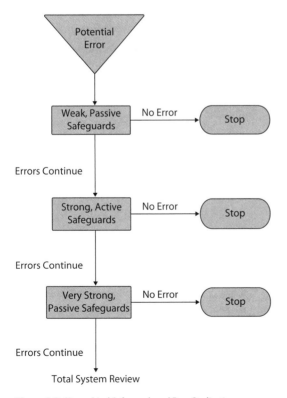

Figure 5.9 Hierarchical Safeguards and Error Realization

The framework of Table 5.7 and Figure 5.9 provides a clear distinction between the types of controls and ranks them on desirability. The continuum from weak to very strong indicates the reliability and effectiveness of the safeguard; the passive-to-active component denotes the level of human involvement required to operate the safeguard.

Physical safeguards, such as locks, walls, specialized gas line fixtures, and electrical plugs are the first choice as they are the most reliable safeguards. These safeguards make it difficult or close to impossible to do things incorrectly by placing physical barriers between the actor and error. One must break a lock to access resources or insert a gas line or electrical cord into a receptacle that it does not fit. Locks, on the other hand, prevent only errors by those who do not have the key (outsiders). Locks will not prevent errors or violations from those given access.

natural safeguards
the insertion of time or distance between an actor and an action

Natural safeguards seek to insert time or distance between an actor and error. Distance (placing things out of reach or contact) and time (limiting availability or exposure) interrupt action and provide an opportunity to reflect on what is being done and whether it is appropriate. Central storage of narcotics and other drugs is an attempt to reduce the probability of the wrong medicine being administered by introducing distance to the process. Nurses will be less likely to administer the wrong drug when they must walk to a centralized storage site than if a variety of medicines are available at the bedside. The insertion of distance and time into the drug administration process allows care givers time to consider their actions. Infusion pumps are another example of a natural safeguard: limits are set on the amount of medication that can be infused in a given amount of time. Recent use of time-out before surgery is an example of forcing an interruption in activity to perform a final review of the situation; is it the correct patient, site, and procedure, and are the necessary equipment and materials at hand?

The very strong, passive safeguards are the most likely to consistently produce the desired result because of the obstacles they create for hasty and ill-conceived action. Physical safeguards present formidable obstacles to sabotage, and the restructuring of processes under natural safeguards ensures that commonly accepted ways of doing things are permanently altered.

Not all potential problems will require or can be controlled through physical and natural safeguards. The strong, active safeguards require more human intervention to be effective, and their effectiveness can be undermined by the willingness of workers to ignore warnings or the unwillingness of managers to monitor processes.

Information safeguards, such as labels, signs, and alarms, caution people about hazards and help people to avoid problems when the message is recognized and understood. CPOE can remedy legibility problems and interact with databases to identify drug allergy and interaction problems. **Information safeguards** are effective by providing real-time feedback to actors on what they are doing. The use of bar codes for patients in VA hospitals has reduced the rate of incorrect medication administrations to 0.007%, or seven medication errors for every 100,000 drug administrations (Nicholson 2006).

information safeguards
alerts given to personnel of potential problems that could arise from an intended action

Measurement, verification, and inspection processes are safeguards designed to ensure that work is performed within safe limits. **Measurement and inspection safeguards** include tests, visual inspections, and other types of data collection. The old adage is "that which is measured, gets attention." When employees know that aspects of their performance will be reviewed or measured, they will be more diligent in their performance. The weaknesses of inspection, whether it be two employee checks or review by a superior, are that it may not be performed or, when performed, the reviewing party may fail to detect errors.

measurement and inspection safeguards
require data collection to ensure work is completed according to generally accepted standards

The safeguards least likely to produce a desired outcome are knowledge and administrative safeguards. Both safeguards depend on employees knowing what is expected and on their willingness to follow directives. Unlike with the strong, active safeguards, there is no point of action warning or review. With a knowledgeable and motivated workforce these safeguards may be appropriate for some types of problems, but management must track outcomes to ensure they are effective. When higher than acceptable error occurs, management must be ready to implement more effective safeguards.

Knowledge safeguards, such as checklists, charts, and posting of information, are designed to ensure that relevant information is constantly available to staff. The problem is attention and overload: Do employees pay attention to posted notices? Is there too much information to digest? One example of an effective knowledge safeguard is the World Health Organization's surgical safety checklist, which has reduced surgical error (WHO). A second type of knowledge safeguard is training; however, the problem with training is that often it may not be effective or it may be provided in advance of need and employees may forget the training by the time they need the information.

knowledge safeguard
definition of performance standards and report performance

The effectiveness of **administrative safeguards**, such as policies and procedures, relies on how well the policies are communicated to employees and the willingness of managers to enforce them. Policies written to comply with externally imposed standards and those not consistently enforced will have little impact on employee behavior. The problem with many organizations is their reliance on policy and procedural announcements rather than on establishing the case for change. Many organizations act as if all promulgated policies and procedures are read thoroughly and internalized by employees when, with the advent of e-mail, many of these pronouncements may end up directly in the recycle bin.

Some safeguards are easier to subvert than others. Administrative safeguards can be easily rendered useless under lax management. Routine violations occur because employees know policies are not enforced—lack of measurement, verification, or inspection. Knowledge safeguards can be undermined by a lack of investment in quality education and continuous training. Measurement safeguards can be circumvented when people falsify data. People can ignore information safeguards and circumvent natural and physical barriers (storing medications at the bedside to increase efficiency or breaking locks). In the case of circumvention of natural barriers, this could be a knowledge problem. An employee striving to increase the timeliness of care may believe it is appropriate to store medication at the bedside for ease of access without realizing that easy access increases the probability of error. Managers must ensure that employees understand the reason for procedures rather than see them simply as obstacles to providing care.

The best systems incorporate multiple safeguards to prevent and catch error. Strong systems are built around policies and procedures that are communicated to employees through training sessions and bulletin boards and incorporate physical and natural barriers to reduce the probability of error. The effectiveness of these five safeguards should be tested and reinforced by periodic assessment that checks whether policies and procedures are being followed, how many errors occur, and whether errors are increasing or decreasing. The results of periodic assessment should be fed back to employees so they can recognize and reinforce successful actions and focus on and improve actions that have not produced the expected changes.

In well-designed systems error occurs only when multiple conditions coexist. For example, simple ignorance of a policy by an employee who received no training should not produce ongoing errors if work is measured and managed. A policy or procedure violation should be discovered and corrected quickly (the employee should be trained on the appropriate behavior), if management is monitoring work. A communicated policy will not be effective if management does not enforce it. Similarly, physical and natural safeguards will be ineffective if the safeguards are not used (storage areas are left unlocked) or circumvented (materials are not returned to central storage). The task of management is to determine if the designed safeguards are being used (how often are physical safeguards rendered inoperable?), and if they are effective.

Defense in depth is designed to reduce error by relying on the idea that all safeguards will not fail simultaneously. Weak, passive safeguards work when employees internalize the aim of these defenses, but problems arise when the aim is not internalized or conflict arises. For example, a hospital may institute a policy to prevent misidentification of patients by requiring that two identifiers be checked before a medication, treatment, or procedure is given, but employees may feel that the policy is unnecessary or that staffing has been reduced to a point where meeting the policy is impossible. Given a choice between providing patient care and checking two identifiers, it is likely that employees will choose patient care.

It may also become common knowledge that despite policy, training, and informational signs that violations of policy will be overlooked. Many initiatives have a short half-life; new policies are frequently promulgated after an adverse event and monitored for a short period of time before the process returns to its prior state. When employee actions return to previous ways of working, measurement, natural, and physical safeguards are ignored to quicken the delivery of care or to minimize staff workload. When the aim of patient safety initiatives is not understood or internalized, the opposite of defense in depth is the result. A failure of one safeguard is not independent of the failure of other safeguards; ignoring one safeguard often predicts the circumvention of other systems.

Carroll, Rudolph, and Hatakenata (2002) point out that the lack of something is seldom the root cause of error. Explanations pointing to of lack of training, management, and so on are often given, but they short-circuit the identification of causes and may derail effective corrective action. These types of causes are also narrowly focused; they conclude that an employee or a group of employees requires training rather than that a system is poorly designed or understood. Similarly, lack of leadership, supervision, or inspection is often cited as a root cause, but other industries have long abandoned the idea that quality can be inspected into a product. Quality must be built into the product, and when quality is the job of every employee, inspection and supervision can be reduced.

Cases and Applications

Single-Event Analysis: The Wrong Patient

One of the least defensible medical errors is performing a procedure on the wrong patient. These events are the result of human error, as previously discussed, but consideration of environmental factors is also warranted. Gray et al. (2006) concluded in an NICU more than 50% of patients were at risk of misidentification due to shared surnames, similar surnames, or similar medical record numbers. Chassin and Becher (2002) provide an insightful review of a situation in which one hour into an invasive electrophysiology study the medical team discovered that the adult patient undergoing the procedure did not need it and was not scheduled for it. Their account is discussed in three parts: data collection, data analysis, and corrective or preventive actions.

Data Collection

The event began with the admission of two patients with similar names; the pseudonyms Joan Morris and Jane Morrison were used. Morris was a direct admission to the telemetry unit and Morrison was a transfer. Morris was subsequently transferred from telemetry to oncology.

On the day of the procedure, electrophysiology telephones telemetry seeking Morrison, but an unidentified telemetry staff member incorrectly reports that she has been transferred to oncology, mistaking Morris for Morrison. Electrophysiology telephones oncology seeking Morris, and Ms. Morris's nurse agrees to transport her to electrophysiology for the procedure despite the lack of a written order. Ms. Morris states that she does not want to undergo the procedure.

Ms. Morris and her chart are delivered to electrophysiology. Given the patient's reluctance to undergo the procedure, the attending is called and despite having met Jane Morrison, the scheduled patient, the prior evening, the attending does not recognize that Morris is not Morrison. The attending instructs the nurse to prepare Morris for surgery and states that she has agreed to surgery.

An electrophysiology nurse notices the consent form is missing although the daily schedule reports that it has been obtained and notifies the fellow scheduled to do the procedure. The fellow notes a lack of pertinent information in the patient chart but proceeds to discuss the procedure with Morris and obtains her consent.

Approximately 45 minutes after Morris was transported to electrophysiology, an oncology resident discovers she is not in her bed and has been transported for a procedure. The resident goes to electrophysiology to determine why she has been transported there. Informed that she had been previously scheduled for the procedure, the resident assumes the attending has simply failed to inform him and he leaves the unit satisfied.

Approximately one hour and 15 minutes after transport, the procedure begins on Morris. Forty minutes later, a second nurse calls from telemetry to inquire why Morrison, the scheduled patient, has not been called to electrophysiology. At approximately the same time, the charge nurse in electrophysiology notices that Morris's name does not match any name on the daily schedule. Neither discovery results in recognition of the misidentification. The telemetry nurse is told to send Morrison to the unit, and the charge nurse's discovery is relayed to and dismissed by the fellow, who was at a demanding part of the procedure.

Approximately one hour after beginning the procedure, an interventional radiology attending goes to check Morris and is told she has been transported to electrophysiology. He follows up with electrophysiology, where the attending maintains that Morris is in fact Morrison. At this point, the charge nurse informs him that Morris is on the table and a review of patient chart bears this out. The procedure is stopped and the patient returned to oncology. The attending subsequently explains the error to the patient and her family.

Data Analysis

Chassin and Becher note that 17 active errors contributed to the misidentification of the patients and surgery on the wrong patient. The timeline, Figure 5.10, is invaluable in understanding the sequence of events as well as the dynamics of the situation.

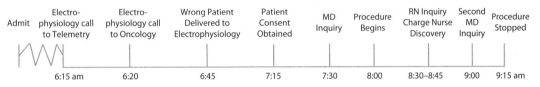

Figure 5.10 Timeline of Events

From Chassin and Becher's chronology of events, it is clear that the initial error occurred when an unknown telemetry staff member mistakenly informed electrophysiology that the scheduled patient had been transferred to oncology when the patient was still on the unit. The initial misidentification began a cascade of errors but was insufficient by itself to result in surgery on the wrong patient. Multiple individuals, including physicians and nurses, failed to correctly identify the patient. Care givers were unreceptive to the patient's objections to the procedure as well as undeterred by the lack of documentation to support the procedure. Multiple warning signs were ignored and a number of individuals had the ability to recognize the patient identification error before the procedure had been in process for more than an hour.

The identification of latent errors shifts gears and examines the features of the system that contributed to the error. Were there systemic reasons why after the initial misidentification subsequent care givers did not recognize that the patient transferred to, prepared for, and undergoing a procedure was not the correct patient? In identifying latent errors, the concern is less with the actions taken or not taken than with why these actions occurred or did not occur. In this case, the actors and actions are known. But if other people had been involved, would the outcome have been different?

Answering this question requires understanding organization practices and the larger health care delivery system. Health care delivery is built on professional sovereignty, clear lines of authority, specialization, and teamwork. The sovereignty and authority of physicians is based on their competence and ability to select the best course of treatment for patients as well as to monitor the quality of care provided. The downside of professional sovereignty, specialization, and authority is that the health care industry has not developed fail-safe communication, monitoring, and accountability systems. The need for teamwork and faith in the ability of others, in this case and other cases, results in an unwillingness to question the actions of other health care providers.

Poor communication was a systemic problem between staff and nurses, nurses and other nurses, nurses and doctors, and doctors and doctors. Although the patients' names were similar, the event progressed without anyone recognizing the difference. A second problem was that much of the communication regarding the patient was transacted without using the patient's name. A third systemic problem was the willingness of staff to proceed without proper documentation. The lack of written orders or informed consent was not seen as a red flag but simply something to be worked around. This speaks to the fact that many organizations have policies, such as documentation requirements, that have little impact on day-to-day processes.

Fourth, once the process was set in motion, there was a reluctance to stop it despite a dearth of information. This may be the result of an unwillingness to fall behind schedule, overconfidence in the abilities of coworkers, or complacency with the process. In many organizations, standard operating procedures rise to such a high level of regard that employees do not want to be seen as upsetting the system instead of focusing on their duty to protect the interests of their patients. Finally, the case shows this institution had no standardized patient identification protocol.

The authors concluded that environmental pressures contributed to the error; that is, reduced staffing, the desire for rapid treatment and discharge, and increasing subspecialization put more emphasis on getting things done and undermined a more deliberative approach to care. The major systemic problems appear to be lack of sensitivity toward patients, poor communication, overconfidence in the abilities of others, and an expectation that system deficiencies were common and should be worked around.

Implementing Corrective Action

After this incident, the organization mandated that multiple patient identifiers be checked prior to care. The emphasis on ensuring the correct identity of the patient (verification) is valuable; care givers should not assume they have the correct patient. Will multiple identifiers correct the problem? The problem was not that two identifiers needed to be checked, but that care givers did not check a single identifier, the patient's name, after the initial misidentification occurred. A second problem is the inability of enforcing this policy. Will hurried professionals check a second identifier when they have verified one? Probably not. Will hurried professionals indicate that they have checked two identifiers for documentation purposes but only review one? Probably.

The second corrective action implemented appears to be more substantial. A policy was promulgated that no transport was to take place without a signed order. This places informational, measurement, and natural safeguards into the system. The informational safeguard is the order, the measurement safeguard is verification of another party, and the natural safeguard is the time (time-out) imposed on action by this requirement.

Multiple-Event Analysis: Patient Falls in VA Facilities

Multiple-event analysis uses a different set of skills than single-event analysis to achieve improvement. Multiple-event analysis incorporates more than a single case and covers an extended time period during which causes as well as the impacts of corrective actions can be evaluated. The Veterans Administration (VA) initiated a multiple-event analysis to gain insight into patient falls and the effectiveness of its prevention activities. The VA collected RCAs from 97 sites, for a total of 176 studies that analyzed 10,701 falls (Mills et al. 2005).

Data Collection

Multiple-event RCAs differ from single-event RCAs in that each site had summarized data from a number of events. In this study, each aggregate RCA studied 63.6 falls on average. This study focused on identifying causes and determining what actions had been taken to reduce the number and severity of falls and the factors that increased or decreased the effectiveness of these interventions.

Data Analysis

Descriptive statistics, including bar charts and frequency tables, were created on the type of root causes (see Table 5.8), action plans implemented to reduce patient falls, and facilitators and barriers to success.

Table 5.8 Root Causes Contributing to Patient Falls

1.	Policies and procedures	44%
2.	Communication problems	23%
3.	Insufficient training	16%
4.	Environmental	13%
5.	Fatigue/scheduling	4%
	Total	100%

Implementing Corrective Action

A total of 745 interventions were suggested, of which 61% were fully implemented and 21% were partially implemented. The recommended actions were divided into three categories: policy changes, 301 (40.4%), clinical changes, 241 (32.4%), and education and training, 202 (27.1%). The number of interventions, however, is not a measure of success, and the authors undertook further work to determine if the number of falls or the injury resulting from falls had decreased. Table 5.9 shows the reported reductions in the number of falls and injuries across facilities studied.

Table 5.9 Outcomes Achieved for Fall Prevention at VA Hospitals

Falls	Percent
Reduced falls	34.4
No change	43.8
Too soon to tell	20.8
Do not record	1.0
Major Injuries	
Reduced injury	38.9
No change	26.3
Too soon to tell	31.6
Do not record	3.2

Given the outcomes, why did 34.4% of facilities report reductions in falls while 64.6% were unable to document reductions in falls? The authors surveyed patient safety managers to determine what factors they believed contributed to reducing the number of falls or their severity. Six factors were noted by more than 50% of managers: persistent follow-up, staff feedback before implementation, leadership and staff support, use of same team to identify causes and implement action, and good tracking systems. Only two barriers to success were noted by more than 50% of the surveyed managers:

not enough time to improve between reporting periods and insufficient resources committed to support change. The authors note that in the VA system multiple-event RCAs are performed every three months, which may explain why 43.8% and 20.8% of reported falls had not been reduced or it was too soon to tell (as well as the similar results for reductions in injuries). The three-month gap between reports may also explain why more than 50% of managers thought not enough time had passed to successfully implement and evaluate action.

This study concludes that direct clinical changes are required to reduce falls and injuries, but that changes in policy and staff education had little impact. Their conclusion highlights the chasm between desired action, clinical change, and implemented action, since the majority of interventions involved policy changes and education. The study illuminates the difficulty that health care providers face in improving care and reducing injury. The VA achieved commendable reductions in the number of falls and injuries. Some may be disheartened by the degree of improvement: falls declined by 34.4% and injuries by 38.9%, hence up to 65% of the time intervention did not reduce the number of falls, and up to 60% of the time injuries were not reduced (pending results from the "too soon to tell" category).

The outcomes remind us that not all adverse events can be prevented. Adverse drug reactions (ADR) provide insight. Initial ADR may not be preventable, but ADR should not reoccur after an allergy has been identified. Likewise, health care facilities cannot restrain every patient, and patient behavior will ensure that falls will not be eliminated.

The VA study focuses our attention on what should and should not be the goal of quality improvement efforts. Effective interventions were environmental assessment, toileting interventions, specific clinical changes, and establishing defined responsibility. There was no association between simple implementation of changes and decreases in injuries or falls. A scattershot approach emphasizing multiple actions may be less effective than an approach that focuses on a limited number of clinical changes. Their research also found an adverse result for employee education; actions that specified staff education were negatively correlated with falls. An approach focusing on training, policy, and management has intuitive appeal and is easy to formulate, but as this study shows, the results may not only be less than desired but may produce the opposite result. Approaches centering on education, policy changes, and managerial oversight will always depend on whether the proposed change addresses the problem and whether it is implemented successfully, neither of which can be assumed.

There is an obvious paradox in efforts to reduce medical error. That is, individuals make errors and will continue to do so, but current thought emphasizes systemic change. While improvement requires system change, we should not be blind to the fact that individuals have slips and make mistakes and are willing to violate promulgated policies and procedures. Evidence is required to determine when individuals should receive training or other action due to the frequency of their errors. Broad-brush approaches that assume everyone requires training will be less than effective if not out-right counterproductive when a specific individual or group of individuals should be targeted for attention. We should not let a misdirected concern for employee sensitivity undermine quality improvement. Credibility and employee support will be increased only if quality improvement programs are focused on root causes. In many cases, this will be the system, but when individuals routinely err, the program must identify these individuals and implement effective corrections to ensure that future patients are not injured. Proposed solutions that ignore obvious problems or have little probability of changing existing clinical practices will not be embraced by employees.

Summary

Root cause analysis is an investigation into an undesirable event or events. In the case of a single event, the investigation often requires asking why the event occurred and comparing the event to other opportunities where the same result could have occurred but did not. When RCA is applied to a group of events, the investigation becomes a data analysis exercise to identify common factors across adverse events. Both types of RCA seek to identify the primary reason or reasons for a system failure.

Finding the primary reason for an undesirable outcome is only the beginning of the improvement process. The more challenging part of the process is to improve the system. Any changes designed to prevent reoccurrence of undesirable outcomes should be reliable and effective; they should consistently produce the desired results. A hierarchy of safeguards based on their reliability and effectiveness and on the level of human effort was presented to challenge the reader to consider both factors when developing safer systems. The nature of the threat will determine whether weak or very strong safeguards are required and what level of human involvement should be applied to the system to reduce or eliminate error.

This chapter dealt with how to analyze an undesirable event retrospectively, that is, after it has occurred. Chapters Six through Eight will introduce the tools necessary to monitor processes on an ongoing basis (statistical process control).

KEY TERMS

Active error

Administrative safeguards

Adverse event

Aggregate root cause analysis

Cognitive error

Consensus

Control group

Deductive approach

Error of commission

Error of omission

Exceptional violation

Experimental group

Five Whys

Heinrich triangle

Hindsight bias

Inductive approach

Information safeguards

Is–Is Not matrix

Lapse

Latent error

Knowledge safeguards

Measurement and inspection
   safeguards

Mistake

Natural safeguards

Near-miss event

No-harm event

Physical safeguards

Root cause analysis

Routine violation

Sabotage

Sentinel event

Slip

Statistical analysis

Swiss cheese model

Technical safeguards

Violation

Why-Why diagram

REVIEW QUESTIONS

1. Explain the insight that the Heinrich triangle provides into the relationship between injury and unsafe practices.

2. Explain the differences among skill-, rule-, and knowledge-based errors.

3. Explain the difference between active and latent error.

4. What is the difference between single-event and multiple-event RCA? Which skills are needed to successfully conduct each?

5. Create a Why-Why diagram analyzing why patients fall (or why they contract postoperative infections, pressure ulcers, or another issue of your choice).

PROBLEMS

1. Administration decides that the focus of the patient falls analysis should be only falls that resulted in injury and time from registration. Using the Data Set of Adverse Events, Chapter05.xls, Figure05–07 tab, prepare a frequency table and column chart using only falls that produced major or minor injury. Would this change in focus alter the direction of the RCA?

2. Using the Data Set of Adverse Events, Chapter05.xls and the Figure05–07 tab, determine if there is any relationship between patient falls and patient age and gender.

3. Prepare an analysis of medication errors using the Data Set of Adverse Events, Chapter05.xls and the Figure05–07 tab, that focuses on location. Prepare a frequency table and column chart showing which locations have the highest rates of medication errors.

4. Prepare an analysis of treatment errors using the Data Set of Adverse Events, Chapter05. xls and the Figure05–07 tab, focusing on the day of the week on which the error occurs. Prepare a frequency table and column chart showing the days with the highest rates of treatment errors.

5. Add the following six cases to the Data Set of Adverse Events, Chapter05.xls and the Figure05–07 tab. Prepare a frequency table and column chart. Does adding these cases alter the frequencies of events?

Date	Patient Age	Gender	Meds	Days after Reg.	Shift	Injury	Event
01/01/13	76	M	Non-narc	2	Day	Major	Med Error
01/03/13	34	F	Narcotic	0	Evening	Minor	Med Error
01/03/13	52	F	Narcotic	0	Evening	No Harm	Infection
01/04/13	40	F	Non-narc	1	Night	No harm	Med Error
01/06/13	71	M	Non-narc	2	Night	Minor	Infection
01/06/13	68	F	Non-narc	0	Day	No Harm	Med Error

References

Bates DW, Pruess K, Souney P, and Platt R, 1995, Serious Falls in Hospitalized Patients: Correlates and Resource Utilization, *American Journal of Medicine* 99 (2): 137–143.

Bates DW, Spell N, Cullen DJ, Burdick E, Laird N, Petersen LA, Small SD, Sweiter BJ, and Leape LL, 1997, The Costs of Adverse Drug Events in Hospitalized Patients, *JAMA* 277 (4): 307–311.

Batty L, Holland-Elliott K, Rosenfeld D, 2003, Investigation of Eye Splash and Needlestick Incidents from an HIV-Positive Donor on an Intensive Care Unit using Root Cause Analysis, *Occupational Medicine* (London) 53 (2): 147–150.

Beckford J, 1998, *Quality: A Critical Introduction*, Routledge, New York, NY.

Carroll JS, Rudolph JW, and Hatakenata, S, 2002, Lessons Learned from Non-Medical Industries: Root Cause Analysis as Culture Change at a Chemical Plant, *Quality and Safety in Health Care* 11, 266–269.

Chassin MR, and Becher EC, 2002, The Wrong Patient, *Annals of Internal Medicine* 136 (11): 826–833.

Decision Systems Inc., 2005, *Reason 6.5 Root Cause Analysis Software*, New York, NY.

Dew JR, 2003, Using Root Cause Analysis to Make the Patient Care System Safe, *ASQ Health Care Division Newsletter*, Spring 2003.

Garnerin P, Schiffer E, Van Gessel E, and Clergue F, 2002, Root-Cause Analysis of an Airway Filter Occlusion: A Way to Improve the Reliability of the Respiratory Circuit, *British Journal of Anaesthesia* 89 (4): 633–635.

Gosbee J, and Anderson T, 2003, Human Factors Engineering Design Demonstrations Can Enlighten your RCA Team, *Quality and Safety in Health Care* 12, 119–121.

Gray JE, Suresh G, Ursprung R, Edwards WH, Nickerson J, Shiono PH, Plsek P, Goldmann DA, and Horbar J, 2006, Patient Misidentification in the Neonatal Intensive Care Unit: Quantification of Risk, *Pediatrics* 117 (1), e43–e47.

Grenier-Sennelier C, Lombard I, Jeny-Loeper C, Maillet-Gouret M-C, and Minvielle E, 2002, Designing Adverse Event Prevention Programs Using Quality Management Methods: The Case of Falls in Hospitals, *International Journal for Quality in Health Care* 14 (5): 419–426.

Heinrich HW, 1959, *Industrial Accident Prevention: A Scientific Approach*, 4th ed., McGraw-Hill, New York, NY.

IOM (Institute of Medicine), 2004, *Patient Safety, Achieving a New Standard for Care*, National Academy Press, Washington, DC.

Joint Commission, 2010, *Comprehensive Accreditation Manual for Hospitals*, Oakbrook Terrace, IL.

Joint Commission, 2013, Sentinel Event Data: Root Causes by Event Type, 2004–2012, http://www.jointcommission.org/assets/1/18/Root_Causes_Event_Type_04_4Q2012.pdf, accessed March 12, 2013.

Kaplan HS and Fastman BR, 2003, Organization of Event Reporting Data for Sense Making and System Improvement, *Quality and Safety in Health Care* 12 Suppl 2, ii68–ii72.

Kepner CH and Tregoe BB, 1965, *The Rational Manager*, McGraw-Hill Book Company, New York, NY.

Knudsen P, Herborg H, Mortensen AR, Knudsen M, and Hellebek A, 2007, Preventing Medication Errors in Community Pharmacy: Root-Cause

Analysis of Transcription Errors, *Quality and Safety in Health Care* 16 (4), 285–290.

MMS (Massachusetts Medical Society), 2001, Case Studies and Root Cause Analysis of Adverse Events, *Workshop Leaders Guide.*

Mills PD, Neily J, Luan D, Stalhandske E, and Weeks WB, 2005, Using Aggregate Root Cause Analysis to Reduce Falls and Related Injuries, *Journal on Quality and Patient Safety* 31 (1): 21–31.

NHS Institute for Innovation and Improvement, *Root Cause Analysis Using Five Whys,* http://www.institute.nhs.uk/creativity_tools/creativity_tools/identifying_problems_-_root_cause_analysis_using5_whys.html, accessed July 8, 2013a.

NHS (National Health Service), *Root Cause Analysis (RCA) Tools: Analysing to Identify Contributory Factors and Root Causes,* http://www.nrls.npsa.nhs.uk/resources/?entryid45=75605, accessed July 8, 2013b.

Nicholson RJ, *USA Today,* July 31, 2006.

Perkins JD, Levy AE, Duncan JB, and Carithers RL, 2005, Using Root Cause Analysis to Improve Survival in a Liver Transplant Program, *Journal of Surgical Research* 129, 6–16.

Reason JT, 1990, *Human Error,* Cambridge University Press, New York, NY.

Ricci M, Goldman AP, de Leval MR, Cohen GA, Devaney F, and Carthey J, 2004, Pitfalls of Adverse Event Reporting in Pediatric Cardiac Intensive Care, *Archives of Disease in Childhood* 89, 856–859.

Rooney JJ and Vanden Heuvel LN, 2004, Root Cause Analysis for Beginners, *Quality Progress* 37 (7): 45–53.

Schwendimann R, Milisen K, Bühler H, and De Geest S, 2006, Fall Prevention in a Swiss Acute Care Hospital Setting: Reducing Multiple Falls, *Journal of Gerontological Nursing* 32 (3): 13–22.

Shojania KG, Duncan BW, McDonald KM, and Wachter RM, 2001, *Making Health Care Safer: A Critical Analysis of Patient Safety Practices, Evidence Report/Technology Assessment,* No. 43, Agency for Healthcare Research and Quality, Rockville MD.

Statistical Abstract of the United States, 2000, http://www.census.gov/compendia/statab/.

Van Vuuren W, Shea C, and van der Schaaf, 1997, The Development of an Incident Analysis Tool for the Medical Field, Eindhoven University of Technology, The Netherlands, http://alexandria.tue.nl/repository/books/493452.pdf, accessed December 18, 2012.

WHO (World Health Organization), Surgical Safety Checklist, http://www.who.int/patientsafety/safesurgery/tools_resources/SSSL_Checklist_finalJun08.pdf, accessed December 19, 2012.

Vincent C, Adams S, Chapman J, Hewett D, Prior S, Strange P, and Tizzard A, 1999, A Protocol for the Investigation and Analysis of Clinical Incidents, Department of Psychology, University College London and ALARM (Association of Litigation and Risk Management), London, UK.

CHAPTER 6

STATISTICAL PROCESS CONTROL FOR MONITORING SYSTEM PERFORMANCE

Introduction

Root cause analysis (RCA) is a major feature of current quality control efforts given that the Joint Commission requires accredited health care organizations to conduct such an analysis on systems and processes when a sentinel event occurs. RCA is a comprehensive examination of an adverse event with the goal of reducing harm to patients by preventing the reoccurrence of the event. RCA, however, is limited by the fact that it does not focus on the everyday operation of systems and that it is sometimes carried out on only a single event. RCA is often concerned with discovering the cause of a specific event and is less focused on identifying systemic weaknesses. If a system weakness had no effect on an event being investigated, it might not be explored or corrected. In contrast, statistical process control (SPC) is less concerned with single events and concentrates on the day-to-day operation of a system.

To improve a system we must first understand its operation. If we do not know how a system operates, we cannot predict how a modification will affect a system, let alone hope that it will improve performance. While Chapters Four and Five demonstrated how to assess performance, Chapters Six through Eight ask what we can expect a system to produce. The two main issues are what range of output is produced, and does the output meet expectations?

SPC monitors the regular operation of a system by examining multiple events to determine if a process is consistently producing output that satisfies customers or that meets technical standards (or both). In health care, SPC

LEARNING OBJECTIVES

1. Understand when systems should be modified or corrected

2. Review the statistical concepts underlying statistical process control

3. Recognize the difference between natural and special cause variation

4. Understand how performance targets are established

5. Construct and interpret control charts for system performance

6. Avoid tinkering with stable systems

can be used to determine if the health care delivery system will produce safe and effective patient outcomes. Rather than concentrating on one event, SPC examines multiple events and uses averages to determine the attributes of a process or its outcome. The difference between SPC and multiple-event RCA is that RCA is always a retrospective examination of problems whereas SPC can be a real-time or prospective tool for proactive quality improvement. That is, in addition to identifying problems, it can be employed to prevent problems and errors from occurring. While success in an RCA may be the discovery of a single event that produced a problem, success in SPC requires continuous monitoring of the system to ensure it is operating as expected and is not heading toward a problem. SPC can identify changes from past performance that may not currently affect patient care but that could negatively impact future outcomes if the trend continues.

Similarly, SPC can monitor the outcomes to determine if a process is meeting expectations; that is, does a high mortality rate or long average length of stay (ALOS) indicate a troubled health care delivery system? With regular monitoring, deviations from desired performance can be identified and corrected before the system produces a defective or unsafe outcome.

In arguing for a broader approach than RCA, researchers have noted that "when multiple sources of variation are present, isolated observations provide insufficient information on which to base objective decision making" (Wadsworth, Stephens, and Godfrey 1986, 4–12). Health care managers are faced with multiple sources of variation, including the patient, the patient care team, treatment methods, supplies, equipment, and environmental factors. The recognition that multiple factors are always present propelled the shift of quality management from narrow, blame-placing efforts toward strengthening systems. While an organization may be able to pinpoint the source of an error, its goal should be to quickly identify and correct the problem and rebuild the production process to reduce the probability of errors reoccurring. SPC is a tool to broaden the organization's perspective toward monitoring a system rather than responding to specific errors. As SPC is examined in these chapters, the reader will see that it does not focus on specific persons or events but tracks the performance of processes that are the result of the interaction of multiple persons and tasks.

The first question that must be asked is: Is performance acceptable or as good as it can be? If the question is answered affirmatively on either score, the organization and its employees may do nothing more than to continue monitoring system performance. When performance is neither acceptable nor as good as it could be, employees need to assess their work to determine how to improve performance.

Why Don't Systems Produce the Expected Output?

Every time an error occurs, a system has produced an output other than the one it was expected to produce. Why don't systems produce the expected output? This question can be answered broadly: either the people operating the system don't know how the process should work (lack of design) or they don't know how the system is actually working (lack of oversight and control). If a good or service is not adequately designed (what attributes should the desired product have?), or the system created to produce the product is not adequately planned (what should take place and when it should occur?) it is likely that the outcome produced will be different than the one envisioned by the producer and expected by the consumer.

Even if adequate planning of the final product and the production system has taken place, the output may still fail to meet its design specifications or satisfy its consumers. The second requirement to ensure that a system is operating at its capacity is to monitor it in action. Well-planned systems can fail to produce what they are capable of producing if good procedures are poorly executed, if there are inadequate preventive measures to guard against degraded performance, or if there is an inability to recognize or correct errors when they arise. A large part of the challenge in monitoring a system and initiating corrective action is determining when a system requires change. **Tinkering** with a system that is functioning correctly can be as bad as failing to correct a poorly operating system. Change is a constant in all systems, so the challenge in quality management is detecting when systems need correction and when a system is operating within acceptable limits.

Tinkering
unwarranted modification to a stable system

When Is Corrective Action Required?

Think about the human body as a system. Its normal temperature is 98.6°, but how far away from 98.6° will we permit a person's temperature to move before we take her to the doctor or hospital? Science tell us that human temperature fluctuates in a given day by 0.5°, reaching a low point approximately two hours before we wake and hitting its daily high between 4:00 and 6:00 PM. We know that how and where we take a temperature affects the reading, oral temperature being lower than temperature taken in other body cavities. We also know that temperature varies by individual and is affected by outside, environmental factors. Based on normal fluctuations, minor deviations in temperature are nothing to be concerned about, but how high (or low) should we allow temperature to go before corrective action is initiated?

We need to know the point at which we move from no concern to recognizing when a person may be entering into trouble. Hyperthermia occurs at 105.1° and requires immediate attention, but at this point the damage has been done. What we need to know is the range in which nothing needs to done and the threshold at which we should alter behavior before hyperthermia is reached and outside assistance is needed. If we can recognize when our temperature is moving into a dangerous range we can take corrective action. Assume you are working outside on a hot day; as long as your temperature remains below 101° you may choose not to alter your behavior. Once your temperature tops 101° you may choose to relax in an air conditioned room and drink water. If your temperature tops 102° this may signal the end of outdoor physical activity for the day. Above 102° active cooling activities, such as immersion in a bath, should be undertaken to reduce body temperature and avoid the need for more dramatic intervention.

Figure 6.1 describes the potential states of a system and operator response. Monitoring is essential. First we must know the condition of the system, for example, what the temperature is. Second, we must decide what should be done based on the state of the system. If temperature exceeds 101.0°, what actions should be taken to lower the temperature or return the system to a safe operating range? Monitoring and making effective adjustments in response to changes in system performance minimizes problems and avoids costly corrective action.

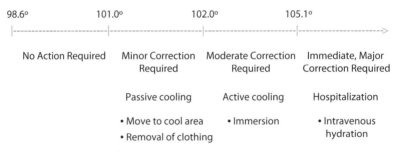

Figure 6.1 Temperature and Response

Statistics Review

continuous data
measures events that can assume any value

discrete data
records events that can only assume a finite number of values

The events to be monitored and how they are measured determine what type of analysis can be performed. There are two basic types of data: continuous and discrete. **Continuous data** encompasses events that can assume any value; these events can be measured on a continuous scale. Examples of continuous data include temperature, weight, time, and distance. **Discrete data** is characterized by gaps in the values that can occur. Discrete data is further broken into two groups: categorical data and count data. **Categorical data** describes events that either do or do not meet a standard. Examples of categorical events are a live birth or a stillbirth, a positive or negative test, an error or nonerror, or performance that meets or does not meet a standard. **Count data** describes the number of occurrences, for example, the number of errors in a medical record, the number of patient falls, or the number of arrivals at an emergency room. Unlike continuous data, counts cannot be measured in fractions, and unlike categorical data, count data can measure more than one occurrence. Half of a patient fall or one-third of a postoperative infection does not constitute a data point, but more than one of these events for a patient can be recorded.

categorical data
divides events into groups

count data
records the number of occurrences of an event

Continuous and discrete data describe different aspects of system performance. Variables that can be measured on a continuous scale record how a system is operating. Continuous variables are vital when excess or deficiency can adversely affect outcomes. Discrete data records either something that was done or whether an event occurred (categorical) or how many events occurred (count). Categorical data can be used to describe a process when the primary concern is to ascertain whether treatment rendered (rather than how it was rendered) or to describe an outcome, for example, whether a treatment was successful or whether a patient lived. The prime goal of categorical variables is to record the existence or absence of an attribute. Counts are concerned with the number of events that arise and are used when multiple occurrences can arise in a single case. Unlike categorical data, which might track whether a patient contracted a single type of infection, counts record how many infections a patient contracted. Chapters Seven and Eight examine how SPC monitors categorical events and counts.

There are three types of statistics: descriptive, inferential, and test statistics. SPC is built on **inferential statistics**, that is, drawing conclusions on a large body of data from looking at a subset, a sample. In statistics, *population* refers to the universe of all events or observations; but it is often prohibitively expensive and time consuming to examine each event to understand the characteristics of all events. Inferential statistics is based on making decisions about a large group by examining a subset of the group. In most cases when larger samples are drawn, the subset yields more accurate information on the characteristics or performance of the population. However, greater accuracy must be weighed against the higher cost of acquiring larger samples.

inferential statistics
the use of statistics to draw a conclusion on a large body of events by examining a small group of events

Assume that you want to determine the effectiveness of blood sugar management in a group of 100 patients. A sample of five patients would provide the average blood sugar level in the subgroup and allow us to infer if the larger group is well or poorly managed. A sample of ten would generally provide a better estimate of the blood sugar level in the larger group as it is less likely to be skewed by drawing a disproportionate share of patients

descriptive statistics
the use of statistics to summarize or describe a set of events

mean
a measure of central tendency that totals the sum of all observations and divides it by number of observations to determine the group average

standard deviation
a measure of dispersion that calculates how far each observation lies from the group mean

with high or low blood sugar levels. When small samples are used to study a population, larger fluctuations in performance are accepted before we conclude that a system is unstable and needs examination and potential correction. When larger samples are drawn, the range of acceptable variation is reduced. The greater accuracy of larger samples reduces tolerance, and less variation is accepted before investigation is initiated.

Calculating **descriptive statistics** is a means of converting data into information. The two primary descriptive statistics are the **mean** and **standard deviation**; these two statistics provide great insight into the underlying characteristics of a group of events. The mean, also known as the average, is a measure of central tendency and tells us the most likely result from a set of data. In SPC, the mean is used to determine if performance meets the desired standard; that is, does the average output of a system meet a target or goal?

The mean for a sample is calculated as:

6.1

$$\overline{X} = \sum x_i/n$$

The mean ($\overline{X}$) equals the sum (Σ) of the sampled observations (x_i) divided by the sample size (the number of observations in the sample) (n). If Excel is used to record data, the mean can be found by entering **=AVERAGE(range of observations)**.

Say you draw a sample of ten babies from all the babies delivered at a particular hospital in a given month and want to know if the babies are underweight. You would add up the weights of the ten babies and divide by ten to determine their "average" weight and compare this number against the threshold defining low birth weight. The average birth weight in the United States is approximately 3,175 grams (7 pounds). It is unlikely that your sample will equal the expected target, but SPC is not concerned with an exact match. Rather, it asks, is the difference between the sample and the target too large? We want to know if your sample of ten indicates that the babies born at the hospital are severely underweight or overweight and whether they might thus face greater health challenges than normal weight babies. The March of Dimes considers babies under 2,500 grams (5 pounds, 8 ounces) to be low birth weight. Thus we want to know how far away from the target the sample average is and whether we should be concerned with the difference. As long as a sample average did not fall more than 675 grams (1 pound, 8 ounces) below the average U.S. birth weight, we would conclude that the sample is normal. The question statistics seeks to answer is: When does a difference make a difference? How far away from an expected value will we permit a sample to be before we anticipate problems?

Using the mean to describe a set of data ignores the variation in the data. To fully understand a phenomenon, the standard deviation must be calculated. If five babies weigh 2,400 grams each and the other five weigh 3,000 grams each, the average is 2,700 grams. It thus appears that the average baby weighs more than 2,500 grams (the amount that defines low birth weight) despite the fact that 50% of the babies are below the recognized low birth weight threshold. A high standard deviation means that a large number of observations are far from the mean, and it reduces our ability to accurately predict performance. Standard deviation is the commonly used measure to determine how much variance there is in data or how far away from the mean we expect events or observations to occur.

Standard deviation for a sample is calculated as:

$$s = \sum \sqrt{(x_i - \overline{X})^2 / n - 1}$$

6.2

Standard deviation (s) is the square root of the squared sum of the differences between the sampled observations (x_i) and the mean ($\overline{X}$) divided by sample size minus 1. If Excel is used to record data, the standard deviation can be found by entering **=STDEV (range of observations)**.

When 50% of babies weigh 2,400 grams and the remaining five weigh 3,000 grams, the standard deviation is 316.23 (square root (5 × *(2,400 − 2,700)^2 + 5 × *(3,000 − 2,700)^2 ÷ 9). The "5" preceding the difference between x_i and $\overline{X}$ accounts for the five observations above and the five observations below the mean.

To determine when we should be concerned that baby weights are too low, we use the normal distribution. Statistics tells us that 50% of all events are above the mean and 50% are below. While this observation is not terribly enlightening, when we add the standard deviation to the normal distribution we get a good picture of average performance and how far away from the mean we can expect performance to fall. Within one standard deviation of the mean we should observe 68.3% of all activity. In the above example, we would expect 68.3% of babies to fall between 2,384 and 3,016 grams (2700 ± 316). The lower limit of 2,384 grams indicates that a substantial number of babies may weigh less than the low birth weight threshold of 2,500 grams (since approximately 16% will occur under 2,384, one standard deviation below the mean) and that action to increase baby weights may be warranted. Knowing that 2,500 grams defines low birth weight, we can calculate the percentage of this population that may fall under 2,500 grams given a mean of 2,700 and standard deviation of 316.

The Excel formula is = **NORMDIST (x, mean, standard deviation, cumulative)** where x is the value to evaluate (what percentage of the sample will fall below this value) and *cumulative* indicates whether the user wishes to see everything below this value (cumulative = 1) or the percentage of the sample at this point (cumulative = 0).

Entering **=NORMDIST(2500,2700,316,1)** returns 26.3%, so despite the fact that the mean exceeds the low birth weight threshold, the standard deviation predicts that more than one out of four babies will have birth weights under 2,500 grams. There are two possible indicators of trouble in this example: a mean under 2,500 grams (not present) or a large standard deviation (present).

Figure 6.2 displays the normal distribution and highlights the 68.3% of observations that fall between plus one and minus one standard deviations from the mean. Within two standard deviations we expect to observe 95.5% of all observations and between three standard deviations 99.7%. SPC relies on the normal distribution to determine expected performance and identify unexpected events that require investigation. For example, beyond two standard deviations 4.5% of activity is expected to occur, while at three standard deviations only 0.3% of activity is expected to be observed.

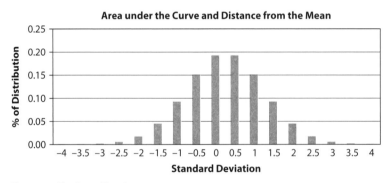

Figure 6.2 The Normal Distribution

upper control limit

the maximum possible value for a sample before investigation is initiated to determine if a system is stable

lower control limit

the minimum possible value for a sample before investigation is initiated to determine if a system is stable

SPC typically uses three standard deviations to establish control limits, that is, the maximum or minimum thresholds (the **upper control limits** and **lower control limits**) that, when exceeded by a process or an output, warrant investigation. Keep in mind that SPC uses an average versus a single event to determine if a system exhibits sufficient change to warrant investigation. The goal of the investigation is to determine if the system is operating up to the desired performance or if performance has deteriorated to the point at which the quality may be adversely affected. Based on the normal distribution, a normally operating system will produce a sample statistic outside three standard deviations approximately three times in every 1,000 opportunities ($p = 0.003$). This level of variation from average is deemed sufficient to warrant investigation. Conversely, a poorly functioning system producing low-quality outputs would frequently be expected to produce a sample statistic outside three standard deviations.

Some quality analysts establish control limits at two standard deviations as an early warning system, but the trade-off is that a normally functioning system will breach these levels approximately one time for every twenty samples drawn ($p = 0.045$). These tighter limits provide faster recognition of a deteriorating system but are also more likely to trigger unnecessary investigation and possibly undesirable intervention in the systems operation.

Inferential statistics is designed to draw conclusions about a population by examining a small portion of the group. Statistics, unfortunately, can also lead us to the wrong conclusion. A system is either working properly or it is not, and the statistic drawn from the sample will lead us to conclude that the system is operating properly or not. The problem is that the signal obtained from a sample may not correspond with the actual performance of the system. Table 6.1 displays the four situations that can arise.

Table 6.1 Statistical Inference and System State

	SYSTEM STATE/PERFORMANCE	
Sample Statistic Indicates	**Operating within Standard**	**Operating outside Standard**
Stable/In-control <continue>	Correct, system should not altered	Incorrect, should fix system but no action taken Type II error
Unstable/Out-of-control <fix>	Incorrect, fix undertaken when not required Type I error	Correct, system requires fix and action taken

Table 6.1 illustrates that we want to be operating in cells one or four, where the sample statistics lead us to make a correct inference about the state of the system and take correct action when needed. In cell one, the system is operating up to standard; the system should be allowed to run and any change could lower performance. On the other hand, when the system is not meeting standards (cells two and four) changes should be made to move the system toward the desired level of performance (cell four).

If a nonrepresentative (or bad) sample is drawn, it may lead to the wrong conclusion. In cell two, the sample statistic falls within the upper and lower control limits, indicating the system is performing properly when it is not, a type II error. The problem is, based on the sample we will let the system run without change when changes are needed to improve performance. In cell three, the sample statistic falls outside the control limits indicating the system is not operating properly when in fact it is, a type I error. In cell three the problem is that time will be spent investigating and fixing a system that does not need adjustment and if a change is made there is a possibility that it will not improve the system but rather reduce performance.

The SPC conclusions parallel the decisions a jury can reach in the criminal justice system. A defendant is either innocent or guilty, and the jury can find the defendant guilty or not guilty. Problems arise when a jury finds the innocent to be guilty or when the guilty are set free, as illustrated in Table 6.2.

Table 6.2 Jury Verdict and Innocence or Guilt

Jury Decision	Innocent	Guilty
Not guilty	Correct, innocent goes free	Criminal goes free
\<freed\>		Type II error
Guilty	Innocent is imprisoned	Correct, criminal is imprisoned
\<incarcerated\>	Type I error	

type I error
rejecting the null hypothesis, the assumption that the system is operating within standards, when it is true

type II error
accepting the null hypothesis when it is false

natural variation
the ever-present factors in a process that produce deviation in performance

special cause variation
the emergence of new factors in a process that cause performance to deviate beyond previously observed limits

common cause variation
see *natural variation*

inherent variation
see *natural variation*

The goal of the judicial system is to arrive at the correct decisions, freeing the innocent and imprisoning the guilty. The American legal system attempts to limit the number of innocent imprisoned (a **type I error**), by requiring a unanimous guilty verdict from twelve jurors. Similarly, SPC wishes to avoid fixing systems that are not broken and generally relies on a three standard deviation threshold to initiate action. A properly functioning system will only be investigated (type I error) 0.3% of the time. Reducing the probability of type 1 error, requiring unanimity of a jury or using more than a three standard deviations threshold, increases the probability of releasing a criminal or failing to detect a broken system (a **type II error**). The U.S. criminal justice system operates on the principle that it is better to let ten criminals go free (type II error) than to falsely imprison one innocent person (type I error). Quality management operates on the same premise: it is better to let a system run poorly than to stop a properly functioning system. Harrison states "the fact that it is usually more expensive to look for problems that do not exist than to miss some small problems is the reason that the $\pm 3\sigma$ limits are usually chosen" (Juran and Godfrey 1999).

Types of Variation

Walter Shewhart was instrumental in developing SPC and identifying **natural variation** and **special cause variation**. Natural variation (also called **common cause variation** or **inherent variation**) recognizes that output and performance will fluctuate due to phenomena that are always active in a system. Human beings, machines, and systems will not always produce the same outputs due to time of day, day of week, temperature, lighting and other factors. It is unreasonable to expect any process to produce identical output over any period of time, so we need to establish a range of acceptable variation. Natural variation accounts for changes in output due to things we cannot control or do not want to control.

Natural variation is predictable on a probabilistic basis. Based on its history, we know the range of outcomes a system has produced. The question is, what constitutes excessive variation? One can think of natural variation as the probability of obtaining a head in a coin toss. The outcome is a product of chance. The probability of tossing a head (H) or a tail (T) is 50%, but probability does not mean we will observe H, T, H, and T in a series of four tosses. The probability of obtaining H, T, H, T is the same as tossing four heads in a row, 6.25%. When examining a production system we expect performance to fall within a range set by historical experience. When only natural variation is occurring, we say the system is **stable** or **in-control**; however, this may not mean performance is acceptable. A system could be consistently producing poor-quality outputs with little difference between current and historical performance.

Special cause variation (also called **assignable variation** or **noninherent variation**) signals the emergence of new phenomena in a system. Special cause variation is inherently unpredictable. One can think of this type of variation as attempting to predict when a breakthrough on a disease or process innovation will occur. Special cause variation moves the system beyond historical experience and could indicate either improved or poorer quality. For example, when a new employee is hired, the person could have comparable skills to current employees and the level of quality will be consistent with historical performance, or the employee could have higher (or lower) skills and quality will improve (or fall).

SPC typically identifies performance beyond three standard deviations from the mean as indicating the potential emergence of special cause variation (or nonnormal operation). Based on the normal distribution, normally operating processes have an extremely low probability of producing outputs in this range. When outputs are observed more than three standard deviations from the mean, we assume the system has changed enough to warrant investigation and possibly require correction. We cannot assume that correction is actually required, because normally operating systems will produce outputs outside three standard deviations three times in every 1,000 opportunities. SPC thus establishes the threshold on how far from historical performance a sample average can fall before investigation is required.

stable
systems where performance falls within a range set by historical experience

in-control
see *stable*

assignable variation
see *special cause variation*

noninherent variation
see *special cause variation*

When special cause variation arises, workers should be capable of identifying the factor responsible for the change (for example, new employees, impaired employees, mismatch between workload and resources available to complete work, new system or change in procedure). It is the job of management to be cognizant of system changes, able to distinguish when correction is required, and able to implement timely and effective correction when necessary.

unstable
a system where performance falls outside a range set by historical experience

out-of-control
see *unstable*

A process that is operating with only normal variation is called stable or in-control. Processes that are affected by both normal and special cause variation are described as being **unstable** or **out-of-control**. An important point to remember is that in an unstable process it is impossible to predict what future output will be. In this book the term *stable* is used to describe normally operating systems, because describing a system as *in-control* can be misinterpreted as good or acceptable performance. Similarly, Shewhart described a stable system as "controlled within limits," which does not imply acceptable performance ([1931] 1980, 25).

Setting Performance Targets

Systems can be stable without meeting generally accepted standards or satisfying patients. The idea of what is acceptable, or what the goal of the organization should be, can arise from three sources: the consumer, the industry, or the organization. When *consumer expectations* are used to establish performance goals, the organization is simply asking what failure rate is acceptable to their customers. This type of information can be gathered through surveys. In health care, the use of patient expectations may be problematic as patients may not understand controllable and noncontrollable risks, or they may be unwilling to accept any failure. Malpractice experience shows that more cases are filed based on poor outcomes than medical negligence. Acceptable performance in health care is typically determined by providers because of their greater familiarity with medical science.

There are two types of *industry information* that can be used to establish performance targets. The first is best practice: What level of performance is achieved by the outstanding performer in the industry? While many people hold that every organization should aspire to match the performance of the top performer, this often is not achievable given the combination of human and other resources that may be required to reach the highest level of performance.

The most relevant target may be the performance of organizations in head-to-head competition with the organization, a local standard. Unlike the best practice standard, the immediate goal of the organization should be to be the best in their market. Competitor performance information is closely guarded and may not be obtainable since it could provide a competitive advantage to the top performer in a market. A second problem with industry information is different organizations may measure phenomena differently. For example, one hospital might record every patient fall while others record only the falls that result in injury. When different organizations measure the same phenomena differently, it results in an invalid apples-to-oranges comparison and could produce inaccurate conclusions of performance.

Establishing performance goals based on the *organization* involves examining past history and using prior performance as a standard. The advantages of historical data are that the organization can readily obtain the information, and what it measures should be understood by staff. Historical performance is the default standard when customer expectations, local standards, or best-in-class is not known. When using historical information, the organization can determine if its performance is improving, deteriorating, or constant across time. Regardless of what target is adopted, the goal of every organization should be continuous improvement, exceeding their past performance.

Table 6.3 highlights the two essential operating characteristics of a process: Does the average output from the system satisfy established standards, meet customer expectations, or match historical performance, and is it stable?

Table 6.3 Expected Performance and Variation

	Stable	Unstable
Average performance meets expected standard	Goal: No Defects	Occasional Defects
	Consistently good performance	Occasionally bad performance
Average performance does not meet expected standard	Worst Case: All Defects Consistently bad performance	Frequent Defects
		Occasionally good performance

For example, if we are monitoring in-hospital bariatric mortality rates and have a target of 0.5% or less, our sample average is either less than or equal to this standard (good) or above it (bad). While the average may be better or worse than our target, SPC is also concerned with the consistency of performance. If the process is stable, it will consistently perform around its historical level. When it is unstable, history cannot predict future performance. In Table 6.3, the best possible situation (cell 1) is that mortality rates are stable and less than or equal to 0.5%. The next best case (cell 2) is that average performance is at or less than 0.5% but the system is unstable because there are samples where the mortality rate has exceeded 0.5%. The third best situation (cell 4) is that average performance is greater than 0.5%, but the system is unstable so there are periods when the mortality rate drops below 0.5%. The worst case (cell 3) is when the mortality rate is stable and consistently higher than the desired rate.

Table 6.3 highlights the need for organizations to improve their performance if it is below target or unstable (cells 2, 3, or 4). If a process is consistently producing outputs that meet expectations, the system should be allowed to run. Changes to stable systems that are meeting targets can disrupt performance rather than improve it. In cell 2 the problem is that the process occasionally produces unacceptable outputs. When unacceptable samples are identified, managers need to identify when they arose and the factors present that may have reduced performance. In cell 2 we would expect that the periods of unacceptable performance would be limited, as average output meets expectations.

Conventional wisdom would identify the worst situation as poor and inconsistent performance (cell 4). Poor and inconsistent performance may be the most difficult situation to remedy because two problems are apparent: not only does the system regularly fail to meet targets but it is impossible to predict when it will and will not fail. Poor and inconsistent performance may arise from the same cause. For example, it may involve a single employee; when that employee works, the output is less than expected and variability increases. If a single cause is responsible, fixing the situation may be easier than remedying consistently poor performance. When there are times a process works as expected, these periods can be used as a benchmark to contrast against the times when the process does not meet expectations. While average performance may be poor, the question is: What is occurring in the periods when acceptable output is produced? If employees can identify when the process works and when it does not work—a situation appropriate for the use of an Is–Is Not Matrix—they may be halfway to establishing consistently good performance.

The worst position is cell 3, consistently poor performance; the system never meets expectations, and SPC cannot identify a starting point for investigation. Workers will be unable to identify any internal reference point when the process was meeting expectations to start an investigation. The manager may want to seek external information on systems that meet expectations as a starting point for redesigning the entire process. When a system is unstable (cells 2 and 4), SPC will highlight the periods when problems occur, making it easier to identify the factors affecting production at that point of time. When every period is bad and even the "best" performance fails to meet expectations, employees will have to start from scratch to improve the system.

Statistical Process Control for Continuous Data: $\bar{X}$ and R Charts

SPC is a tool that defines how performance is measured, what quality is, and when investigation and possibly correction should occur. SPC, once understood, empowers the doctor, nurse, department manager, and other health care workers to enter into the quality management process on a more equal basis with those trained in quality management techniques.

The three major difficulties in advancing health care quality are the lack of specificity in defining health care processes and outcomes, establishing performance standards, and measuring compliance with standards after they are defined. Attempts to improve processes and outcomes are difficult, if not impossible, when standards and measures are ill-defined or absent. Efforts to define medical processes continue to be hotly debated. Opponents argue that there is too much variation in medical practice (often arising from differences in the conditions of patients) to establish one way of treating patients and that dictating to physicians will not improve patient care and may hurt patients. On the other hand, myriad research has been done to define proper medical practice; much of this work is amendable to and should be tracked using SPC to improve health care outcomes. For example, McGlynn et al. (2003) reported that patients received 54.9% of recommended care, and the treatment standards they document could easily be tracked using SPC.

Other industries recognize that poor performance is the result of variation; that is, deviations from proper procedures adversely impact outcomes. Controlling variation is the key to process improvement. Health care providers are arguably saddled with more sources of variation than producers of other goods and services, but the issue remains: Is there too much variation in treatment, and will a more systematic approach to health care delivery improve outcomes? SPC is a tool that health care workers can use to determine when variation is a routine part of patient care, necessary and beneficial for patients and the health care system, and when variation is excessive and potentially harmful. Armed with this information, it is the duty of providers to reduce inappropriate variation.

SPC is a broader approach than RCA in that it continuously examines processes to identify undesirable trends in performance and initiate corrective action before harm arises. The Joint Commission (2001, LD.5.2) recognizes that sentinel event analysis is reactive and does not fully meet the intent of its patient safety standards. SPC supplements RCA by adding continuous monitoring of performance to providers' quality toolbox, enabling them to identify changes in system performance before problems arise.

The goal of SPC, as envisioned by Shewhart, is to determine when a system is unstable and requires adjustment to improve its performance. A stable system simply indicates it is operating close to its historical performance; stability does not guarantee the system is meeting generally accepted standards or customer expectations. An unstable system indicates that performance is significantly different from historical performance; this deviation could signify either better or worse outcomes. The goal of SPC is to identify when performance deviates sufficiently to endanger quality, and given this information, workers should take the necessary steps to improve performance and outcomes.

Shewhart's second goal was to devise a quality monitoring and improvement system that could be operated effectively by workers whose expertise lies in areas other than statistics. An effective monitoring and control system requires clear signals to indicate when system performance fluctuates too much and must be easy to use. Shewhart created SPC in a manufacturing environment for those trained in engineering, and it is also applicable to service industries and those trained in medical sciences. The SPC process can be described and completed in six steps, as show in Table 6.4.

Table 6.4 The Six Steps of Statistical Process Control

1.	Collect data
2.	Calculate descriptive statistics
3.	Calculate control limits
4.	Graph actual and expected performance
5.	Interpret performance
6.	Investigate instability and improve as needed

SPC can be used to monitor the behavior of any system that produces outputs that can be measured numerically. This chapter focuses on output characteristics measured on a continuous scale, while Chapter Seven examines categorical data, such as the percent of defects in a sample, and Chapter Eight tackles count data, the number of defects in a sample.

Step 1: Data Collection

SPC requires employees to routinely collect simple performance measures to monitor quality. For continuous data, this could include charges, costs, LOS, time to start or complete a procedure, dose strength, range of motion, and other performance measures. Data collection is the most time-consuming part of the SPC process (once the control limit calculation and graphing is understood). The health care worker wanting to assess performance using SPC must determine the desired sample size, the frequency with which samples are to be drawn, the procedures for ensuring that the samples are random, and the personnel responsible for data collection. Juran and Godfrey (1999) note that sample sizes typically are between four and five observations for variables.

The data users must realize that they face a trade-off between the cost of collecting data (sample size and sampling frequency) and the accuracy of information obtained from the collected data. Larger samples typically produce more accurate information but are more costly and time consuming to collect. The events sampled must be randomly drawn to ensure that the sample is not biased. Information gained from the sample must be representative of the larger population for it to accurately reflect the characteristics or performance of the unsampled phenomena. The procedures and responsibility for data collection should ensure that the data collector has no incentive to collect either favorable or unfavorable performance. After the data is collected, it should be recorded in a spreadsheet or database.

Step 2: Calculation of Descriptive Statistics

After the data is recorded, descriptive statistics are calculated. Descriptive statistics provide the information necessary to understand how the system is operating.

The two primary statistics are the mean (the measure of central tendency) and the standard deviation (the measure of variation). For example, if the effectiveness of medication administration is the target for quality improvement, the mean can be used to determine if patients received the specified dose—a larger or smaller dosage may be a problem. Likewise, science and common sense dictate that medicine is most effective when delivered at the appropriate time; medicines delivered too early or too late may not serve the purpose for which they were prescribed.

Rather than using standard deviation to measure variation, the second statistic often is the range (R). Range is easier to calculate as it is the highest value in the sample minus the lowest value. Range is also easier to understand than standard deviation. Excel can calculate the range in a series of numbers by identifying the highest and lowest values and subtracting the minimum from the maximum. The range calculation can be performed in Excel by entering the following command:

= MAX(range of observations) − MIN(range of observations)

The importance of understanding mean and range can be demonstrated with an example of a prescribed dose of a pain medication: 325 mg, four times a day. Patients and their doctors prefer the dose and timing be strictly adhered to; if the average administered dose is 250 mg, the patient may be in unnecessary pain. If the average dose is 400 mg, withdrawal difficulties could develop. However, a process that produces an average dose of 325 mg may nevertheless fail to achieve the efficacy of the medication.

Given inherent variation, it is unlikely that each dose will be exactly 325 mg; some will be more and others less. A process that delivers 50% percent of medication at 320 mg and the remaining 50% at 330 mg is preferred to one that dispenses two doses of 500 mg and two doses of 150 mg. The average dosage, $\overline{X}$ (Xbar), is the same 325 mg—(320 + 320 + 330 + 330) ÷ 4 and (500 + 500 + 150 + 150) ÷ 4—but the first process has a 10 mg range (330 − 320 mg) while the second has a 350 mg range (500 − 150 mg). The problem is the lack of predictability in the second process. The medication was prescribed to provide continual relief to the patient, and double doses at one scheduled administration and skipping the next dose does not provide the treatment of four even doses. Processes with the narrowest range of performance are generally superior.

Table 6.5 demonstrates that medication delivery regime A fully meets the prescribed physician order; the patient receives the prescribed dosage at the prescribed time (mean = 325; range = 0). Regime B fails to deliver the recommended dosage but provides the same amount of medication at each prescribed time (mean = 250; range = 0). Under regime B the patient may experience a continual low level of discomfort due to the lower-than-prescribed dose.

Table 6.5 The Importance of Calculating the Mean *and* the Range

	A	B	C	D
Dose 1	325	250	650	725
Dose 2	325	250	0	75
Dose 3	325	250	650	725
Dose 4	325	250	0	75
Mean	325	250	325	400
Range	0	0	650	650

Regime C delivers the total daily recommended dosage but fails to deliver the recommended dosage at each administration (mean = 325; range = 650). The patient receives twice the recommended dose at the first and third administration and zero medication at the other two points. The problem is the spikes and valleys; the patient is overmedicated half the day and may experience intense pain in the intervening time. Regime D fails to delivered the total daily recommended dose and the administrative process is inconsistent (mean = 400; range = 650). The patient receives more medication than prescribed and also experiences regular periods of discomfort. Table 6.5 demonstrates why care givers must monitor both the mean and the range (variability) of a process to provide quality care.

Process improvement is built on meeting a desired standard and reducing variation in performance. Workers must monitor performance on an ongoing basis using the mean and range to ensure that performance targets are met. $\bar{X}$ **charts** monitor how average sample performance varies from historical performance, while **R charts** measure uniformity—the difference between the variability observed in the sample and the historical variability. Both charts are used to identify when performance should be investigated. Does observed performance deviate significantly from historical performance? Is the sample average close to the desired target and is performance consistent? The key question is: By how much do the average and the range deviate from historical performance?

$\bar{X}$ charts
charts that track performance that can be measured on a continuous scale using sample averages and establish upper and lower control limits

R charts
charts that track the uniformity of performance that can be measured on a continuous scale using sample ranges (the difference between the maximum and minimum) and establish upper and lower control limits

Step 3: Calculation of Control Limits

The calculation of control limits requires four formulas and provides a quantitative answer to how much variance will be accepted before a process is investigated. There are two formulas for the $\bar{X}$ chart and two for the R chart. The formulas for the upper control limit (UCL) and lower control limit (LCL) of the $\bar{X}$ chart are:

$$\textbf{LCL } \bar{X}: \quad \bar{\bar{X}} - (\textbf{A} * \bar{R})$$

6.3

$$\textbf{UCL } \bar{X}: \quad \bar{\bar{X}} + (\textbf{A} * \bar{R})$$

6.4

The terms in these formulas are:

: the grand average, the average performance across all samples ($\bar{\bar{X}} = \sum \bar{X}_i \div k$); this is the average of sample averages.

k: the number of samples.

$\bar{R}$: the average range across the samples ($\bar{R} = \sum R_i \div k$).

A: the control chart factor.

$\bar{\bar{X}}$ and $\bar{R}$ establish the historical performance against which individual samples will be judged. $\bar{\bar{X}}$ documents the average performance achieved over a large number of samples or extended time period and $\bar{R}$ defines the average range of performance (average variation) across the same samples or time. The control chart factor, A, is multiplied by the average range, $\bar{R}$, to determine the acceptable range of average performance. Acceptable variation in sample averages is a multiple (A) of the historical range in performance.

The magnitude of the control chart factor A is determined by sample size, that is, by the number of observations (n) in a sample. A larger sample size generally produces more accurate statistics, and consequently the control chart factor is reduced, producing tighter control limits, as shown in Table 6.6. When identifying a control chart factor, it is a common mistake for students of SPC to confuse the number of samples (k) taken with the sample size (n)— control chart factors are determined by the sample size, the number(n) of observations in a sample, rather than the number of samples drawn (k).

Table 6.6 Control Chart Factors for $\overline{X}$ and R charts

Sample Size	Mean	Lower Range	Upper Range
n	A	D_3(LCL)	D_4(UCL)
2	1.880	0.000	3.267
3	1.023	0.000	2.575
4	0.729	0.000	2.282
5	0.577	0.000	2.116
6	0.483	0.000	2.004
7	0.419	0.076	1.924
8	0.373	0.136	1.864
10	0.308	0.223	1.777
20	0.180	0.414	1.586
25	$\sqrt{n}$ 0.153	0.459	1.541

Source: N Gaither and G Frazier, 2002, *Operations Management*, 9th ed., Southwestern Thomson Learning, Mason: OH, 671.

The product of the control chart factor and the average range is added (or subtracted) from the historical performance (the average of the averages) to determine the upper (or lower) control limit. For example, when samples of five are drawn, the average output of a process is expected to fluctuate by ±57.7% of its average range ($\pm 0.577 \times \overline{R}$). One can see the impact of drawing a larger sample size; when samples of 25 are collected, the average output of a process is expected to fluctuate around its historical performance by only ±15.3% of its average range ($\pm 0.153 \times \overline{R}$)

The $\overline{X}$ chart identifies when a process should be allowed to run and when investigation is required. When a sample of five is drawn, we expect average performance for any sample to lie within ±57.7% of its historical average. As long as the sample mean falls within this range, the process is judged to be stable and no investigation or correction is required. Sample means above or below 57.7% of historical average should initiate investigation, and the findings of the investigation will determine if corrective action is needed. When a sample of 25 is drawn, the stable range is greatly reduced. As seen in Table 6.6, the amount of variation allowed before investigation is initiated is ±15.3% of the historical range.

It is not sufficient to monitor only the sample mean, because high and low values can produce an average that makes the system appear to be meeting its targeted goal when individual members of the sample are far from the desired performance. R charts must be created to monitor the variability (consistency) of performance by examining the difference between the highest and lowest values in each sample. The upper and lower limits for the R chart require two formulas:

$$\text{LCL}_R: D_3 * \bar{R} \qquad\qquad 6.5$$

$$\text{UCL}_R: D_4 * \bar{R} \qquad\qquad 6.6$$

D_3 and D_4 are control chart factors (see Table 6.6) used to establish the thresholds in which the sample range should fall, and, similar to A, these factors produce tighter control limits as sample size increases. When samples of five are drawn, the sample range could be up to 111.6% above or below the average range ($\pm 2.116* \bar{R}$) before investigation is warranted. Using a sample of 25, acceptable variation is reduced to 54.1% above or below the average range ($\pm 1.541* \bar{R}$). Investigation and potential corrective action is required when a sample range exceeds an upper or lower control chart limit.

Standard deviation and an s chart can also be used to gauge variation. Standard deviation, rather than range and an R chart, is used because of its better properties. Standard deviation uses all members of the sample to assess variation, while range uses only the maximum and minimum values in the sample. The upper and lower limits of an s chart are calculated using two formulas:

$$\text{LCL}_s: B_3 * \bar{s} \qquad\qquad 6.7$$

$$\text{UCL}_s: B_4 * \bar{s} \qquad\qquad 6.8$$

where $\bar{s}$ is the average standard deviation across samples, and B_3 and B_4 are control chart factors (not provided in Table 6.6), and similar to A these factors produce tighter control limits as sample size increases. When samples of two are drawn, B_4 is 3.27 times average standard deviation, $\bar{s}$, while the factor for a sample of five is 2.09.

Step 4: Graphing Performance

The creation of control charts requires graphing the information assembled in steps one through three. Step one compiled actual performance, and steps two and three supplied the sample mean, range, and control limits. The sample means (or ranges) are graphed as scatter (or XY) charts with the x-axis defining when the sample was collected (reported in chronological order) and the y-axis recording the value of the sample mean or range. The **center line** (CL), $\bar{\bar{X}}$ or $\bar{R}$, and the upper and lower control limits are graphed to provide the baselines against which actual performance is evaluated. Routine monitoring of performance, after the control limits are established, requires the relatively simple task of collecting data, calculating the sample mean and range, and charting the values for new samples.

center line

average performance as established by a series of samples

Step 5: Interpreting Performance

Step five is the examination of actual and expected performance to determine if the process is stable. A stable process is one in which actual performance, $\bar{X}$ and R, falls within the control limits with data points lying on either side of the center line, without exhibiting a trend or pattern. When dealing with continuous data, users must determine if average performance (the mean) *and* its variability (the range) fall within the calculated control limits. We want to avoid a situation in which the mean meets the expected standard but conceals the fact that a large percentage of sample elements have measurements that are too high or too low. Assessing the performance of processes measured using continuous data requires examining both the $\bar{X}$ and R charts.

Figure 6.3 presents four possible scenarios dealing with the Medicare Quality Initiative for Surgical Care Improvement Project, which specifies that prophylactic antibiotics should be started one hour before surgery. A hospital would want to measure the average lapse time between surgery and antibiotic administration on a $\bar{X}$ chart and the difference between the shortest and longest time for patients in a sample using an R chart. Figure 6.3 shows the four conditions that can occur: both charts can be stable, neither chart is stable, or one is stable and one unstable.

The $\bar{X}$ and R charts are stable if the sample means and ranges fall within the control limits, as seen in Figures 6.3a and 6.3b. The average patient receives his antibiotic within 60 minutes of surgery, and delivery time is consistent across patients in the sample. If the $\bar{X}$ chart is unstable, Figure 6.3c, and the R chart is stable, Figure 6.3b, we have a consistent delivery process that fails to achieve the expected performance. Delivery time is consistent across patients but patients do not always receive their antibiotic on time.

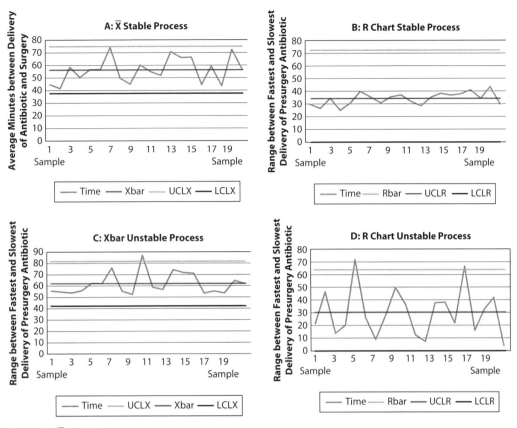

Figure 6.3 $\bar{X}$ and R Charts

If the $\bar{X}$ chart is stable, Figure 6.3a, but the R chart is unstable, Figure 6.3d, we have a process that on average meets expectations but has sporadic performance problems. Average delivery time meets the desired standard, but the R charts tell us that groups of patients are not receiving their antibiotics on time. The final possibility is that both charts are unstable, 6.3c and 6.3d, and average performance and the variation in performance are unacceptable. Average delivery time does not meet the expected timeliness, and the process is inconsistent, resulting in long and short delivery times for patients.

Figures 6.3a and 6.3b show a stable process; data points do not breach the upper or lower control limits and are randomly distributed around the center line. Figures 6.3c and 6.3d present the classic unstable processes in which one or more sample values (sample 10 on the $\bar{X}$ chart and 5 and 16 on the R chart) breach the established control limits. Besides a breach of a control limit, there are four other situations that signal an unstable process, but due to the length of this chapter the discussion of these four conditions will be undertaken in Chapter Seven.

Figure 6.3 provides two examples of process problems: poor performance and erratic performance. When these signals are received, the workers' first responsibility is to determine whether the system has changed. Users of SPC charts must understand that a breach of a control limit is not conclusive proof of a system change. As noted earlier, there is a small chance that a nonrepresentative sample has been drawn from a normally functioning process. The sample statistics may not represent the parameters of the population from which it was drawn. For example, the sample mean may be substantially different than the population mean. Second, after confirming that a change has occurred, the user must determine why the change occurred and whether the change improved or reduced system performance—what effect did the changes have on patients? Once the change and its effects are understood, users need to institutionalize changes that improve outcomes or initiate corrective action for those that reduce the effectiveness of health care processes.

Step 6: Investigate Instability and Improve as Needed

Steps one through five are necessary to identify when a process should be reviewed; control charts indicate when a limit is exceeded, but they do not identify what has changed or the effect of the change on patients. Step six is the most challenging part of the process: Does breaching control limits indicate that the process is unstable and requires correction (or does it signal improved performance)? Additionally, in the absence of limit breaches, is a process meeting expected standards?

The answers to these two questions are not straightforward, because the nature of sampling ensures that occasionally nonrepresentative samples are drawn. A particular sample may include a disproportionate number of high (or low) values and breach an upper (or lower) control limit, indicating a process change when no change has occurred. The first task that should be undertaken after a control limit is exceeded is to determine if the system is truly unstable or if a nonrepresentative sample has been drawn.

When a sample statistic exceeds a control limit (Figure 6.6, charts c and d), the first step in the investigation may be to draw a larger sample to determine if the out-of-range result holds after more observations are examined. Larger samples are more expensive to collect, but often the additional cost and effort will be lower than implementing unnecessary corrective action. The first step is to verify the unstable result; if the expanded sample produces a mean or range that falls within the control limits, employees can assume the process is stable, resume monitoring, and avoiding tinkering with the system. One of the primary goals of SPC is to focus employee effort on areas that have significant variation and may need correction and on documenting stable processes that can be left alone.

If the control limit continues to be breached after the sample size is increased, workers can assume nonrepresentative sampling did not produce the out-of-range result. The harder task of determining why performance has changed now arises. Breaches of control limits are designed to be rare events so users will not spend significant amounts of time or efforts investigating trivial variation in performance. SPC can maximize the effectiveness of improvement efforts by concentrating user efforts toward special cause variation and controllable causes and away from stable processes.

Given the rarity of breaches of control limits indicating that processes are not functioning as they have in the past, the users' job is to pinpoint the causes of change when it occurs and enact corrective action if the change impairs outcomes. SPC enhances employees' ability to pinpoint causes by providing a detection system to identify performance that is inconsistent with historical performance. Prompt identification of change may enhance employees' ability to pinpoint the cause of change, while operating conditions are fresh in their minds.

The uses to which SPC can be applied in health care are numerous: Are generally accepted standards of care being followed? Is health care provided differently to different populations? Are waiting times appropriate? Does performance vary with the personnel delivering care, the location of service, or the time or day of service? The next section applies the six-step process to a set of hypothetical data to illustrate the SPC technique. Readers are encouraged to calculate the descriptive statistics and control limits and create the control charts for themselves.

Emergency Room Wait Time Example

Quality medical care requires meeting technical standards and customer expectations. The director of an emergency room known for high-quality care but oft-criticized for its long waiting times wants to reduce wait times to improve patient satisfaction. The ER director has set a goal that the average patient time (defined as the time between when the patient is registered and her first contact with a physician) should be 30 minutes or less, and no patient should wait more than one hour.

Step 1: Collect Data

The director has collected a random sample of five patients per week for the last 20 weeks to assess wait times, for a total of 100 observations (5 patients * 20 weeks) and recorded the data in a spreadsheet, shown in Table 6.7. A copy of this complete data can be obtained online in the Chapter06.xls file under the Figure06–04 tab.

Table 6.7 ER Wait Times, January–May 2012

Patient	Week					
	1	2	3	4	. . .	20
A	32	61	10	70		83
B	9	88	8	30		57
C	87	61	31	70		6
D	79	72	38	27		2
E	5	8	12	20		28

Step 2: Calculate Descriptive Statistics

The first week produced an average wait time of 42.4 minutes, (32+9+87+79+5) ÷ 5 or **=AVERAGE(C6:C10)**. Once the Excel formula is entered, it can be copied to the remaining columns (through column V) to calculate average wait time for each week. The performance of the first week can be contrasted against the minimum average wait time of 19.8 minutes achieved in week 3 and the highest average wait time of 67 minutes in week 19. The average time across the 20 weeks, $\overline{\overline{X}}$ the center line, is 43.93 minutes. The Excel formula is **=AVERAGE(C12:V12)**. As stated earlier, an industry average or patient expectation, if known, could be used to establish expected performance.

Week 1 has a range between the longest and shortest patient wait of 82 minutes, 87 − 5. The Excel formula is **=MAX(C6:C10)-MIN(C6:C10)** and must be copied to all the columns up through column V to calculate the range for each week. Week 1's range of 82 minutes is the highest difference over the 20 weeks sampled and can be contrasted with the shortest range of 30 minutes, in week 3. The average range between the shortest and longest wait time for patients across the 20 samples is 61.5 minutes. The average and the range indicate that average ER wait time is 43.93 minutes ± 30.75 (61.5 ÷ 2) minutes, or actual wait times range from 13.18 to 74.68 minutes.

Step 3: Calculate Control Limits

The descriptive statistics make it apparent that the ER director's goals are not being met, but is the process stable? Are wait times within their historical range of performance and subject to only natural variation, or is wait time unpredictable due to the presence of special cause variation? The control limits calculated below show the acceptable range of variation based on a sample of five.

$$\overline{X} \text{ UCL: } 43.934 + (0.577 * 61.5) = 79.42 \text{ minutes}$$

$$\text{Center line (the grand mean)} = 43.93 \text{ minutes}$$

$$\bar{X} \text{ LCL: } 43.934 - (0.577 * 61.5) = 8.44 \text{ minutes}$$

$$\text{R UCL: } 61.5 * 2.116 = 130.13 \text{ minutes}$$

$$\text{Center line (the average range)} = 61.50 \text{ minutes}$$

$$\text{R LCL: } 61.5 * 0.00 = 0.00 \text{ minutes}$$

Enter the $\bar{X}$ control limits and center line directly below the calculation of the average wait time in the spreadsheet and copy across all columns. Similarly, the R chart limits and center line should be entered and copied below the range for each sample.

The control limits indicate that if the patient intake process is stable, average wait time will fluctuate between 8.44 and 79.42 minutes. If the process is unstable, the average of one or more samples will breach the control limits. Similarly, the range between the shortest and longest time for a patient to be seen by a physician in any sample should fall between 0.00 and 130.13 minutes. If any sample breaks these limits, the process may be unstable and require correction. Breaches of the upper limits indicate deterioration in performance (longer wait times), while downward breaches may indicate positive changes in the process and improved performance. Downward breaches are still a concern as they indicate system performance is unpredictable.

Step 4: Graph Actual and Expected Performance

Once the averages and ranges for each sample have been calculated and the upper and lower control limits and center lines are entered, Excel can create control charts through the **Insert** function. After Insert is selected, the user selects **Chart** and **Line** (type of chart) and enters the desired Data Range for the $\bar{X}$ chart. The data range entered must include the mean for an $\bar{X}$ chart, or the range for the R chart, the upper and lower control limits, and the center line. In Figure 6.4, the x-axis of each chart reports the week the sample was collected.

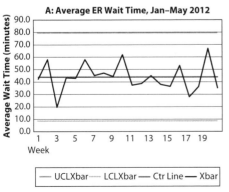

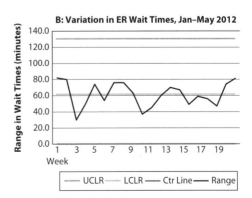

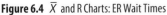

Figure 6.4 $\bar{X}$ and R Charts: ER Wait Times

Step 5: Interpret Graphs

The $\overline{X}$ and R charts demonstrate that average wait times and the difference between the shortest and longest wait time both fall within the calculated control limits. The ER intake process is stable and operating within its historical limits.

Step 6: Investigate Instability and Improve as Needed

Control charts do not judge performance; both charts indicate that investigation is not required as the patient intake process is stable. However, at the beginning of the case, a 30-minute average wait and a maximum wait time of one hour were desired. The control charts indicate that the process is operating within its historical parameters but that neither performance goal is being reached. The $\overline{X}$ chart shows that average wait time is more than 12 minutes above the targeted time, and two samples have average wait times in excess of 60 minutes. Similarly, the R chart shows that the average difference between the patient seen the fastest and slowest is more than one hour. Given the center line on the R chart is 65.07 minutes, each sample on average has at least one patient who waits more than one hour.

The director must assess this information to determine if changes are required. Is a 42.40 minute wait to see the doctor acceptable? How are competitors performing? Do patients expect faster service? The director must determine if performance is acceptable and whether wait times can be reduced, given the resources at her disposal. The director must also recognize that attempts to decrease wait times could disrupt the process and produce longer wait times.

The lack of special cause variation may be seen as simplifying the improvement process. If the process was unstable, the first task would be to eliminate the factors creating the excess variability and then recalculate the control limits to see if the process is stable after corrections have been made. In this case, the process is stable and the director can institute any change that she believes may reduce waiting times.

Medication Management Example

Effective medication requires that drugs be administered on a timely basis. Recognizing timeliness is a key determinant of effectiveness. A hospital has set a performance standard requiring that medicines be administered within one hour, plus or minus 30 minutes, of the prescribed time. Rather than examining every dose delivered, SPC allows the use of a sample of a small number of drug administrations to determine if the system is stable: Is it meeting the one-hour window, or is it out of compliance? A 100% sample may not be particularly informative as it is unlikely that 100% of drugs are delivered within one hour since natural variation is at work; for example, patients have and exercise the right to refuse medication or the patient may be receiving other treatments and be unavailable for medication. A 100% sample would also be arduous, if not impossible, to collect, considering that a 500-bed hospital may dispense 160,000 medications in a month.

The previous example examined the waiting time for an ER; this case presents several factors that complicate the analysis. The first is that time can be either positive or negative: a drug can be given too early or too late. Second, the sample is taken from three shifts during which different processes may be in place. Finally, samples are drawn on a daily basis and the process in place Monday through Friday may differ significantly from weekend performance. To analyze the medication management process, the six-step SPC technique is again followed.

Step 1: Collect Data

A random sample of 20 medications was drawn for each shift—day, evening, and night—every day for a month for a total of 1,860 observations (20 medications * 3 shifts per day * 31 days) and recorded in a spreadsheet. The sample size of 20 was arbitrarily determined. It is hoped that a sample size of this magnitude would persuade skeptical employees that the data were valid. As the validity of the SPC process is demonstrated, the sample size could and should be reduced. *Technical note:* with a sample size greater than ten, an $\bar{X}$ and s (standard deviation) chart is recommended, but this case will use the more understandable R chart. A copy of the case data can be obtained online in the Chapter06.xls file, under the Figure06–05 tab.

Step 2: Calculate Descriptive Statistics

The first sample (Day 1, Day Shift, Monday) produced an average delivery time of 14.00 minutes, **=AVERAGE(B8:B27)**. This result, however, is deceptive as the positive and negative values are cancelling each other out. It would be incorrect to assume that all medications were delivered within 14 minutes of the prescribed time. The simple average indicates more drugs are administered after the prescribed time than before the prescribed time. Due to the presence in the data set of negative values, drugs delivered prior to the prescribed time, an average based on the absolute value must be calculated. The user must enter: **=AVERAGE(ABS(B8:B27))**.

The ABS function converts negative values to positive values to determine the average deviation regardless of whether the drug was administered before or after the prescribed time. After entering the function, the user must hit **Ctrl+Shift+Enter** to calculate the absolute deviation. If the user hits the correct sequence, the cell content will change to {=AVERAGE(ABS(B5:B24))}. The addition of the brackets indicates that

Excel processed the data as an array. The output of this transformation is 53.70, indicating that medications are delivered on average 54 minutes before or after their prescribed time.

Once the Excel formula is entered, it can be copied to the remaining columns (through column CP) to calculate average administration time for each shift each day. The performance of the first sample can be contrasted against the most timely average delivery time of 16.35 minutes (#62), and the least timely, 66.65 minutes (#3). The average time between the prescribed medication time and the actual administration of medicines for all 93 samples, $\overline{\overline{X}}$, is 34.71 minutes. The Excel formula is **=AVERAGE(B30:CP30)**, and the center line is established at 34.71 minutes based on historical performance.

Sample #1 has a range of 157 minutes between the most premature and delayed delivery of medicine, **=MAX(B8:B27)-MIN(B8:B27)**. This formula must again be copied to each column up through CP to calculate the range for each shift each day. Sample #1's range of 157 minutes can be contrasted with the low of 57 minutes (#41) and the high of 165 (#5). The average time between the earliest and latest medication administration for the 93 samples is 107.32 minutes. The average and the range indicate that average medication administration time is 34.71 minutes ±53.66 (107.32 ÷ 2), and the actual administration of medicine ranges from −18.95 to 88.37 minutes before or after the prescribed time.

A cursory review of performance, based on the descriptive statistics, provides a manager with a good idea of where he should devote his attention. For example, the highest mean delivery time and greatest range in performance occur on Monday and Tuesday, and drugs administered on Friday through Sunday are the most timely and consistent. There is dramatic difference in performance across shifts. The highest mean delivery time and greatest range in performance occur on the second shift, while the first and third shifts have similar performance. Is this performance acceptable? Should the manager devote his time and energy to investigating the delivery processes on these shifts? SPC will answer these questions. At this point the high mean and wide range suggest that desired performance is not being achieved and action may be needed.

Step 3: Calculate Control Limits

$$\overline{X} \text{ UCL: } 34.71 + (0.18 \times 107.32) = 54.03 \text{ minutes}$$

$$\text{Center line (the grand mean)} = 34.71 \text{ minutes}$$

$$\overline{X} \text{ LCL: } 34.71 - (0.18 * 107.32) = 15.39 \text{ minutes}$$

$$\text{R UCL: } 107.32 * 1.586 = 170.21 \text{ minutes}$$

Center line (the average range) = 107.32 minutes

R LCL: 107.32 * 0.414 = 44.43 minutes

Enter the $\bar{X}$ control limits and center line directly below the calculation of the average medication time in the spreadsheet and copy across all columns. The R chart limits and center line should be entered and copied below the range for each sample.

The control limits indicate that if the medication process is stable, average medication time should fluctuate between 15.39 and 54.03 minutes before or after the prescribed time. The range, the difference between the most premature and delayed administration, should vary from 44.43 to 170.21 minutes. If these thresholds are exceeded, SPC indicates that the process may be unstable; in other words, it indicates a potential change in performance that requires investigation. Breaches of the upper limit indicate less timely administration of medicines while downward breaches may indicate positive changes in the process and improved performance.

Step 4: Graph Actual and Expected Performance

Once the averages and ranges for each sample have been calculated and the upper and lower control limits and center lines are entered, Excel can create control charts through the Insert function. After **Insert** is selected, the user selects **Chart** and **Line** (type of chart) and enters the desired Data Range for the $\bar{X}$ chart; the data range entered must include the mean for an $\bar{\bar{X}}$ chart, or the range for the R chart, the upper and lower control limits, and the center line. In Figure 6.5, the x-axis reports the sample number, 1 through 93.

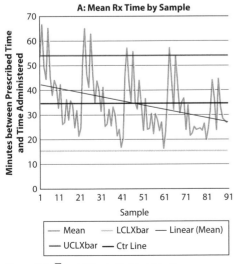
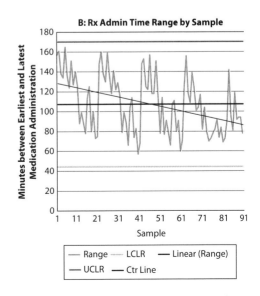

Figure 6.5 $\bar{X}$ and R Charts: Rx Administration

Step 5: Interpret Graphs

The $\overline{X}$ chart demonstrates that medication is routinely delivered outside the desired one-hour window and breaches the control limits. The sample means reveal that average performance ranges from 16.35 to 66.65 minutes before or after the prescribed time. The R chart shows wide differences in delivery times, but no control limits are breached. The R chart demonstrates that on one shift there is a 165-minute range: one patient received his or her medication 103 minutes after the prescribed time, while another patient in the sample received his or her medicine 62 minutes before the prescribed time. The best-performing shift had a 57-minute range.

Given average performance of 34.71 minutes and the average range of 107.32 minutes, patients are receiving their medication between 18.95 minutes before and 88.37 after the prescribed time. The reader should see SPC is a potent tool to evaluate how a process has been and is operating. Is the medication administration process operating acceptably? Despite the fact that the lower control limit is set at 15.39 minutes, the organization should be striving to reduce its average medication time below the current 34.71 minutes. Control charts provide an early detection device for identifying changes in system functioning over time. More (or less) timely delivery of medication and more (or less) consistent delivery of medicines should be reflected in the sample average and range, thus allowing employees to recognize positive or negative changes in their operations.

In this example the process is unstable: the $\overline{X}$ chart shows many breaches of the upper control limit and there are clear patterns in the data. The manager should explore both issues. The sample ranges on the R chart lie within their control limits, but many samples are located around the upper and lower control limits. The data points appear to form a pattern, suggesting the need for investigation. Further investigation will reveal that there are systematic differences in average performance and that the range between the most on-time and the least on-time administrations is based on day of the week and shift. These differences provide valuable information for understanding system performance: which shifts provide the most on-time delivery of medicines, and whether differences in performance are related to the day of the week.

Step 6: Investigate Instability and Improve as Needed

Control charts do not judge performance but rather indicate when investigation is required. The charts suggest that the medication administration system is unstable: the upper control limit on the $\overline{X}$ chart shows that medicines are routinely not administered within the desired one-hour window. Once this signal is sent, it is the responsibility of workers to determine if the system requires improvement. The first question that should be asked is: What factors prevent the timely administration of medicines? This is an open-ended question, but SPC can make identifying the causes easier by examining performance on different days or shifts, that is, by stratifying the data.

Diagnosing and improving a system is easier when substandard performance can be isolated to a particular shift, day, or unit. If differences in performance can be detected between shifts and days, this information can be used to diagnosis the performance issues. Are there particular days of the week that demonstrate consistently high performance, or are there days with low performance? An old adage, which may or may not have merit, is that people should avoid purchasing automobiles built on Friday or Monday. Workers on Friday were too focused on the weekend to do a good job while on Monday they were recovering from their weekend exploits. One of my colleagues swears she never schedules a medical appointment on Monday or Friday for similar reasons.

Diagnosing the Problem

Medication times are failing to meet the desired standard, so the question is, what is wrong? Are there unique factors occurring on different shifts or days that prevent timely administration of medicines? The manager could decide to draw a larger sample to see if the results persist, but given a sample of 20 it is unlikely that a new sample will produce different results. We will assume that the findings are valid and proceed to diagnosing the problem.

Sorting the data allows the performance of individual shifts or days to be graphed against the established control limits. The data can be sorted by shifts. Use the Excel Sort function: **Data, Sort, Options, Orientation, Left to Right**, row seven (day, evening, and night shifts). Then the charts in Figure 6.6 can be created. The x-axis now reports the day of the month, 1 through 31, rather than the sample number since only one shift per day is graphed.

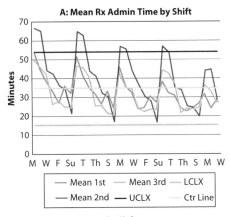

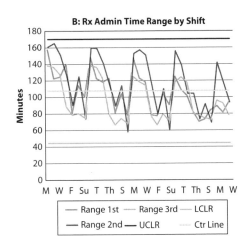

Figure 6.6 Performance by Shift

First Shift

Medications are routinely delivered in less than the average of 34.71 minutes on the first shift. There are only nine samples (out of 31 opportunities) in which the medication time is above the center line, that is, above the historical average. Performance according to the $\overline{X}$ chart meets the established standard, yet the R chart raises concern. The upper range limit is 170.21 minutes, almost three hours. On the first shift, the average range is 104.94 minutes, but ten samples exceed 120 minutes, suggesting a consistency problem. The wide range indicates that individual patients routinely receive their medications beyond the desired one-hour window. The greatest variation occurs on Mondays and Tuesdays, while performance on Fridays through Sundays is more uniform. What factors are different between the start and the end of the week that could account for this difference in performance?

This finding demonstrates the need for both control charts: the $\overline{X}$ chart *may* show that performance lies within the calculated control limits, but performance may still be unacceptable if the range is wide. Assume that one-half of patients receive their medication 30 minutes after their prescribed time and the other half in 90 minutes; the $\overline{X}$ chart would report an acceptable average of one hour, but one-half of the patients would not be receiving their medication within the target window.

Second Shift

Analysis of the $\overline{X}$ chart shows that drug administration times for the second shift routinely breach the upper control limit of 54.03 minutes and miss the targeted 60-minute window. The eight breaches of the upper control limit occurred on Mondays and Tuesdays in the first four weeks samples were drawn. This should be the chief concern of workers as the process is unstable and not meeting expected standards.

The R chart reinforces the performance concern as it shows that the difference between the most timely and least timely delivery of medicines often exceeds 140 minutes. No samples breach the upper control limit of 170.21 minutes, but 14 samples on the second shift had ranges greater than 120 minutes and these breaches occurred every Monday and Tuesday. Further analysis demonstrates that the second shift achieves superior performance at the end of the week; the most consistent and on-time delivery of medicines occurs on the weekends during the second shift. As in the analysis of the first shift, the question is: What factors can account for the different performance of the evening shift between weekdays and the weekend? After isolating evening shift performance, it is clear that the performance of the second shift is not meeting established targets and further investigation is needed.

Third Shift

The third shift has the most punctual medication times, with all samples lying close to the center line. The $\overline{X}$ chart shows an interesting pattern in that average administration time is above the center line on Monday and Tuesday and below it for the remaining days of the week. The third shift has the lowest and least fluctuation for average administration times. The R chart shows a similar pattern; this shift has the smallest range and is more consistent in the drug delivery process.

  While on-time delivery of medication is a goal of the organization, the lack of consistency between the shifts indicates an unstable process. Instability means an inability to predict outcomes; the organization cannot predict when medications will be delivered given the differing performance across shifts. The manager should explore the reasons for inability of the second shift to deliver medicines within historical limits or within the targeted one-hour window. There appears to be at least one factor that accounts for the lack of on-time administration during the second shift and wide range in delivery times. Potential factors include patient volume, staffing, or the assignment of duties.

Comparing Performance across Shifts

Analyzing performance across shifts indicates that there are one or more factors that explain the different performance of the first, second, and third shifts. Average medication time is 32.5 on the first shift and 31.7 minutes on the third shift, while second shift is substantially higher at 39.9 minutes. The second shift has average administration times approximately 24% higher than those achieved on the first and third shifts. The range shows less pronounced differences in each shift: 96.3 minutes on third shift, 104.9 on first, and 117.5 on second. The second shift demonstrates consistently poorer performance in on-time delivery of medicines and uniformity than the other two shifts.

Performance across Days

The $\overline{X}$ and R charts in Figure 6.7 display only the performance of the process on the days where the process is operating at its extremes. Monday and Tuesday show medicines are delivered the furthest from their prescribed times while Sunday deliveries are most timely. The inclusion of Wednesday through Saturday, four additional lines, would obscure rather than illuminate performance. In the first two weeks, drugs are delivered between 45 to 65 minutes off their prescribed times. Improvement has been made but only four times (out of 15 opportunities) did performance fall below average. The

R chart shows similar results; Monday and Tuesday have the highest range in performance, with often more than 120 minutes separating the most premature and delayed delivery of medicine.

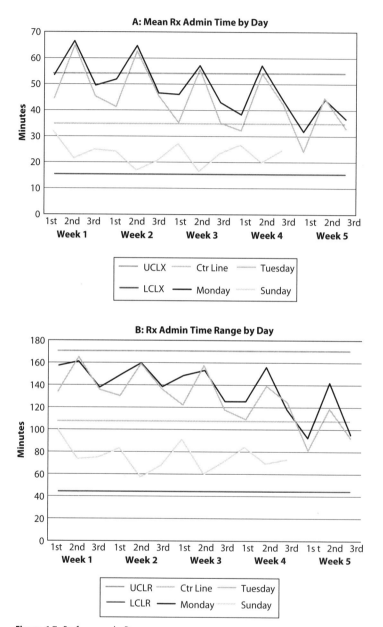

Figure 6.7 Performance by Day

Sunday provides an example of superior performance: every shift delivers medicines within 16.4 to 31.8 minutes of the prescribed time, and all sample averages fall below the center line of 34.7 minutes. The range on

Sundays varies from 57 to 100 minutes (versus 81 to 165 on Mondays and Tuesdays) and every sample range lies below the center line of 107.3 minutes. While improvements in timeliness have been achieved over time, the processes on Monday and Tuesday are dissimilar to Sunday, suggesting that different processes are at work.

The reasons for the differences in performance across shifts and days must be understood in order to improve performance. The reasons may be wholly or partially due to the distribution of nursing and pharmacy duties between shifts or different staffing levels or patient loads. The stratification of the data by shift and day makes it apparent that investigation should begin by contrasting the medication delivery process occurring on the evening shift on Mondays and Tuesdays, the least timely samples, against the Sunday night shift, which has the most on-time performance.

Identifying the Major Causes of a Problem

The first task in improving outcomes is to identify an area for improvement. SPC was used to recognize the untimely delivery of medications on the second shift on Mondays and Tuesdays. The next task is to explore and identify the potential causes of substandard performance. Why is performance routinely failing to meet expectations? Cause and effect diagrams (Chapter Four) can be employed to explore the potential causes of performance problems. Cause and effect diagrams begin the exploration process by identifying the major causes—manpower, materials, methods, machines, and environment—to determine why unacceptable performance could occur. Each cause should be explored to identify specific organization practices (sub-causes) that could contribute to the problem. For brevity, untimely administration of medications may be the result of four major causes: nurse staffing (manpower), patient case load (materials), process design (methods), and pharmacy (materials).

After the major causes are identified, employees should explore the issues within each major cause to identify if, why, and how it affects the delivery of medicines. Examining the effect of nurse staffing on the timeliness of medication should lead to investigating staffing levels, employee qualifications and training, productivity of personnel, and other staffing issues. Examining patient case load requires determining if the number of patients or the intensity of care affects timely administration of drugs. Questions of process design may explore job assignments and scheduling (admissions, surgeries, ancillary tests, discharges, and housekeeping duties), and, finally, pharmacy issues may include the delivery of medications from the pharmacy, medication errors (dosage or type), illegibility of orders, and adverse drug reactions or contraindications.

One role of the unit manager, quality improvement director, and other members of the health care delivery team is to evaluate and eliminate the causes identified on the cause and effect diagram, Figure 6.8, until the most probable factors are identified and corrective action taken. The identification process may involve reaching consensus among the involved parties or running investigations and tests.

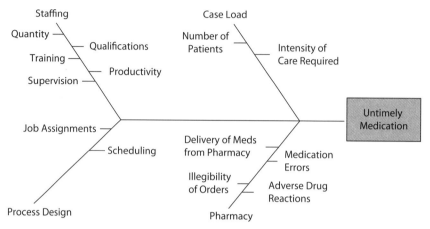

Figure 6.8 Cause and Effect Diagram

After the most likely cause is identified and corrective action taken, SPC should be used to determine if the action produced the intended effect. Were medications delivered more on time more often? If timeliness does not improve, then further review is required: Was the correct cause identified? If the correct cause was identified, was an effective correction proposed? If an effective solution was proposed, was it implemented and maintained? On the other hand, if the corrective action is successful in improving performance, monitoring must be continued to ensure that improvement is not lost over time and as a base for initiating a CQI cycle.

The implemented solution may have addressed the wrong or a trivial cause. If the problem continues, the improvement team should return to the cause and effect diagram to explore other likely causes. The cycle of analysis, modifying the process, and review of results should continue until performance meets expectations.

SPC improves management by setting clear performance standards for employees, establishing a consistent evaluation standard for managers and employees to use, and providing a tool to monitor processes. Managers have the ability to monitor second and third shift and weekend processes in spite of the fact they may work the first shift Monday through Friday.

Tinkering

The point has been made that stable systems should not be altered. Some find this conclusion counterintuitive and believe that systems should be optimized; that is, if performance is not exactly what is desired, then adjustments should be made. Table 6.8 and Figure 6.9 demonstrate that adjustments to stable systems may not improve performance but can make the system more erratic and unnecessarily consume resources.

Assume a person is measuring his blood pressure (BP) and has collected the data in Table 6.8. The desired BP is less than 120, and we will assume upper and lower control limits of ± 20 points (100 to 140). Blood pressure is affected by medication (ace inhibitors, alpha and beta blockers, and diuretics) and lifestyle factors (obesity, smoking, diet, alcohol, heredity, disease, age, race, and use of other medications). Column 2 shows the unmanaged systolic BP readings; the readings fluctuate around the desired 120 level and reflect normal variation.

Table 6.8 Blood Pressure

	Systolic	Tinkered
Day 1	105	104*
Day 2	121	120*
Day 3	124	123*
Day 4	122	121*
Day 5	119	118*
Day 6	115	114*
Day 7	130	129*
Intervention→ Day 8	111	102
Day 9	126	136
Day 10	110	106
Day 11	124	129
Day 12	108	99
Day 13	110	125
Day 14	123	121
Average	117.7	118.1
Standard Deviation	7.8	11.3

*For display purposes, BP was reduced by one unit to produce two distinct lines on Figure 6.9, but the average was calculated using the actual figures.

Assume the individual decides on day seven that his reading is too high at 130 and he increases his medication on day eight to move his BP closer to 120. He decides he will continue to follow the rule of increasing his next day's medication if BP > 120 and reducing his medication when BP < 120. The only situation in which his level of medication will stay the same is when BP = 120. Column 3 shows the "tinkered" readings.

BP was going to fall on day eight due to normal factors (column 2) but his attempt to optimize his reading by increasing his medication exacerbates the fall. On day eight, he reacts to his low reading by reducing his medication and this change again reinforces the natural tendency to move to the average. The reduction in medication propels his BP to a level higher than it otherwise would have been if the use of medication had been constant. This process of changing the level of medication based on the prior day's readings exacerbates the naturally occurring changes and worsens, rather than improves, his BP readings. Figure 6.9 demonstrates that tinkering with a stable process may produce the opposite result: a less stable, and perhaps more dangerous, situation than one anticipates.

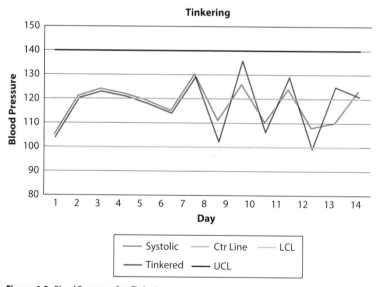

Figure 6.9 Blood Pressure after Tinkering

Figure 6.9 shows that the peaks and valleys have been increased rather than reduced due to the attempt to obtain a perfect reading of 120. The mean and the standard deviation (in Table 6.8) present a different picture; the optimization attempt has marginally increased the average BP reading from 117.7 to 118.1, but more importantly the standard deviation shows that variability has increased from 7.8 to 11.3. The average is closer to 120, but it masks the fact that this result is due to more extreme readings in each direction. The attempt to optimize has not improved the system but has made it less stable and predictable.

Cases and Applications

The medical literature has many examples of applications of SPC; however, its use and potential to improve patient care remain largely untapped. The following applications demonstrate the uses to which SPC can be put and the results achieved.

SPC and Cardiac Surgery: Application 1

One of the best examples is provided by Shahian et al. (1996), examining cardiac surgery. Their study did an outstanding job collecting information, applying SPC tools, and demonstrating positive improvement in cardiac care delivery. $\bar{X}$ and s charts were used to analyze LOS and demonstrated that postoperative surgical stays were unstable, as shown in Figure 6.10.

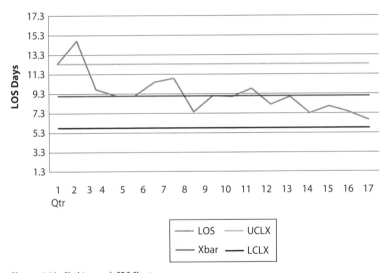

Figure 6.10 Shahian et al. SPC Chart

The $\bar{X}$ chart shows a breach of the UCL in period 2 and their s chart (not shown) shows breaches of the UCL in periods 1 and 2. Because of the instability in the process, changes were instituted in their practice pattern, clinical pathways were established, and staff was hired. Average LOS over 17 quarters was 9.1 days. In the first seven quarters LOS never fell below the average of 9.1 days, and after the changes were instituted, the last four quarters never saw LOS exceeding the average.

Besides examining LOS, the number of total and major complications and the occurrence of adverse events were analyzed. The number of total and major complications is count data and was examined using u charts (covered in Chapter Eight). Total and major complications were unstable in the second quarter and were reduced as the study progressed. While the count of complications provided understanding of how complications were changing over the study period, it was insufficient to direct corrective action. P charts, which are useful in analyzing categorical events and are covered in Chapter Seven, were used to analyze the eight major adverse events. Two of the eight adverse events, post-op bleeding and leg wound complications, were determined to be unstable. Changes were instituted in coagulation management to reduce post-op bleeding, and different harvesting and closing procedures were introduced to reduce leg wound problems. Although the other six adverse events were stable, all showed improvement over the course of the study.

The outstanding points of this article were the authors' ability to apply SPC to various cardiac surgery processes and outcomes. First, they identified the state of the process: the average LOS, the number of complications, and the frequency with which the adverse events arose. After assembling this data, they selected the appropriate SPC tools to use. After creating their control charts, they were able to drill into the data to recognize which processes had high variability. Recognizing that surgical complications were unstable was the starting point. Once instability was recognized, they collected specific information on which particular adverse events had the highest variability and potentially could be improved. Finally, they demonstrated that given the appropriate information, they could institute changes in processes that would improve health care outcomes.

SPC and Hip Replacement: Application 2

Multiple studies have shown that physicians will alter their practice patterns based on credible information on clinical practice. Johnson and Martin (1996) developed a physician education program on elective hip replacement and used SPC to determine if the program altered clinical practice. Physicians received surgeon-specific data on LOS, charges, readmission rates, complication rates, and infection rates. Johnson and Martin used $\overline{X}$ charts to examine LOS and total billed charges and p charts for readmissions, complications, and infections.

Between January 1992 and March 1993, before the intervention, LOS averaged 13.7 days; from April 1993 through December 1993, after the intervention, it was 9.9 days (see Figure 6.11). As expected with a drop in days hospitalized, billed charges decreased from $22,103 to $18,607.

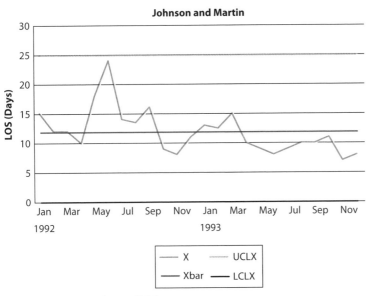

Figure 6.11 Johnson and Martin SPC Chart

Control charts showed LOS and charges were routinely above the center line prior to education and below it in the last nine months of the study. The p charts did not indicate any significant changes in the other factors analyzed. Johnson and Martin demonstrated that credible information can alter practice patterns, and SPC is tool that can document success and be used to provide feedback to practitioners show their efforts bore fruit.

SPC and Door-to-Needle Time: Application 3

Bonetti et al. (2000) sought to reduce delays in the treatment of patients with acute myocardial infarction by examining coronary thrombolysis. They examined "door-to-needle time" (DTNT) for 37 patients, and although they found significant reduction in the timeliness of care, they remained skeptical of the overall impact on care. This study is interesting because the authors used a sample size of one. Each patient was a sample, and the mean and standard deviation (30 minutes and 5 minutes) were not based on historical performance but rather on desired times. The first 16 patients (prior to initiation of their study) had DTNT greater than 30 minutes (see Figure 6.12). This finding resulted in rewriting practice guidelines, training staff, and emphasizing a DTNT goal of 30 minutes or less. During the intervention, all five patient treatment times fell below 30 minutes. The next 16 cases demonstrated an increase in DTNT, and 6 cases exceeded the 30-minute target.

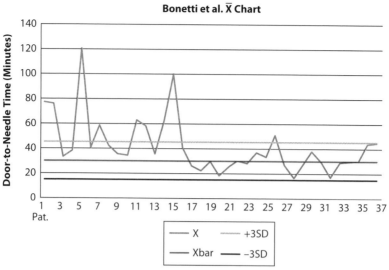

Figure 6.12 Bonetti et al. SPC Chart

Bonetti et al. used a cause and effect diagram to identify delay-causing factors using the major cause categories of equipment, people, methods, and communications. Despite the reduction in DTNT, they were concerned that the increased time among the last 16 patients might indicate that the improvement achieved would not be sustained over time and might be a Hawthorne effect. A **Hawthorne effect** is a reaction to the process of being observed rather than the result of efficacy of the change implemented. A bigger issue noted was that the primary time delay occurs before patients enter the hospital; the 25-minute reduction in DTNT achieved may not have a significant impact on patient outcomes if patient arrival to the hospital is delayed by hours. The delay in seeking treatment points out that factors beyond the control of medical providers may have a greater effect on health outcomes than how, and how quickly, medical care is delivered does.

Hawthorne effect
a change in behavior resulting from the subject being included in a study as opposed to a change resulting from the effectiveness of the intervention being studied

These applications demonstrate the utility of SPC. The researchers were able to institute changes that improved the processes of care and in many cases demonstrate improvements in health outcomes. The commonality in these applications was the willingness of medical providers to collect data and evaluate how they deliver care. After recognizing unacceptable performance, the authors were able to identify special causes that could account for the undesired performance. After causes were identified, they identified and implemented changes to improve performance. These applications also demonstrate how SPC can be employed to analyze the different types of medical events, continuous and discrete, that define health care. This chapter focused on demonstrating how continuous events are analyzed. The next two chapters will focus on discrete events to provide you with the skills required to comprehensively evaluate health care processes and outcomes.

Summary

Improving patient care is a formidable task that should not be hampered by a lack of or misunderstanding of quality management techniques. This chapter reviewed SPC and demonstrated how a widely available spreadsheet package can be used to record data and analyze performance. $\bar{X}$ and R charts can be used anytime a process or outcome can be measured on a continuous scale.

SPC complements and extends current health care efforts to improve health care processes and outcomes. The cases and applications discussed in this chapter demonstrate that SPC provides a wealth of information to understand how current processes are performing and a basis to institute improvement. More important than the information generated is the fact that instilling this way of working (defining, measuring, organizing, and analyzing) into employees can change how they approach their jobs. Recognizing that natural variation is inherent in a process and does not require intervention is essential to minimizing wasted effort and maximizing the effectiveness of corrective actions undertaken. Corrective action should be limited to processes whose effectiveness is being hampered. SPC assists in identifying special cause variation, which should be eliminated.

The cases discussed multiple causes for substandard performance; these causes are not revealed by SPC. SPC simply provides employees with a starting point to apply their analytical and problem-solving skills. Employees will determine how successful quality improvement initiatives will be, and they must see themselves as stakeholders in the process. Health care workers are committed to improving the lives of their patients, but they often lack the perspective and tools to enact effective change. SPC is an easy-to-master yet sophisticated and powerful tool workers can use to quantify performance and identify changes in delivery processes that can improve patient outcomes.

Given the siren song of "quality management," it is important to remember that change must begin with a documented need. As Francis Bacon noted, before we can command, we must obey. In medicine, overtreating a patient can produce worse consequences than letting things be, and overtreating the health care system in response to its perceived deficiencies can produce a less effective system. SPC provides a means to understand current performance and determine when a system should receive "watchful waiting" and when immediate intervention is needed.

KEY TERMS

Assignable variation	Noninherent variation
Categorical data	Mean
Center line	Out-of-control
Common cause variation	R chart
Continuous data	Special cause variation
Count data	Stable
Descriptive statistics	Standard deviation
Discrete data	Tinkering
Hawthorne effect	Type I error
In-control	Type II error
Inferential statistics	Unstable
Inherent variation	Upper control limit
Lower control limit	$\bar{X}$ chart
Natural variation	

REVIEW QUESTIONS

1. Why do systems often fail to produce desired results?

2. What is the difference between continuous and discrete data?

3. Explain the difference between natural and special cause variation.

4. Describe how an organization can establish performance targets.

5. Describe the six-step SPC process.

6. Why can attempts to "perfect" system performance lead to less predictable results?

PROBLEMS

1. Questions have arisen about the strength of IVs. As a result the pharmacy has started randomly testing IVs to determine if they contain the correction proportion of medicine and saline. The pharmacy tests six IVs every day. Assume the recommended mixture is 20 parts medicine to 1,000 parts saline. Samples for the last eight days are shown next.

				SAMPLES				
Observation	1	2	3	4	5	6	7	8
1	12	27	20	18	26	24	27	30
2	18	16	22	17	20	19	16	18
3	20	28	23	22	19	21	23	22
4	24	23	22	28	23	20	22	25
5	14	19	20	23	22	21	23	21
6	13	18	25	23	22	24	23	19

a. Create $\bar{X}$ and R charts.

b. Evaluate both graphs. Are there any concerns that should be explored? Is the IV mixing process performing adequately?

2. One of the quality standards for coronary artery disease is that patients admitted with acute myocardial infarction should receive a beta blocker within 12 hours of admission (unless there are contraindications). The cardiology department wants to know if this standard is being met and has randomly sampled patient records over the last six months. Five patients each month were sampled. If a patient did not receive a beta blocker, or if more than 36 hours transpired between admission and administration of the beta blocker, values of 36 hours were recorded.

Patient	HOURS BETWEEN ADMISSION AND ADMINISTRATION OF BETA BLOCKER					
	Jul	Aug	Sep	Oct	Nov	Dec
1	36 hrs	27 hrs	12 hrs	18 hrs	16 hrs	14 hrs
2	36	16	18	17	10	19
3	20	28	13	12	19	11
4	18	36	14	14	13	10
5	13	18	15	10	12	14

a. Create $\bar{X}$ and R charts.

b. Evaluate both graphs. Are there any concerns that should be explored? Is the quality standard being met?

3. The OR has experienced scheduling problems resulting in surgical delays due to unfinished cases and underutilized surgical suites. Because of this, the OR director has decided to examine surgical times (measured in minutes) over the last month. The Ch06Problems.xls file, Problem 06–03 tab, displays the number of minutes to complete a surgery. Is the process in control?

4. Patients admitted to the hospital for exacerbation of chronic obstructive pulmonary disease (COPD) with a history of coronary disease should have an EKG within 24 hours of admission. To determine if the hospital is meeting the standard, the director of quality improvement samples eight patients per month for ten months. The Ch06Problems.xls file, Problem 06–04 tab, displays the number of lapsed hours between admission and EKG. Create $\overline{X}$ and R charts. Interpret the hospital's performance based on your SPC charts and identify any issues that the director should investigate.

5. Patients admitted to the hospital for pneumonia should be given antibiotics within six hours of arrival. Early treatment with antibiotics has been shown to reduce complications. The top 10 hospitals report a success rate of 100%, and the state average is 95%. To determine if her hospital is meeting the state average, the director of quality improvement has sampled five patients per week over the preceding 25 weeks. The Ch06Problems.xls file, Problem 06–05 tab, records the hours lapsed between admission and recording of antibiotic administration. Create $\overline{X}$ and R charts. Interpret the hospital's performance based on your control charts and identify any issues that should be investigated.

References

Bonetti PO, Waeckerlin A, Schuepfer G, and Frutiger A, 2000, Improving Time-Sensitive Processes in the Intensive Care Unit: The Example of "Door-to-Needle Time" in Acute Myocardial Infarction, *International Journal for Quality in Health Care* 12 (4): 311–317.

Gaither N and Frazier G, 2002, *Operations Management*, 9th ed. Southwestern Thomson Learning, Mason, OH.

Johnson CC and Martin M, 1996, Effectiveness of Physician Education Program in Reducing Consumption of Hospital Resources in Elective Total Hip Replacement, *Southern Medical Journal* 89 (3): 282–289.

Joint Commission, 2001, JCAHO Standards in Support of Patient Safety and Medical/Health Care Error Reduction, http://www.dcha.org/JCAHORevision.htm.

Juran JM and Godfrey AB, 1999, *Juran's Quality Handbook*, 5th ed., McGraw-Hill, New York, NY.

McGlynn EA, Asch SM, Adams J, Keesey J, Hicks J, DeCristofano A, and Kerr EA, 2003, The Quality of Health Care Delivered to Adults in the United States, *New England Journal of Medicine* 348 (26): 2635–2645.

Shahian DM, Williamson WA, Svensson LG, Restuccia JD, and D'Agostino S, 1996, Applications of Statistical Quality Control in Cardiac Surgery, *Annals of Thoracic Surgery* 62, 1351–1359.

Shewhart, WA, (1931) 1980, *Economic Control of Quality of Manufactured Product*, ASQ Quality Press, Milwaukee, WI. Citations refer to ASQ edition.

Wadsworth HM, Stephens KS, and Godfrey AB, 1986, *Modern Methods for Quality Control and Improvement*, John Wiley & Sons, Inc., New York, NY.

CHAPTER 7

STATISTICAL PROCESS CONTROL FOR MONITORING FAILURE RATES

Introduction

Chapter Six demonstrated how control charts can be used to evaluate system performance when the variable of interest is measured on a continuous scale. The variable of interest typically reports on how a process is operating by measuring the inputs used or outputs produced. In health care, continuous variables are used to monitor patients' condition, dosage of medicines, and when medicines, procedures and tests are given. Measurement is simply a means to establish better control over a process by recognizing when intervention is required: when treatment should be delivered, how much care should be delivered, and whether treatment produced the desired result. For example, measuring blood pressure (BP) allows providers to determine when medication should be delivered and how many units should be administered. Subsequent measurement will determine if treatment was successful in reducing the patient's BP.

Many health care events are not amenable to continuous measurement, and the concern may not be with the way something was done but rather with whether treatment was provided, and if performed, what the result was. The process and outcome of care are often dichotomous events; for example, was a test or procedure performed, and was the result successful or unsuccessful? The variable of interest is an either-or proposition and can be measured as one (yes) or zero (no); the variable of interest either meets or does not meet a criterion. The focus is: Does an event meet or fail to meet a standard and was the outcome

LEARNING OBJECTIVES

1. Construct and interpret control charts for system outcomes

2. Identify when a process is unstable

3. Establish valid control limits

4. Compare constant and variable control limits

5. Determine when control limits should be rebased

a success or failure (defective or not defective)? Mortality is the most visible and pertinent binomial variable in health care: Did a patient survive or die after treatment? There are many variables that can be measured dichotomously: was treatment delivered within the prescribed time frame, did the patient contract an infection or experience a complication, were practice standards followed, was treatment successful, and so on.

Chapter Eight will review the other type of discrete data, counts, which examines the number of errors or occurrences. Counts are used when more than one error per event can occur. This chapter tackles issues such as whether a patient contracted a particular infection during her hospital stay. Chapter Eight will ask how many infections a patient acquired, since multiple infections can be contracted. Chapters Seven and Eight are concerned with recording failure rates when a single event defines performance, and the number of nonconformities when a single patient can encounter multiple undesirable events. The same six-step process introduced in Chapter Six will be used to analyze binomial data.

Statistical Process Control for Binomial Data: p and np charts

Binomial data is a subset of discrete data used to record the outcome of events that produce one of only two possibilities. It uses the six steps presented in Chapter Six for tracking continuous data (see Table 7.1), but the first three steps introduce substantial changes in data collection, in the descriptive statistic used, and in control limit formulas. Recognizing the similarities in the process for different types of data will enhance the reader's understanding of the fundamental structure and goals of SPC.

Table 7.1 The Six Steps of Statistical Process Control

1.	Collect data
2.	Calculate descriptive statistics
3.	Calculate control limits
4.	Graph actual and expected performance
5.	Interpret performance
6.	Investigate instability and improve as needed

Step 1: Collect Data

The process for collecting data is similar to the procedure discussed for continuous data: the user must determine the frequency of sampling (daily, weekly, monthly), the sample size, the procedure for drawing the sample to ensure that it is random, and the personnel responsible for drawing the sample. Juran and Godfrey (1999) note that sample sizes typically are between 50 and 100 observations for attributes, and attribute charts may not be based on samples but rather may be based 100% on inspection.

The user must identify the event to monitor, but instead of monitoring performance (how much, how long) the concern is whether a test or treatment was properly performed or whether the outcome was successful. The user must establish the standard against which an event or performance will be judged: What constitutes performance (timing, duration, dosage, completeness), and what constitutes a successful outcome?

The remainder of the chapter discusses binomial events in terms of **conformance**; units or events that meet a defined standard are categorized as conforming while those that do not meet the standard will be called nonconforming. **Nonconformance** covers tasks scheduled but not performed, unacceptable performance, failure to pass a test, or bad outcomes. In some cases there is little or no dispute over the outcome: Did the patient survive treatment? Did the patient contract an infection?

conformance
products or services that meet defined standards and are deemed acceptable for sale or further use

On the other hand, many medical outcomes are subject to interpretation, dependent on determining whether guidelines were adhered to or treatment was delivered at the appropriate time. Problems arise when adherence and timeliness is left to the judgment of individuals whose expectations and standards are not the same. Flight delays in the airline industry are tracked and published, but what constitutes a flight delay? Examining flight delays provides insight into developing a system to track surgical or other medical delays.

nonconformance
products or services that do not meet defined standards and are deemed unacceptable for sale or further use without rework

The Federal Aviation Administration (FAA) provides clear criteria to define a flight delay. First, there is a time element: 15 minutes or more past the scheduled time is considered a delayed flight. Second, there is a definition: *scheduled time* refers to movement to or from the gate. In the case of departing flights, airlines have an incentive to load the flight and push back from the gate within 15 minutes despite knowing that other factors may prevent takeoff. The FAA standard is clear: nonconformance occurs only if a plane is at the gate 15 minutes after its scheduled departure, or not at the gate within 15 minutes of its scheduled arrival (BTS 2013). Airline passengers may define a delayed flight as any flight that does not take off at the designated time, because passengers see little difference between waiting at the gate and being fourth in line for departure on the taxiway. Airline statistics do not record flight delays as commonly understood; rather, they record events that fail to meet two precise criteria.

Those attempting to institute SPC must define as precisely as possible the event they wish to monitor and control; that is, instead of asking whether a treatment adhered to a multifaceted guideline, measurement should focus on one or more critical aspects of the guideline. Instead of attempting to determine compliance across a wide range of recommended tests and procedures, the user should identify the critical tests and procedures, those most likely to affect health outcomes, and monitor the key elements (Did surgery start on time? Was a prophylactic antibiotic administered within two hours of the start of surgery? Was an EKG performed? Was the patient advised to lose weight and quit smoking?). The airline departure performance definition eliminates any discretion in interpretation by defining departure (pushback from gate) and the allowable time between scheduled time and actual time (15 minutes).

After defining the performance standard, data must be collected and assessed, and the outcomes recorded (conforms = 0; does not conform = 1). The second step is to evaluate performance, to determine what the data says about system performance.

Step 2: Calculate Descriptive Statistics

Descriptive statistics provide the information necessary to understand how the system is operating based on the recorded data: conforms = 0, and does not conform = 1. The count of nonconforms divided by total observations provides the failure rate. One of the largest obstacles to quality improvement in health care is the lack of understanding of previously achieved outcomes. There is substantial disagreement on the effectiveness of many medical treatments, and the effectiveness of individual providers is less known because they have a small number of patients and do not have the time and resources to study their outcomes.

The descriptive statistics required to understand binomial data are the nonconformance frequency in a sample (p_x) and the nonconformance frequency across samples ($\bar{p}$). To determine if a system is stable, the performance of a particular sample is compared to average performance across samples (an event's **historical probability**, also known as empirical probability). The formulas for p and $\bar{p}$ are:

historical probability the number of times an event has occurred in the past

| 7.1 |

$$p = \textbf{nonconforming units/sample size } (n)$$

p_x provides the proportion (or rate) of nonconforming events (or failures) in sample x.

| 7.2 |

$$\bar{p} = \textbf{total nonconforming units/total units (N)}$$

$\bar{p}$ describes average performance across all samples; that is, over the period of time studied, how often do nonconforming events occur? What is the average rate of failure? The sample average (p_x) and the nonconformance rate across samples ($\bar{p}$) allow us to determine if the variance in a sample is excessive compared to historical performance.

Step 3: Calculate Control Limits

As seen in Chapter Six, the question is not whether current performance is better or worse than historical performance but rather whether current performance is significantly different from its history and whether corrective is action required. Control limits must be calculated and performance assessed against these limits, but unlike continuous data the user must determine what type of limits to calculate. Binomial data can be presented as nonconformance rates (%) in **p charts** or the number of nonconforming events in an **np chart**.

    The decision to use a p or np chart is based on the sample size; a p chart must be used when sample size varies. A p chart tracks the *proportion* (or percentage) of nonconforming units or events in a sample and accounts for changes in sample size by dividing nonconforming events by the sample size. The np chart tracks the *number* of nonconforming events and can only be used when sample size is constant.

    For example, if the nonconformance rate (p) is 5%, the p chart will report 5% if one nonconformance is found in 20 events or if two events are identified in a sample of 40. On the other hand, the np chart reports the number of events and would report either one or two nonconforming events, creating the impression that the failure rate may have doubled when the increase in nonconforming events is merely the expected result of increasing the sample size. The np chart is easier to understand from a user standpoint since users do not have to convert data from counts to percentages, but its use is limited to applications in which a constant sample size is drawn, for example, 50 surgical cases being reviewed each month. The p chart can be used for either constant or nonconstant sample sizes. A p chart would have to be used if an organization decides it will sample a percentage of all events; for example, 5.0% of surgical cases will be audited to determine if a postsurgical infection arose. Given 1,200 surgeries in January and 900 in February, the sample sizes will be 60 and 45; the number of expected postsurgical infections should vary directly with the number of cases reviewed. A p chart must be created when the sample size varies from period to period.

    The following formulas define the upper and lower control limits for p charts:

$$UCL_p = \bar{p} + 3 \times \sqrt{\bar{p} \times (1 - \bar{p})/n}$$
7.3

$$LCL_p = \bar{p} - 3 \times \sqrt{\bar{p} \times (1 - \bar{p})/n}$$
7.4

p charts
charts that track the rate at which events meet a defined standard and establish upper and lower control limits; must be used when sample size is not constant

np chart
charts that track the number of events that meet a defined standard and establish upper and lower control limits; can only be used when sample size is constant

The np chart may be more desirable than the p chart due to its easier interpretation. The np chart does not require users to make any mathematical calculation but can compare the number of nonconforming items to the upper and lower limits, which are measured in natural units to determine if they fall within the limits. A p chart requires users to determine whether three nonconforming events fall within the control limits. For example, if the upper limit is 15% and the lower limit is 5%, the system will be stable if the sample size is between 20 (3/20 = 15%, equal to the upper limit) and 60 (3/60 = 5%, equal to the lower limit). When sample size is constant and an np chart can be used, the upper and lower control limits are calculated as:

7.5
$$\text{UCL}_{np} = n\bar{p} - 3 \times \sqrt{n \times \bar{p} \times (1 - \bar{p})}$$

7.6
$$\text{LCL}_{np} = n\bar{p} - 3 \times \sqrt{n \times \bar{p} \times (1 - \bar{p})}$$

To make the np chart more intuitive, two formulas for calculating the center line (the historical or empirical probability) are demonstrated:

7.7
$$n\bar{p} = \textbf{total number of nonconforming units or events/number of samples}$$

or

7.8
$$n\bar{p} = \textbf{sample size } (n) \times \textbf{average proportion of nonconforming units or events } (\bar{p})$$

The output of both formulas is the expected number of errors per sample. For example, the mortality rate for cardiac bypass surgery was 2.7% in 2000 in New Jersey. If a hospital in that state recorded four deaths in 20 samples, formula 7.7 predicts that the average number of deaths *per sample* is 0.20 (4/20). Formula 7.8 requires knowledge of the sample size: if $n = 10$ and $\bar{p} = 0.02$ (4/(10*20)) then we should expect this hospital to see 0.20 deaths per sample of 10 patients (or one death for every 50 patients or every five samples).

The preceding example points out the difference between using a p and np chart. To compare a hospital's performance against the New Jersey average, the state mortality rate of 2.7% must be multiplied by the hospital's sample size (0.027*10 = 0.27). If the hospital had the same mortality rate as the state, they would expect 0.27 deaths per sample of ten patients rather than the 0.20 they have achieved. The result of both comparisons is the same: the hospital has a lower mortality rate than the New Jersey average. Using an np chart—tracking the number of nonconforming events—will often require further mathematical computations to compare an institution's performance against commonly reported quality rates.

The names of the binomial control charts are intuitively tied to their function; p = proportion and np = number of nonconforming units or events. Again, the advantage of the np chart over the p chart is that the user does not have to calculate or interpret percentages. The user does not have to convert the number of nonconforming units or events into a percentage (nonconforming events/n [sample size]) and compare it to the calculated control limits. The user needs only to compare the nonconforming units or events in a sample to the control limits; that is, does the number of nonconforming units fall between the UCL and LCL?

Step 4: Graph Actual and Expected Performance

A line chart is used to visually display the actual nonconformance rate (p) or number of nonconforming events (np) against the historical nonconformance rate ($\bar{p}$) or number of events (n$\bar{p}$). The control limits again indicate when there may be a significant change in a process, that is, when nonconforming events (or failures) have substantially increased or decreased relative to past performance. Unlike continuous data, which uses two charts to examine average performance and variability of performance (how the process is operating), binomial data requires one chart to track either the proportion or number of nonconforming events (did the process occur, or did it produce the expected result?).

Step 5: Interpret Performance

The goal of step 5 is to determine if there is a change in system performance that could negatively impact outcomes; that is, is the system stable or unstable? The upper and lower control limits establish the acceptable range of performance in the monitored process or outcome. When a control limit is breached, there is sufficient cause to investigate the process to determine if correction is needed.

Figure 7.1 presents five indicators that a system may not be stable. The outcome being monitored is the rate of AMI patients who do not receive aspirin upon arrival to the hospital. Figure 7.1A demonstrates that historically 8.5% of patients do not receive aspirin within two hours of arrival at the hospital and the system is stable. The percentage of patients not receiving timely aspirin administration ranges from 0.0% to 20.0% and falls within the control limits. While the process is stable, the key issue for the hospital is: Is this acceptable performance when, barring contraindications, the goal is for 100.0% of AMI patients to receive aspirin within two hours of arrival?

Figure 7.1B presents the classic unstable system, in which one or more samples breach a control limit. Again 8.5% of AMI patients do not receive aspirin within two hours of arrival and the upper control limit is set at 27.7%, but sample 3 has a rate of 30.0%, indicating that the system is not operating within its historical range and may be subject to special cause variation. The breach indicates that something out of the ordinary may

trend

a series of points moving in a general direction

pattern

a series of points that form a repeating sequence

have occurred in sample 3 that drove the rate of nonconforming events beyond its historical performance. In addition to control limit breaches, users must be alert to identify **trends**, **patterns**, and series of points that fall on one side of the center line or close to the upper or lower control limits. While each of these indicators is important, users must pay particular attention to indicators suggesting deteriorating performance.

Figure 7.1C shows an upward trend starting in sample 11, and if the trend continues, the UCL will be breached in the future. Some observers may argue that no trend exists as there are three downturns in the nonconformance rate. But the periodic downturns do not offset the overall upward trend. Data analysts should remember that Excel provides a simple-to-use utility function, Add Trendline, which can insert trendlines into a graph if there is doubt whether there is an upward or downward tendency in the data.

The presence of the trend indicates that the process is being affected by more than natural variation and presents an opportunity to improve the performance. If the cause of a trend—worsening performance of labor, a machine, or material—can be identified and corrected, the organization can move its overall outcomes toward the level achieved when superior workers, equipment, or supplies are used.

Figure 7.1D presents a series of points on one side of the center line. (Assume that a series must contain at least six points.) If a process is stable, samples should fall around the center line. When there is a series of points on one side of the center line, it demonstrates a shift, indicating the process has changed or possibly two or more processes are being observed. The performance in samples 1 through 10 differs dramatically from samples 11 through 20. Starting in sample 11, performance improves substantially: the failure rate never exceeds 5.0%. Before sample 11, though, 14.0% of AMI patients did not receive aspirin at arrival.

More difficult to detect are patterns. Figure 7.1E shows that the nonconformance rate is consistently lower in even samples. The question that must be asked is: Why is nonconformance higher in odd samples and lower in even samples? Perhaps the samples are collected weekly and staff scheduling is one-week-on and one-week-off, so the pattern reflects performance of two different medical teams. Or perhaps even samples are collected during the day shift and odd samples are drawn at night, reflecting different treatment processes. Unlike projecting a trend, the sawtooth pattern created by a systematic up and down movement of the odd and even samples may never breach a control limit, but the pattern indicates that the process is being affected by more than natural variation and presents a clear opportunity for improvement. If the cause of a pattern can be identified, the organization can move its outcomes toward those achieved in the higher-performing group.

Figure 7.1F presents a series of points close to the UCL. The concern in this situation is the proximity to breaching the limit. A small change in performance could result in an unacceptable outcome. Employees may want to examine why 20% of AMI patients were consistently not receiving aspirin at arrival in the first six samples. The tracking and investigation of performance in the first six periods may have led to the reiteration of the need to administer aspirin or to a change in procedure, which could explain the improved performance demonstrated in samples 7 through 20. The objective of graphing and interpretation is to identify special cause variation, any change indicating that the system is not performing as it has in the past. Users need to recognize that change is indicated in a variety of ways: control limit breaches, trends, patterns, a series of points above or below the center line or a series of points close to the UCL or LCL.

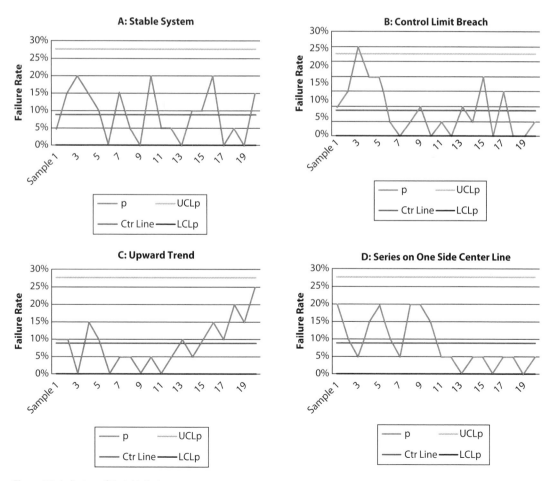

Figure 7.1 Indicators of Unstable Systems

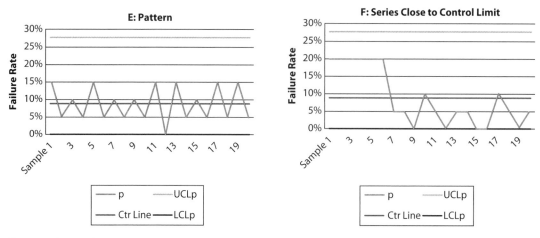

Figure 7.1 Continued

Step 6: Investigate Instability and Improve as Needed

If control limit breaches, trends, patterns, or a series of data points are identified, the user must determine their cause and eliminate the cause if possible. It is easier to identify the indicators of special cause variation (points exceeding control limits or points indicating the start of a trend or pattern) than it is to determine their causes. See Chapter Five, root cause analysis, for a detailed discussion of investigating the source of problems. Control charts provide information on when a breach occurred, or when a trend or pattern began, thus providing a starting point for investigation. But determining what factors affected the process at a particular point of time is a challenging and time-consuming process. Once a cause or causes are identified, correction presents a still more formidable challenge.

Attempts to eliminate special cause variation and change systems frequently run up against inertia and opposition from powerful interests. Systems develop over a prolonged period of time, and attempts to change processes will encounter opposition from those who are content with current procedures. The advocates of change will have to make a persuasive case for change; they will have to demonstrate that poor patient outcomes are directly related to the current process to overcome opposition.

Investigations may identify factors that have little or no impact on performance; that is, the analysis may lead down a blind alley. The quality improvement team must recognize that continuous monitoring is required to determine if outcomes improve. Investigators may not identify the correct cause of a problem in their first attempt, or multiple causes may contribute to the problem. Users must approach change with an open mind, recognizing that mistakes are possible, and adopt a CQI/PDCA cycle mindset. The

PDCA cycle emphasizes continual improvements and starts by identifying a problem or opportunity (special cause variation) and plan for improvement. Users do not assume that the opportunity or the chosen correction is infallible. The second phase of the cycle, Do, is a small-scale test. Users following PDCA precepts do not initiate wide-scale change as they assume all improvements must be tested before they are implemented across an organization. Only if modifications achieve what they were expected to produce (Check) are they rolled out to the entire organization (Act). If the expected results are not achieved, users return to planning and begin the cycle anew. Change is often a trial-and-error process in which various modifications are attempted before the desired outcomes are achieved.

Once special cause variation is eliminated and the system is stable, the PDCA cycle should be used to pursue continuous quality improvement. A stable system is not negatively affected by a particular cause, but overall performance may still be lower than what is achievable, what customers desire, or what competitors offer. The performance of a stable system is predictable, but this does not mean the outcomes cannot be improved. Improving a stable system requires a total process review (versus eliminating one factor responsible for special cause variation) in which every aspect of an operation is studied with an eye toward making it more effective or efficient.

Accuracy of Surgical Coding Example

A hospital wants to track the accuracy of surgical coding. The accuracy of surgical coding affects reimbursement, and errors in coding could substantially inflate or reduce revenue. Both types of errors should be avoided. Coding that understates the level of difficulty of surgery may undermine the hospital's ability to remain open since it may expend more resources to provide care than it can recoup in reimbursement. On the other hand, surgical codes that overstate work performed may attract attention from payers, resulting in audits and substantial civil or criminal penalties if billing codes are wrong. Common surgical coding errors include failure to record a modifier, using overly general CPT or diagnostic codes, or keystroke errors.

Step 1: Collect Data

A sample of 50 surgical cases was collected each month for the past year, and the number of incorrect claims was recorded. When an error was detected, the claim was recorded as a 1 if incorrect or nonconforming, and 0 if correct. Two errors were identified in the January sample of 50 claims; one record had a transposition of numbers, and the second did not include a modifier. The first sample consequently had an error rate (p) of 4.0% (2 ÷ 50). Table 7.2 records the number of errors over one year.

Table 7.2 Errors in Surgical Coding

	Incorrect	Sample	p
Jan	2	50	4%
Feb	3	50	6%
Mar	1	50	2%
Apr	2	50	4%
May	3	50	6%
Jun	1	50	2%
Jul	11	50	22%
Aug	7	50	14%
Sep	5	50	10%
Oct	2	50	4%
Nov	3	50	6%
Dec	1	50	2%
Total	41	600	6.83%

Step 2: Calculate Descriptive Statistics

The number of nonconforming claims in Table 7.2 was totaled and revealed that 41 incorrect claims were submitted to payers from January through December, based on the review of 12 samples of 50, for a total of 600 claims.

$$\bar{p} = 41/600 = 0.0683 \text{ (or 6.83\%)}$$

The average nonconformance rate across all samples is 6.83%; the fourth column in Table 7.2 displays the monthly nonconformance rate (column 2 divided by column 3). Column four highlights two points: the average monthly rate was between 2% and 6% most of the year, and a high number of nonconforming claims occurred in July, August, and September. The question for users is: Would the increase in coding errors in July trigger an investigation and possible corrective action? Considering that the goal of SPC is to improve performance, are the nonconformance rates in July, August, and September sufficiently different from historical experience to signal that the system may have changed?

Step 3: Calculate Control Limits

The appropriate control chart is based on whether the sample size varies or is constant. A p chart must be used when sample size varies, but the user can elect to use either a p or an np chart when sample size is constant. The advantage of the np chart, which reports the number of nonconforming events, is that it is easy for employees to understand. On the other hand, comparisons of results with other organizations favor the use of a p chart, which reports nonconforming rates. Since a constant 50 records per month were reviewed, either a p or an np chart is appropriate. Both charts will be created and the results compared. The p control chart limits are calculated below:

$$\text{UCL}_p = 0.0638 + 3 \times \sqrt{0.0683 \times (1 - 0.0683)/50} = 0.1754$$

$$\text{LCL}_p = 0.0638 - 3 \times \sqrt{0.0683 \times (1 - 0.0683)/50} = -0.0387$$

The center line $\bar{p}$ shows that the average error rate on coding surgical claims during this twelve month period is 6.83%. The lower control limit was calculated to be −3.87%, a negative error rate, but since error rates cannot be less than zero, the lower limit is set to the minimum possible rate of 0.00%. A stable process would produce errors in a range from 0.00% through 17.54%. Given that the lower boundary is 0.00%, the only issue for users is to note when the error rate exceeds 17.54%. When this limit is exceeded, we will conclude the process has changed sufficiently to justify an investigation to determine if the process is unstable (not operating within its historical range) and being affected by special cause variation.

If Excel is used to calculate the control limits, creation of the control chart is a straightforward process. Calculate the nonconformance rate (p) for each sample, the center line ($\bar{p}$), and the upper and lower control limits (=B\$19±3*(B\$19*(1-B\$19)/50)^.5 or =B\$19±3*SQRT(B\$19*(1-B\$19)/50)). Next, set up four columns for the control chart: p (the sample specific nonconformance rate), $\bar{p}$ (the average nonconformance rate for all samples), UCL, and LCL. After setting up the columns, set up a formula to calculate the sample specific nonconformance rate (errors per sample ÷ sample size) and manually enter the control chart limits as values or use a fixed cell reference. When a fixed cell reference is used, insert a **\$** preceding the row number to ensure that if the cell is copied down the worksheet, the cell's row number is not incremented.

The sample specific formula and control limits can be copied to the remaining eleven periods. After copying the formulas, highlight the cells to be graphed (p, $\bar{p}$, UCL, and LCL). Select **Insert**, **Line** (type of chart to produce), and the type of line chart (2d or 3d, stacked or unstacked, with or without markers) to produce the control chart. Format the chart by right-clicking on the chart to bring up a submenu. Click Select Data and Horizontal (Categories) Axis Labels to enter the period labels. On the main menu, click on Chart Layout to enter the desired chart title and axis labels.

Step 4: Graphing Performance

The p chart shows that the coding process was stable in eleven of twelve periods; the only problem occurred in July when the error rate spiked to 22%.

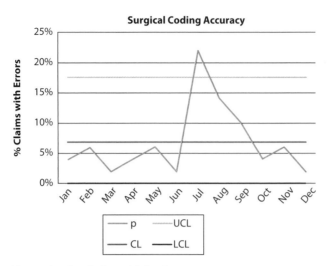

Figure 7.2 p Chart for Surgical Coding Accuracy

The chart demonstrates there were high errors in August (14%) and September (10%), but by October the error rate was equivalent to the rates achieved in January through June. Note that the control limits calculated are not valid due to the presence of special cause variation in July; that is, the coding process is not stable and the variation in performance is increased by the nonrandom variation. Although this point will be ignored, the reader must remember that statistical control can occur only in stable systems, those subject to only normal variation. After the special cause variation is eliminated, the control limits must be recalculated to reflect only normal variation, and the tighter limits will establish the acceptable range of performance before investigation is required.

As stated earlier, a constant sample size of 50 was drawn, so either a p or an np chart is appropriate to analyze performance; np chart limits are calculated as follows:

$$np = 41 \div 12 = 3.417 \text{ (or } n \times \bar{p}, 50 \times 0.0683)$$

Note the change in the denominator. Instead of dividing by total observations, the number of errors is divided by 12, the number of samples. The result of this calculation is the number of expected errors per sample. The average number of incorrect claims expected per sample of 50 is 3.415 and establishes the center line.

$$UCL_{np} = 3.417 + 3 \times \sqrt{50 \times 0.0683 \times (1 - 0.0683)} = 8.77$$

$$LCL_{np} = 3.417 - 3 \times \sqrt{50 \times 0.0683 \times (1 - 0.0683)} = -1.94$$
$$\text{therefore } 0.00$$

The control limit calculations show that based on performance from January through December a stable process may produce up to 8.77 non-conforming events per sample of 50, and the lower limit is calculated to be −1.94, so it will be set at 0.00. A stable coding process would produce errors in a range from 0.00 through 8.77. The advantage of using the np chart is apparent: users do not have to calculate percentages but need only count the number of incorrect claims in a sample and compare this number with the control limits. Investigation is needed only if nine or more incorrect claims are identified.

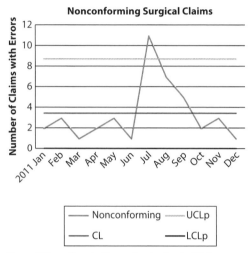

Figure 7.3 np Chart for Nonconforming Surgical Claims

Step 5: Interpreting Performance

The p and np charts are similar, with the sole difference being the y-axis. Unlike the nonconformance *rate* on the p chart, the np chart displays the *number* of nonconforming claims per sample. The interpretation of the chart is the same as the p chart: the coding process was unstable in July, but errors fell the next two months and by October the process was operating below the center line.

Step 6: Investigate Instability and Improve as Needed

The easy part of using control charts is creating and interpreting the charts. The difficult task is to identify the real-world variables that explain fluctuations in performance. In this example the question is, what occurred in July to increase the error rate beyond prior experience? The breach of the UCL may have occurred due to the hiring of a new employee who was unfamiliar with the organization's coding practice and made significant errors until he mastered the coding process. If this was the cause, the chart suggests that the employee's performance improved rapidly (or perhaps the employee was not retained as a coder) as errors fell dramatically in two months.

A second possibility is that given the timing of the spike, the summer months, one or more coders were on vacation. There could have been the same amount of work as prior months but fewer employees. To adapt to the higher level of work per employee, employees may have attempted to work faster to complete their jobs during their standard work week, thus reducing time per claim and inadvertently increasing their error rate. On the other hand, time per claim may have been maintained but the work week could have been expanded through the use of overtime and the additional hours may have produced fatigue among the staff and thus higher errors.

Other changes that could account for the higher error rate include implementation of a new coding system or process, a regulatory change in how procedures should be coded, or the introduction of a new surgical procedure. These changes would require staff to adapt to a new system, learn how to code according to a revised set of standards, or learn the code for a new or previously unused medical technique. Any of these changes would produce a period of learning and transition. Regardless of the cause of the increase in coding errors, the charts show the problem had been rectified by October.

Heart Failure and Smoking Cessation Counseling Example

gaming the data
the manipulation of data to present information in the best possible light to enhance mediocre performance or conceal poor performance

Although it was impossible in the coding example to breach the lower limit, if a nonzero lower limit was established and broken, the cause could be an improvement in the process. On the other hand, dramatic improvement may indicate problems with data collection or intentional **gaming of the data**. Table 7.3 and Figure 7.4 examine the percentage of heart failure patients receiving smoking cessation counseling. Samples of 20 were drawn from January 2011 through August 2012 and reveal that the average percentage of smokers who did not receive counseling is 38%, but starting in July 2012, 100% of patients were reported as receiving cessation counseling. Does the data document that the organization has achieved perfect performance, or does it indicate that employees are simply noting every patient received counseling whether or not it was actually provided?

The question is, does the reported data reflect an improvement in the process or a change in data collection? While we want to believe the change reflects improved health care delivery, investigation is still required. A reduction in the nonconformance rate may be due to honest data entry errors or a failure to detect errors. A dramatic fall in reported errors could also signal manipulation of data, including a deliberate failure to report nonconforming events or selecting a favorable sample unlikely to have errors.

Table 7.3 Heart Failure and Smoking Cessation

Sample	p	Ctr Line	UCLp	LCLp
Jan 2011	0.50	0.3800	0.7056	0.0544
Feb	0.45	0.3800	0.7056	0.0544
Mar	0.60	0.3800	0.7056	0.0544
Apr	0.55	0.3800	0.7056	0.0544
May	0.40	0.3800	0.7056	0.0544
Jun	0.55	0.3800	0.7056	0.0544
Jul	0.45	0.3800	0.7056	0.0544
Aug	0.50	0.3800	0.7056	0.0544
Sep	0.40	0.3800	0.7056	0.0544
Oct	0.30	0.3800	0.7056	0.0544
Nov	0.35	0.3800	0.7056	0.0544
Dec	0.40	0.3800	0.7056	0.0544
Jan 2012	0.30	0.3800	0.7056	0.0544
Feb	0.45	0.3800	0.7056	0.0544
Mar	0.35	0.3800	0.7056	0.0544
Apr	0.40	0.3800	0.7056	0.0544
May	0.25	0.3800	0.7056	0.0544
Jun	0.40	0.3800	0.7056	0.0544
Jul	0.00	0.3800	0.7056	0.0544
Aug	0.00	0.3800	0.7056	0.0544

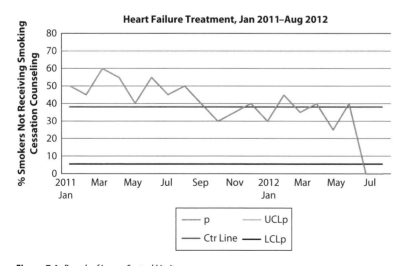

Figure 7.4 Breach of Lower Control Limit

Manipulation of data may occur if an employee's compensation or job is based on achieving a certain level of performance. Dramatic decreases in nonconforming rates must be investigated in the same manner as increases. Achieving and maintaining quality products and services requires employees to know if the process has changed and why it has changed. If the number of smokers with heart failure who do not receive cessation counseling suddenly falls to zero, the user should audit the records to ensure that the information is error-free, verify with patients that they received cessation counseling, draw a new sample to see if the results are maintained in a larger sample, or monitor future patient counseling sessions.

The goal of any organization should be to continually improve its performance. Organizations must be on constant alert to identify opportunities for improvement that will make their products and services more appealing to their customers. These opportunities may emanate from changes in patient needs and desires, technological change, or changes in the offerings of competitors, so driving the nonconformance rate to zero should be the goal of every organization.

Establishing Valid Control Limits

The coding and smoking cessation examples demonstrate one of the primary confusions arising from the use of control charts: control limits are not valid when special cause variation is present. Both examples suggest special cause variation is present as each breaches its control limits. The goal of SPC is to establish control limits that identify when processes are operating outside their historical performance. SPC is based on identifying deviations from historical performance, but valid control limits cannot be calculated if the process under examination is unstable. There are two primary ways of establishing valid control limits when special cause variation is present.

The first requires identifying samples in which special cause variation is present, identifying its cause, and eliminating it. When the special cause variation is eliminated, users will have to collect new samples without special cause variation and calculate new limits using only the postcorrection samples.

A second method would be to eliminate the samples with special cause variation and calculate new control limits based on the remaining data. In the surgical coding example, this would require eliminating July and calculating the control limits using January through June and August through December.

Recalculating the control limits without the eleven errors in July produces a center line ($\bar{p}$) of 5.45% versus 6.83%. Eliminating high-error samples makes intuitive sense, as it would be inappropriate to establish "normal" performance thresholds when there is an obvious problem in the system.

In the coding example, if a new employee must learn how to code, we would not want to establish control limits based on the period of time when he or she is learning and making errors. The time to establish performance standards is after an employee has mastered a skill.

Using $\bar{p}$ = 5.45% reduces the upper control limit on the p chart to 15.09% (vs. 17.54%) and does not affect the lower limit, which had been set to 0.00%. The new control limits can be used to monitor and control the coding process as they reflect the expected variation when the process is stable. Figure 7.5 demonstrates the difference between the center lines and control limits when the system is stable (valid) and unstable (invalid), that is, excluding and including the 22% nonconformance rate in July.

The recalculated limits are narrower and would indicate that investigation is required for performance with error rates between 15.09% and 17.54%, which would have been acceptable within the prior limits. The lower center line and UCL reflect the expected deviation in performance when the billing process is subject to only natural variation, that is, when definable factors that negatively impact performance are absent.

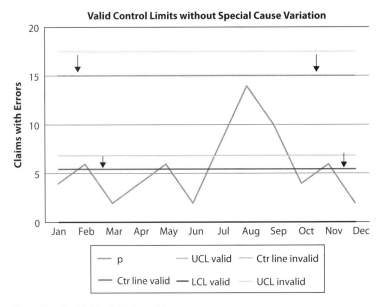

Figure 7.5 Establishing Valid Control Limits

The goals of quality improvement are perfectly demonstrated by the recalculation of control limits; organizations should strive to reduce nonconformance rates (the center line) and narrow the variation in performance (the control limits). The lowering of the center line does not reflect a reduced failure rate but rather the level of performance that should be expected in the absence of unusual events. Lower nonconformance rates and narrower control limits are the tools with which organizations can measure their goal of improving performance.

Constant and Variable Control Limits

variable control limits
control limits that widen when a small sample is drawn and narrow as larger samples are drawn

When an organization decides it will sample a percentage of events each period, the sample size will likely vary from period to period. When sample size varies, a p chart must be used, and it is common to see control charts with nonconstant control limits. These **variable control limits** are the result of the incorporation of the sample size into the control limits calculation:

$$\text{UCL}_p/\text{LCL}_p = \bar{p} +/- 3 \times \sqrt{\bar{p} \times (1 - \bar{p})/n}.$$

There are two primary ways of handling the changing sample size. The first is to calculate an average sample size for the entire study period and use the average in the control limit calculations. As seen in previous SPC charts, using average sample size produces constant or unvarying control limits.

The second method uses the period-specific sample size in calculating control limits and produces variable limits (data set: Chapter 07.xls, Figure 07–06 tab). In Excel, the user would enter a relative cell reference for the sample size, =B$19+3*(B$19*(1-B$19)/C23)^0.5, for the UCL and copy the formula across all periods. The formula uses the center line (B$19—note the $ in front of the row number) and a relative cell reference for the sample size (C23) that can change from sample to sample. The data in this example is the same as Table 7.2 and Figure 7.2, with the exception of different sample sizes (n), and consequently the proportion of errors per period (p) changes. Table 7.4 provides the control limits using the average and period-specific sample sizes.

The reader will note that the main differences between Figure 7.2 and Figures 7.6 A and B are minor changes in the period-specific nonconformance rate, p, between Figure 7.2 and 7.6A, and minor changes in the upper control limit between 7.6 A and B. This first change was the result of the use of the period-specific sample size, n, to calculate p. The center lines are identical since $\bar{p}$ is the same and $\bar{n}$ equals n.

When the control limits are dependent on the sample size, as seen in Table 7.4 (B), the limits narrow as sample size increases and widen when the sample is small, reflecting the fact that information obtained from larger samples is generally more reliable than smaller samples. In this case, the difference between the highest upper limit (obtained when the sample size was 44, in June) and the lowest upper limit (February, when the sample was 55) is only 1.2%.

Table 7.4A Constant Control Limits Based on Average Sample Size

Month	Errors	n	p	Ctr Line	UCLp	LCLp
Jan	2	45	0.0444	0.0683	0.1754	0.0000
Feb	3	55	0.0545	0.0683	0.1754	0.0000
Mar	1	50	0.0200	0.0683	0.1754	0.0000
Apr	2	48	0.0417	0.0683	0.1754	0.0000
May	3	52	0.0577	0.0683	0.1754	0.0000
Jun	1	44	0.0227	0.0683	0.1754	0.0000
Jul	11	52	0.2115	0.0683	0.1754	0.0000
Aug	7	53	0.1321	0.0683	0.1754	0.0000
Sep	5	51	0.0980	0.0683	0.1754	0.0000
Oct	2	48	0.0417	0.0683	0.1754	0.0000
Nov	3	52	0.0577	0.0683	0.1754	0.0000
Dec	1	50	0.0200	0.0683	0.1754	0.0000
Total	41	600				
Average	3.417	50				

Table 7.4B Variable Control Limits Based on Period-Specific Sample Size

Month	Errors	n	p	Ctr Line	UCL	LCL	
Jan	2	45	0.0444	0.0683	0.1812	0.0000	
Feb	3	55	0.0545	0.0683	0.1704	0.0000	Min
Mar	1	50	0.0200	0.0683	0.1754	0.0000	
Apr	2	48	0.0417	0.0683	0.1776	0.0000	
May	3	52	0.0577	0.0683	0.1733	0.0000	
Jun	1	44	0.0227	0.0683	0.1824	0.0000	Max
Jul	11	52	0.2115	0.0683	0.1733	0.0000	
Aug	7	53	0.1321	0.0683	0.1723	0.0000	
Sep	5	51	0.0980	0.0683	0.1743	0.0000	
Oct	2	48	0.0417	0.0683	0.1776	0.0000	
Nov	3	52	0.0577	0.0683	0.1733	0.0000	
Dec	1	50	0.0200	0.0683	0.1754	0.0000	
Total	41	600					
Average	3.417	50					

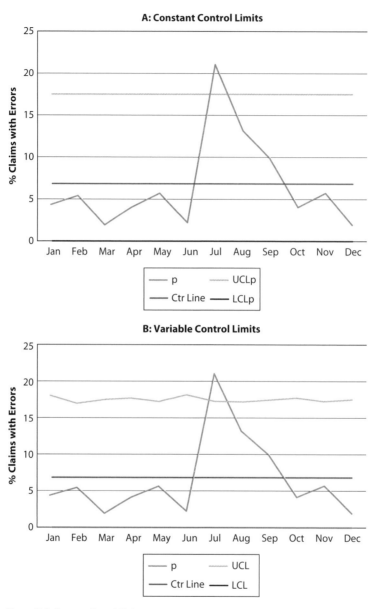

Figure 7.6 Constant Control Limits

The only difference between Figure 7.6 A and 7.6 B is the UCL, which is narrower when sample size is large and wider when the sample is small. The choice of how to handle nonconstant samples is left to the user. Users who believe that presenting employees with consistent performance targets is preferable may wish to use the average sample size. Those desiring greater accuracy or those who have large swings in sample size may elect to incorporate the period-specific sample size into their control limit calculations. Constant and variable limits will reach the same conclusion on performance in the majority of cases.

Rebasing Control Limits and Monitoring Changes over Time

The goal of quality management is to improve performance. If this is achieved, historical control limits will be outdated. If nonconformance rates have been systematically reduced, new sample statistics will consistently fall below the historical center line, indicating a change in the process. As a process is improved, it would be inappropriate to judge current performance against the standards established before improvement occurred. Once improvement is achieved, expectations and standards should be raised, and employees must be diligent to ensure that performance does not revert to preimprovement levels. **Rebasing** control limits provides employees with the tool to identify declining performance and undertake prompt corrective action.

Rebasing recalculation of control limits to recognize changes in process capability

One of the standards for treating AMI is that patients should be given aspirin within two hours of arriving for treatment unless contraindicated. A hospital has recognized that it can improve its delivery of cardiac care without substantially increasing expenses by adhering to this practice standard and has set a target of 95% compliance. The manager of cardiac care has collected aspirin administration data over 16 months—8 months prior to emphasizing the standard and 8 months after. Table 7.5 displays the data.

Table 7.5 Aspirin Administration among AMI Patients

Month	Not Given	N	p	Ctr Line	UCL	LCL
Jan	2	10	0.2000	0.1688	0.5241	0.0000
Feb	3	10	0.3000	0.1688	0.5241	0.0000
Mar	2	10	0.2000	0.1688	0.5241	0.0000
Apr	4	10	0.4000	0.1688	0.5241	0.0000
May	3	10	0.3000	0.1688	0.5241	0.0000
Jun	3	10	0.3000	0.1688	0.5241	0.0000
Jul	2	10	0.2000	0.1688	0.5241	0.0000
Aug	3	10	0.3000	0.1688	0.5241	0.0000
Sep	1	10	0.1000	0.1688	0.5241	0.0000
Oct	0	10	0.0000	0.1688	0.5241	0.0000
Nov	1	10	0.1000	0.1688	0.5241	0.0000
Dec	1	10	0.1000	0.1688	0.5241	0.0000
Jan	0	10	0.0000	0.1688	0.5241	0.0000
Feb	1	10	0.1000	0.1688	0.5241	0.0000
Mar	0	10	0.0000	0.1688	0.5241	0.0000
Apr	1	10	0.1000	0.1688	0.5241	0.0000
Total	27	160				

The table shows on average that 16.88% (27 ÷ 160) of patients did not receive aspirin within two hours of arrival over the 16-month period. The control limits indicate that a stable process will occasionally experience periods where up to 52.41% of patients may not receive aspirin within two hours. The system may be stable, but when it operates at a level where more than half its patients might not receive care according to generally accepted medical practice, it is not meeting the goal of the organization. Figure 7.7 graphs performance and the control limits.

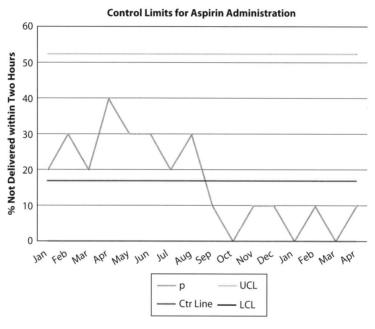

Figure 7.7 p Chart for Aspirin Delivery to AMI Patients

Figure 7.7 indicates that performance is within the established control limits before and after aspirin delivery was emphasized. On first inspection, it may appear the system has not changed. Closer examination reveals that after initiation of the aspirin program in September, the averages for all eight samples are under the center line, indicating a change in the process. To determine the magnitude of the change and the implication for future operations, control limits were recalculated for January through August 2008 (before the change) and September 2008 through April 2009 (after the change).

From January through August 2008 the average number of patients who did not receive aspirin within two hours of arrival was 27.5% (22 ÷ 80).

This is substantially higher than the 16.88% calculated over the entire 16 month period. The UCL is also higher:

$$0.2750 + 3 \times \sqrt{0.2750 \times (1 - 0.2750)/10} = 0.6986$$

From September 2008 through April 2009, after the treatment rule was emphasized, the average number of patients who did not receive aspirin within two hours was 6.25% (5 ÷ 80) and the UCL is lower:

$$0.0625 + 3 \times \sqrt{0.0625 \times (1 - 0.0625)/10} = 0.2914$$

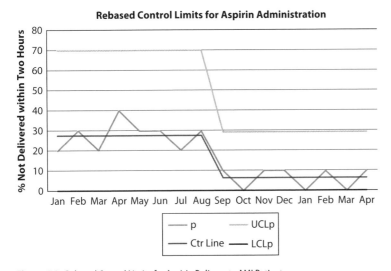

Figure 7.8 Rebased Control Limits for Aspirin Delivery to AMI Patients

Figure 7.8 differentiates the phases of the process before and after initiation of the aspirin program. Before the program began, approximately one in four patients did not receive aspirin within two hours; afterward only six of every 100 did not. The chart with rebased control limits demonstrates that the process was stable before and after the program. In both periods, actual performance revolves around the center line without breaching the control limits or exhibiting any pattern.

The implications of rebasing the control limits with the narrower limits calculated after the program began will require investigation whenever a sample of ten finds three or more patients do not receive aspirin. Under the original limits, investigation would not start until a sample identified six or more missed aspirin administrations. The tighter limits should ensure the improvements achieved are not lost by slippages in performance. The goal of the organization was 95% compliance, so the nonconformance rate of

6.25% indicates that the organization still is above its target. Since the process is stable, further reductions to the nonconformance rate will require a total process review since special cause variation has been eliminated.

Cases and Applications

SPC and Cardiac Rehabilitation Guidelines: Application 1

Peek, Goud, and Abu-Hanna (2008) used SPC to examine adherence to practice guidelines in cardiac rehabilitation. Guideline adherence covers a multitude of medical services over an extended time period, so their first task was to define adherence. The guideline they selected prescribed exercise, relaxation, education, and lifestyle change therapy for patients. Their study included 3,957 patients and eight clinics—five clinics (the intervention groups) began using practice guidelines software and three control groups did not.

The motivation for the study was the introduction of the computerized decision support system in the five intervention clinics. The research question was: Would guideline adherence be greater in the clinics using the new software? P charts demonstrated that adherence increased, but that there was a gradual drop in adherence over time. After the software was installed, three clinics reported higher patient adherence to exercise therapy; however, only one of the three clinics demonstrating higher adherence had installed the software.

Five clinics reported higher patient adherence to relaxation therapy, but only two of these clinics had installed the software, whereas all three control clinics had higher patient adherence. Two clinics experienced reduced adherence to relaxation therapy, and both decreases occurred in the clinics introducing the software. One control clinic saw higher adherence in education while two intervention clinics and one control clinic saw declines. Increases in patient adherence to recommended lifestyle changes occurred in two of the control clinics only.

The Peek et al. study documented little improvement in guideline adherence arising from the introduction of practice guidelines software; in fact the control clinics demonstrated better patient adherence across all four measures. The study documented declining patient adherence over time, noting a common problem with quality improvement: initiatives are often enthusiastically embraced, but compliance and effectiveness decline with time. Both results need to be stressed: first, programs designed to improve quality may not achieve the desired results, and second, early gains may be lost as the novelty of an initiative fades.

SPC and Thyroid Surgery Complications: Application 2

Duclos et al. (2009) used p charts to monitor the outcome of thyroid surgery. Their variables of interest included complications after surgery involving recurrent laryngeal nerve palsy and hypocalcemia. Their research question was: Would the introduction of control charts reduce the rate of postsurgical complications? They studied 1,114 surgeries between January 2006 and December 2007. They found no significant change in the rate of recurrent laryngeal nerve palsy. In the base period, 2004–2005, this complication occurred in 6.4% of patients. After control charts were introduced, the rate of complication increased to 7.4%. They attributed the lack of significant change to the fact that dissection of the recurrent laryngeal nerve is a long-standing technique that "can be performed easily because of an almost uniform anatomy across patients."

On the other hand, they documented a 35.3% reduction in the rate of hypocalcemia, which they attributed to greater variability in practice (more opportunity for improvement), the Hawthorne effect (alteration of physicians' performance due only to the process of being observed), or feedback. The ability of SPC to identify real-time changes in performance was demonstrated. In July 2007 the rate of recurrent laryngeal nerve palsy exceeded a warning limit (a warning limit is lower than a traditional control limit and acts as an early warning system), while the rate of hypocalcemia exceeded a control limit.

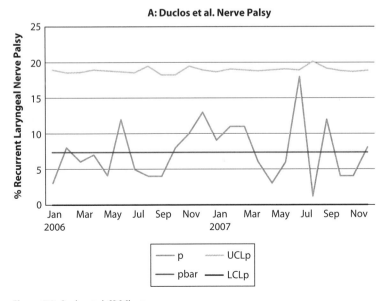

Figure 7.9 Duclos et al. SPC Charts

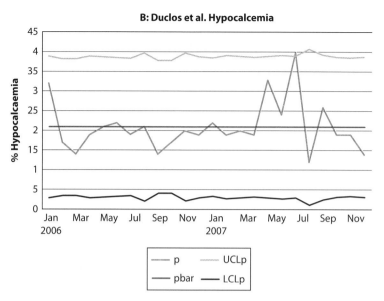

Figure 7.9 Continued

The breaches in July 2007 were traced back to OR renovations that reduced available operating time by 23.8% and the absence of one surgeon. The authors note that patient volumes did not decrease, so all surgeries had to be performed by a single physician. This study was interesting as the researchers established warning limits at two standard deviations, rather than the typical three standard deviations to identify special cause variation, to recognize change sooner.

The adaptation of SPC highlights the fact that SPC can be and is modified to meet the needs and objectives of its users. The increase in postsurgical complications seen in July 2007 attributed to restriction of operating time and the absence of one physician suggests a simple solution. Elective surgeries should not be scheduled when resources are strained because excessive workloads performed under time constraints may lead to higher rates of complications.

SPC and Emergency Room Services: Application 3

In a program to improve quality in emergency room services, Schwab et al. (1999) decided to track the percentage of patients who left without being seen (LWBS). The percentage of LWBS patients is an indicator of dissatisfaction with waiting times and a potential legal risk. During their base period, January 1990 through April 1995, 11.56% of patients left without being seen, with an UCL of 21.76% and LCL of 1.36%. The system was deemed stable as the p chart did not indicate any instances of special cause variation.

To reduce waiting time and the rate of LWBS, four interventions were introduced: establishment of a specimen transport timer, modification to the medical consult procedure, designation of a staff nurse to control ER admissions and discharges, and assignment of patients to specific physicians. The modifications were introduced from August 1995 through July 1996. After their introduction, 6.88% of patients left without being seen, a reduction of 40.5%. A new UCL was established at 14.75%, and LCL was set to 0.00%. While all the points in the postintervention period fell between the control limits established in the base period, the percentage of LWBS patients in the intervention period was always below the center line, indicating that the interventions reduced the percentage of LWBS patients. This article demonstrates how SPC can be applied to a stable system to document whether clinical operational changes improved care processes.

SPC and Anesthesia Administration: Application 4

Fasting and Gisvold (2003) sought to measure the performance of and improve the quality of an anesthesia process by tracking four types of adverse events: inadequate analgesia during brachial plexus block, emergence from general anesthesia, intubation problems, and medication errors. They examined 65,170 events between 1997 and 2001 and identified adverse events in 18.3% of cases, mostly of lesser severity.

The rate of difficulty in emerging from general anesthesia was deemed too high and a change from long-term to intermediate-acting muscular relaxants was introduced in the first quarter of 1999. The rate of difficulty in the base period, January 1997 through April 1999, was 2.98%. After the switch to intermediate-acting muscular relaxants, the rate was reduced to 2.08%, a reduction of 30.2%. Their p chart demonstrated that there was a significant change in the process. Before the change all but 2 (of 13) points were above the center line. After the change only 3 (of 16) were at or above the mean. Because of the improvement in the process, control chart limits were recalculated based on the improvement in the process.

For the other three adverse events—inadequate analgesia during brachial plexus block ($\bar{p} = 16.1\%$ (358/2,228)), intubation problems ($\bar{p} = 1.5\%$ (429/28,081)), and medication errors ($\bar{p} = 0.12\%$ (81/65,173))—the control charts indicated that the processes were stable from 1997 through 2001. Fasting and Gisvold provide a candid and insightful study of anesthesia care; in their conclusion they note their success in reducing difficulties in emerging from anesthesia and the continuing challenge to supply adequate brachial plexus blocks. The rate of inadequate brachial plexus blocks was recorded to be 16.1%, which was higher than other published studies, but the system was stable. The use of SPC in this study demonstrated

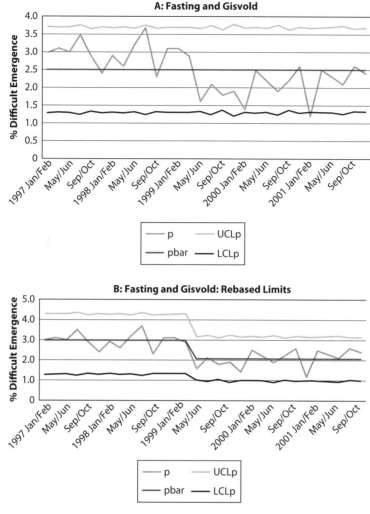

Figure 7.10 Fasting and Gisvold SPC Charts

to providers that they could improve patient outcomes and it encouraged them to tackle more challenging issues.

These four applications—cardiac rehabilitation guideline adherence, thyroid surgery, emergency services, and anesthesia—demonstrate the versatility of p charts. Duclos et al., Schwab et al., and Fasting and Gisvold documented successful changes in medical operations built on SPC. All four articles, including Peek, Goud, and Abu-Hanna's, demonstrate the need to document processes, identify whether a process is stable, and investigate system performance when special cause variation is present. In each case, the introduction of SPC led to a greater understanding of the health care delivery process.

Improving Performance Using SPC

The primary function of SPC is to identify special cause variation, that is, identifying when performance significantly differs from historical performance. Special cause variations are typically indicated by a breach of a control limit. However, users must recognize that trends and patterns may also indicate systemic change. The goal of SPC should be to maintain system stability, and SPC can be used as an early warning system to identify undesirable changes in performance before control limits are breached and patients may be harmed.

If special cause variation is identified, the task of the user is to determine if it can be eliminated. When a user monitors performance in real time, SPC can assist in identifying causes. Investigations should be easier when significant deviations in performance can be promptly identified and operating conditions are fresh in employees' minds. Employees should not have to reconstruct events. When the event is current, they should be able to identify manpower, materials, machines, methods, and environmental conditions that were present when the deviation occurred. After the cause of the deviation is determined, employees must work to eliminate it. If the cause can be eliminated, the organization should rebase the control limits to establish tighter operating parameters.

If the process is stable when data is initially collected or is made stable by the elimination of special cause variation, the organization is at a position where it can manage the process according to the control limits established while the process was stable. Once a system is stable and predictable, users can identify when the process encounters a problem (a breach or pattern) or is heading towards a problem (a trend) by real-time plotting of new data. The real-time plotting of data and identification of problems or potential problems should enhance employees' ability to avoid performance issues or to reduce the length of time performance issues persist.

Following the precepts of continuous quality improvement, organizations should not be content with current performance but continually seek opportunities for improvement. A stable system provides a baseline to introduce and test improvements to a process. SPC can determine if improvements have produced the intended result. Was there a change in the process and have the center line or control limits been reduced? If successful, the improvement should be instituted across the organization and new control limits introduced. Whether successful or unsuccessful, the organization should continue to seek ways of improving its performance and increasing the satisfaction of its patients. The goal of every organization should be to improve its performance (reduce nonconformance rate or increase conformance rates) and provide greater consistency. SPC provides the center line and control limits as an easy-to-understand barometer of each goal.

Summary

This chapter demonstrated how data that cannot be measured on a continuous scale can be monitored using SPC. The chapter focused on events that occur or do not occur or outcomes that meet or do not meet expectations. For either goal, those attempting to improve outcomes must track nonconformance rates using p charts or the number of nonconforming events using np charts. In Chapter Six, performance issues were identified by one or more breaches of a control limit. Chapter Seven introduced four other situations—trends, patterns, a series of points above or below the center line, or a series of points close to a control limit—that could indicate performance problems.

A key issue in managing the use of SPC is determining whether the control limits are valid. Valid control limits require the process under review to be subject to only natural variation. The presence of special cause variation increases variation and results in inflated nonconformance rates and wide control limits. When a process is subject to both natural and special cause variation, its outcomes cannot be predicted. Before valid control limits can be calculated, special cause variation must be eliminated and the process must be measured under normal operating conditions. When a process is subject to only natural variation, we can predict its outcomes, identify when performance is inconsistent with historical performance, and know when investigation and potential corrective action are needed.

The distinction between natural and special cause variation is critical to quality management, as the goal of quality improvement is to fundamentally change systems to improve performance. When an organization has improved a process, control limits should be rebased to reflect its new level of performance to ensure that the system is not allowed to return to its former lower level of conformance or higher rate of variation. SPC's emphasis on measurement focuses provider attention on a specific goal and, when combined with performance standards achieved by industry leaders, can motivate everyone in the organization to higher effort as the goal and performance are clear to everyone.

KEY TERMS

Binomial data	p chart
Conformance	Pattern
Gaming the data	Rebasing
Historical probability	Trend
Nonconformance	Variable control limits
np chart	

REVIEW QUESTIONS

1. Name the five conditions that indicate a process may be unstable.

2. If control limits are not valid due to the presence of special cause variation, how can valid control limits be established?

3. Describe the difference between constant and variable control limits.

4. When can an np chart rather than a p chart be used to monitor system performance? What advantages does an np chart have over a p chart?

5. When should control limits be recalculated or rebased?

6. Explain the three ways SPC can be used to improve performance.

PROBLEMS

1. A hospital is analyzing nosocomial infections and wants to reduce their infection rate below the national average of 2.0%. They have sampled 40 cases every week for the last 20 weeks. The data are shown below. Create p and np control charts. Interpret the graphs. How is the hospital performing in relation to its stated goal?

Sample	Infections	Sample	Infections
1	2	11	3
2	1	12	4
3	1	13	2
4	2	14	3
5	1	15	4
6	1	16	5
7	3	17	3
8	2	18	4
9	1	19	5
10	2	20	6

2. Walter Shewhart ([1931] 1980) presented the following data in his classic *Economic Control of Quality of Manufactured Product*. Create a p chart for each machine. Does either of the two machines show evidence of special cause variation?

Month	MACHINE A Defective	MACHINE A Inspected	MACHINE B Defective	MACHINE B Inspected
Jan	4	527	1	169
Feb	5	610	3	99
Mar	5	428	1	208
Apr	2	400	1	196
May	15	498	1	132
Jun	3	500	1	89
Jul	3	395	1	167
Aug	2	393	2	200
Sep	3	625	1	171
Oct	13	465	1	122
Nov	5	446	3	107
Dec	3	510	1	132
Average	5.25	483.08	1.42	149.33

3. From January 1846 through December 1848 Semmelweis ([1860] 1983) recorded births and the number that resulted in the death of the mother at his hospital. The data is available in the Chapter07.xls file, in the Problem07–03 tab. Create a p chart to analyze performance. Interpret the chart. Was the system stable?

4. Postsurgical infections have been reported to affect 2% to 5% of the 16 million patients who undergo surgery in U.S. hospitals. Infections increase the chance of complications and death. Antibiotics given one hour prior to surgery have been shown to reduce the probability of infection. The director of quality improvement has sampled 20 patients per week over the preceding 25 weeks. The data is available in the Chapter07.xls file in the Problem07–04 tab. The data collected records whether a patient contracted an infection after surgery. Create a p chart to analyze performance. Interpret the hospital's performance based on your control chart and identify any issues that should be investigated. Assuming the average rate of infection is 3.5%, is the hospital doing a good job?

5. Readmission rates within one year for congestive heart failure have been documented at 35%. A local heart program wants to assess its performance against this standard. The program has randomly selected ten patients per month over a 24-month period for review. The data is available in the Chapter07.xls file, in the Problem07–05 tab. Some of the patients were deleted from the sample due to death, relocation, or other reasons that preclude follow-up. Create a p chart. Is the process stable? How is the program performing relative to the documented standard? Since not all months have 10 observations, either use 10 as the sample size or use the average sample size to calculate the control limits.

References

(BTS) Bureau of Transportation Statistics, 2013, Airline On-Time Performance and Causes of Flight Delays, http://www.bts.gov/help/aviation/index .html#q8, accessed May 25, 2013.

Duclos A, Touzet S, Soardo P, Colin C, Peix JL, and Lifante JC, 2009, Quality Monitoring in Thyroid Surgery Using the Shewhart Control Chart, *British Journal of Surgery* 96: 171–174.

Fasting S and Gisvold S, 2003, Statistical Process Control Methods Allow the Analysis and Improvement of Anesthesia Care, *Canadian Journal of Anesthesia* 50: 767–774.

Juran JM and Godfrey AB, 1999, *Juran's Quality Handbook*, 5th ed., McGraw-Hill, New York, NY.

Peek N, Goud R, and Abu-Hanna A, 2008, Application of SPC Methods to Monitor Guideline Adherence: A Case Study, *AIMA 2008 Symposium Proceedings*, 581–585.

Schwab RA, DelSorbo SM, Cunningham MR, Craven K, and Watson WA, 1999, Using SPC to Demonstrate the Effect of Operational Interventions on Quality Indicators in the Emergency Department, *Journal of Healthcare Quality* 21 (4): 38–41.

Semmelweis I, (1860) 1983, *The Etiology, Concept, and Prophylaxis of Childbed Fever*, The University of Wisconsin Press, Madison WI. Citations refer to University of Wisconsin edition.

Shewhart, WA, (1931) 1980, *Economic Control of Quality of Manufactured Product*, ASQ Quality Press, Milwaukee, WI. Citations refer to ASQ edition.

CHAPTER 8

STATISTICAL PROCESS CONTROL FOR MONITORING NONCONFORMITIES

Introduction

In Chapter Seven control charts were created for events in which a process or outcome could be judged acceptable or unacceptable based on a single criterion. This chapter explores events in which more than one defect can occur for a single observation and in which the presence of multiple **nonconformities** may not indicate unacceptable or defective output. These types of nonconformities may be of the near-miss or no-harm variety; that is, they may not produce an adverse outcome but may signal system weaknesses that could culminate in patient injury if left uncorrected.

Chapter Seven was primarily devoted to monitoring events that provide prima facie evidence of poor patient outcomes, such as mortality and infection rates. Chapter Eight is devoted to monitoring nonconformities when more than one can arise in a single case. For example, patient falls could be monitored as a binomial event: a patient either falls or does not fall during a hospital stay or visit. A single patient could fall more than once during an episode of care, so treating patient falls as count data adds information that may increase the organization's understanding of the phenomenon and its ability to reduce future occurrences. Knowing how many times a patient falls may allow the organization to identify high-risk patients, locations, and times. Similarly, if a hospital is concerned about the accuracy of its billing process, it could use p or np charts and ask the question whether a bill is correct or wrong. The problem with a correct/incorrect

LEARNING OBJECTIVES

1. Construct and interpret control charts for nonconformities

2. Implement and monitor the Medicare Hospital Quality Initiative

3. Choose the appropriate control chart for a process

4. Understand the benefits of SPC

5. Identify and overcome the barriers to the use of SPC

6. Identify which processes should be monitored using SPC

7. Understand the difference between stability and capability

nonconformities
one or more deviations of a product or service from defined standards; nonconformities evaluate products and services against multiple standards versus nonconformance, which evaluates a single attribute

approach is that a single bill could have multiple errors. A single bill could contain incorrect patient or insurance information, missed charges, duplicate charges, charges for services delivered to other patients, or missing or incorrect medical record information.

There is a major difference between having an erroneous bill with a single error and a billing system that generates multiple errors per claim. Counting the number of errors illuminates the magnitude of quality problems and allows users to assess their progress. Imagine the disappointment of employees if successful efforts are made to reduce errors but the p or np chart continues to indicate the same percentage or number of defective events since more than one error was originally present.

J.D. Power's Initial Quality Study for automobiles reported there were an average of 118 problems per 100 vehicles in 2008 (J.D. Power). This means there is more than one problem per vehicle. Buick had 118 problems per 100 vehicles (the industry average), Toyota was among the industry leaders with 104 problems, and Volkswagen underperformed at 128. Substantial improvement could be achieved in the auto industry, but on average each vehicle would still have a problem. If Buick reduced its number of problems by 18 for each 100 vehicles (a 15.3% decrease in problems), it would still report 100 problems per 100 cars, an average of one defect per car. If defective cars rather than errors are recorded, the p chart may not register any change.

c chart
a chart that tracks the number of deviations from defined standards for a constant size sample of products or services and establishes upper and lower control limits

Chapter Eight shifts the focus of quality management from nonconforming units—acceptable or unacceptable output—to nonconformities: How many problems or deficiencies are there in the output? Users must analyze the process and available data to select the control chart that will provide the most support for quality improvement. Similar to tracking nonconformance, two different control charts can be produced based on the sample collected. If the sample size is constant, a **c chart** can be used to track the *number* of nonconformities. If sample size varies, a **u chart** must be used to track the *rate* of nonconformities per unit.

u chart
a chart that tracks the number of deviations per product or service and establishes upper and lower control limits; used when sample size is not constant

Statistical Process Control for Counts: c and u Charts

The process for monitoring the number of nonconformities, in which an individual, item, or event can exhibit more than one problem, uses the same six steps presented for continuous and binomial data (see Table 8.1). As we saw for binominal data, the first three steps again introduce substantial changes in data collection, in the descriptive statistic used, and in control limit formulas. Readers will again benefit from recognizing the similarities in the process while extending their ability to track different types of data with SPC.

Table 8.1 The Six Steps of Statistical Process Control: c and u Charts

1.	Collect data
2.	Calculate descriptive statistics
3.	Calculate control limits
4.	Graph actual and expected performance
5.	Interpret performance
6.	Investigate instability and improve as needed

Step 1: Collect Data

The process for collecting data requires the user to determine the frequency of sampling (daily, weekly, monthly), the sample size (is it a constant number or a percentage of activity?), the procedure for drawing the sample to ensure that it is random, and the personnel responsible for drawing the sample. Juran and Godfrey (1999) note that sample sizes typically are between 50 and 100 observations for attributes and that attribute charts may not be based samples but rather may be based 100% on inspection.

Data collection is more difficult and time consuming when counting nonconformities per unit than determining whether an observation meets a standard. Nonconformity is any deviation in a unit or event from a desired standard. Unlike nonconformance, which is judged against a single criterion, a single observation can have multiple nonconformities, as discussed with billing errors. Before data collection can begin, all potential nonconformities must be defined. After nonconformities are defined, each observation must be thoroughly reviewed to identify and record all deviations, including repeated occurrences of the same nonconformity. Data collection for nonconformities is more labor intensive than collecting nonconformance data; in the latter case a single deviation from a desired standard provides all the information needed for analysis—the observation does not meet the standard. When counting nonconformities, on the other hand, the inspection process must continue until all opportunities in which a deviation from a desired standard could arise are reviewed. After the data is collected, the number of errors and the sample size should be recorded in a spreadsheet.

Step 2: Calculate Descriptive Statistics

Descriptive statistics provide the information to evaluate system performance. For the c chart, the required information is the number of nonconformities that are typically observed in a sample. The c chart, like the np chart, has the advantage that users are working with whole, natural units—the number of nonconformities. A user needs only to count the number of nonconformities in a sample and compare the number to the average nonconformities across multiple samples to gain a general understanding of how a system is performing.

The calculation of the descriptive statistics for counts requires the introduction of new symbols and formulas:

8.1
$$c_i = \text{count of nonconformities in sample i}$$

8.2
$$\bar{c} = \frac{\text{total number of nonconformities}}{\text{total number of samples}}$$

There are times when equal size samples cannot be drawn, so a simple count of nonconformities may not provide accurate information on error occurrence. The expected number of nonconformities per sample, $\bar{c}$, should change proportionately with the number of observations in the sample. Large samples should have more nonconformities than smaller samples. A fixed nonconformity count is therefore inappropriate when sample size varies. The unit of comparison should be the number of nonconformities per unit, which is independent of sample size. If the average number of nonconformities is 118 per 100 autos, then in a sample of 50 we would expect 59 nonconformities; the rate of error in both samples is 1.18 nonconformities per vehicle.

8.3
$$u_i = \text{count of nonconformities per sample}/n_i$$

8.4
$$\bar{u} = \frac{\text{total number of nonconformities}}{\text{total units or events}} = \frac{\sum c}{\sum n}$$

The names of the control charts can again be intuitively tied to their function: the c chart focuses on the count of nonconformities per sample, and the u chart monitors the per-unit rate of nonconformities. The advantage of the c chart over the u chart is that the user does not have to calculate or interpret percentages based on sample size. The advantage of the u chart is ease of comparison across organizations since the per-unit rate is independent of sample size.

Step 3: Calculate Control Limits

The decision to use a c chart or u chart is based on sample size. When the same number of observations are included in every sample drawn, either a c chart or u chart can be created. When sample size varies, the u chart must be used. The c chart tracks the number of nonconformities per sample and it is possible that the number of nonconformities may exceed the sample size. The u chart tracks the number of nonconformities per unit or event, and each unit or event can have more than one nonconformity.

Calculating control limits for c charts or u charts requires two formulas. The good news is that the formulas for the upper and lower limits are the most straightforward of the formulas introduced in Chapters Six through Eight, and like previous formulas the difference between the upper and lower control limits is a simple sign change.

$$\text{UCL}_c = \bar{c} + 3 \times \sqrt{\bar{c}} \qquad\qquad 8.5$$

$$\text{LCL}_c = \bar{c} - 3 \times \sqrt{\bar{c}} \qquad\qquad 8.6$$

The formulas for the u chart limits differ from the c chart by focusing on the number of errors per unit (versus per sample) and the incorporation of the sample size to recognize that sample sizes may be different. The incorporation of the sample size in the denominator shows the control limits will tighten as larger samples are drawn.

$$\text{UCL}_u = \bar{u} + 3 \times \sqrt{\bar{u}/n} \qquad\qquad 8.7$$

$$\text{LCL}_u = \bar{u} - 3 \times \sqrt{\bar{u}/n} \qquad\qquad 8.8$$

Step 4: Graph Actual and Expected Performance

A line chart is again used to visually display the actual number of nonconformities per sample (or per unit) against $\bar{c}$ (or $\bar{u}$), and the control limits indicate the level of variation that will be accepted before investigation is initiated. Monitoring system performance using counts, like binomial events, requires only one chart.

Step 5: Interpret Performance

The goal of step 5 is to determine whether there is a change in system performance that could negatively impact outcomes. Users must analyze the control charts to determine if control limits are breached or if trends, patterns, or series exist.

Step 6: Investigate Instability and Improve as Needed

When special cause variation is identified by control limit breaches, trends, patterns, or a series of points above or below the center line or close to the upper or lower limits, the user must determine if this variation indicates a change in system performance. If it is determined to be a change in system performance, the user must determine the cause and whether it reduces performance and should be eliminated, or improves outcomes and should be preserved.

Medical Record Coding Example

The chief of the medical staff at a hospital is concerned about the accuracy of medical record information and the potential effect on physician revenue. The chief wants the director of medical records to track the total number of documentation errors, including missing, incomplete, or incorrect surgical coding, physician and nursing notes, medication notes, and lab and pathology reports to determine if improvements are needed. Given the multiple errors that can arise in a single record, c and u charts will elicit the greatest amount of information from the data.

Step 1: Collect Data

The director reviewed ten medical records each week over a ten-week period and recorded the number, the count, of errors in an Excel spreadsheet. In the first sample of ten, ten nonconformities per sample (c) were identified, an average of one per medical record (u) (see Table 8.2).

Table 8.2 Medical Record Errors

	Errors per sample (c)	Errors per record (u)
Week 1	10	1.0
Week 2	20	2.0
Week 3	15	1.5
Week 4	12	1.2
Week 5	22	2.2
Week 6	21	2.1
Week 7	18	1.8
Week 8	16	1.6
Week 9	15	1.5
Week 10	14	1.4
Total	163	16.3
Average	16.3	1.63

Step 2: Calculate Descriptive Statistics

The number of nonconformities was summed across the ten samples, resulting in a total of 163 errors. Based on past history, the system is expected to produce 16.3 errors per sample or 1.63 per record.

$$\bar{c} = 163/10 \text{ samples} = 16.3$$

$$\bar{u} = 163/100 \text{ records (10 samples} \times 10 \text{ observations)} = 1.63$$

Step 3: Calculate Control Limits

Given the constant sample size, a c chart or u chart can be used to analyze performance; both approaches will be demonstrated. The control limits for the c charts are calculated as follows:

$$UCL_c = 16.3 + 3 \times \sqrt{16.3} = 28.41$$

$$LCL_c = 16.3 - 3 \times \sqrt{16.3} = 4.19$$

Average performance leads the director to expect 16.3 nonconformities per sample of ten records, and the control limits are established at 12.11 nonconformities above and below the center line. The number of nonconformities in a sample performance can vary from 4.19 to 28.41 before the process will require investigation. While it is easy to see the problem when too many errors are identified, if identified errors fall to 4.0 or less, it may signal a failure to identify and report nonconformities rather than improved performance.

Step 4: Graph Actual and Expected Performance

Figure 8.1 graphs the errors per sample from Table 8.2 with the center line and control limits.

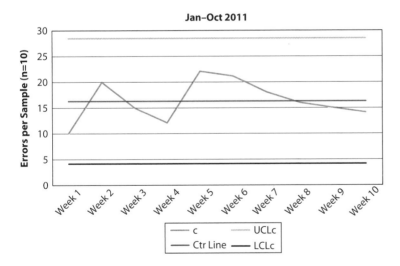

Figure 8.1 c Chart for Medical Record Errors

If the director elected to monitor nonconformities using a u chart, the control limits would be:

$$UCL_u = 16.3 + 3 \times \sqrt{16.3/10} = 2.84$$

$$LCL_u = 16.3 - 3 \times \sqrt{16.3/10} = 0.42$$

Average performance leads the director to expect 1.63 nonconformities per medical record, and the control limits are established at 1.21 nonconformities above and below the center line. The number of nonconformities in a sample performance can vary from 0.42 to 2.84 before the process will require investigation. Figure 8.2 graphs the errors per medical record from Table 8.2 with the center line and control limits.

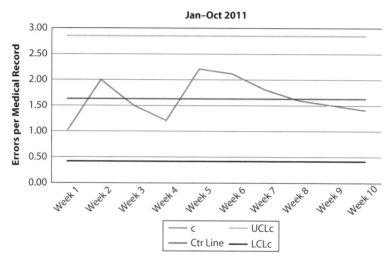

Figure 8.2 u Chart for Medical Record Errors

Step 5: Interpret Performance

The only difference between the c and u charts is the y-axis. The c chart documents errors per sample, and the u chart errors per medical record. The number of errors stays between the upper and lower control limits, but starting in week 5 there is a pronounced downward trend. Given a rule of six points establishing a trend, this series of points indicates a need for investigation. It is hoped that the trend indicates improved coding, but it could also signify missed errors.

Both charts have a nonzero lower control limit, indicating that users must recognize when errors fall significantly below historical performance. An LCL breach, similar to the trend noted above, could signify improvement in the coding process or a problem in the data collection process. The power of SPC is its ability to identify changes in performance. Systems operating at one level of performance, in this example, 1.63 errors per record, are equally unlikely to leap to an error rate of 2.81 errors or more *or* to drop to 0.41 errors or less. Dramatic improvement or deterioration in performance is unlikely without a change in the system.

Step 6: Investigate Instability and Improve as Needed

After investigation, the director concluded that the identified trend reflects improved coding and that no system change is needed. In spite of concluding that no change is required, the director may want to see this trend continue and should attempt to determine what occurred in week 5 that began the downward trend in errors and continued through week 10. If the downward trend continues, the director should recalculate the control limits to institutionalize the improvement. In light of the recent improvement, the hospital still must decide if 16.3 coding errors for every ten records, or 1.63 errors per record, are acceptable. In setting a performance target, the director should consider how the hospital's error rate compares against that of other organizations.

Dietary Concerns Example

The director of nutrition services decided to proactively collect patient complaints about food service at her hospital. The director decided to contact 2.0% of inpatients on a daily basis to record their concerns about the meals they received. The multiple concerns a patient could express (for example, meal is cold, late, unappetizing, did not match the meal order) and the variation in number of patients hospitalized on any given day (the number of complaints should increase as more patients are seen) require that a u chart be used for monitoring.

Step 1: Collect Data

The director surveyed 2% of hospital patients over a 31-day period in December 2009. Patients' concerns over meals were recorded in an Excel spreadsheet. On December 1 six patients were surveyed, and they cited a total of 14 concerns with their meals, or 2.33 concerns per patient (see Table 8.3).

Table 8.3 Dietary Concerns, December 2009

Day	Date	c	n
Tuesday	1	14	6
Wednesday	2	12	6
Thursday	3	15	6
Friday	4	11	5
Saturday	5	12	4
Sunday	6	13	4
Monday	7	14	6
Tuesday	8	13	6
. . .	. . .	. . .	. . .
Thursday	31	11	4
Total		389	157

Step 2: Calculate Descriptive Statistics

A total of 389 concerns were expressed by 157 patients from December 1 through 31, resulting in an average of 2.48 concerns per patient.

$$\bar{u}, \text{ center line} = 389/157 = 2.48$$

The number of concerns ranged from a low of 1.83 per patient on December 16 to a high of 5.00 on December 25.

Step 3: Calculate Control Limits

Given the variable sample size, a u chart must be used to analyze performance. The subscript 1 indicates that these are the control limits for December 1, when six patients were surveyed; other days may have a different sample size based on changes in inpatient occupancy.

$$\text{UCL}_{u1} = 2.48 + 3 \times \sqrt{2.48/6} = 4.41$$

$$\text{LCL}_{u1} = 2.48 - 3 \times \sqrt{2.48/6} = 0.55$$

Average performance demonstrates that the director should expect 2.48 concerns per patient. Normal fluctuation suggests that concerns can vary from 0.55 to 4.41 when six patients are surveyed (n = 6) before the director should investigate. Investigation is warranted if the average number of dietary concerns exceeds 4.41 (too many) or falls below 0.55 (too few). Assuming the rate of nonconformities is relatively constant, the control limits will decrease if more than six patients are surveyed and increase when fewer than six patients are surveyed.

Step 4: Graph Actual and Expected Performance

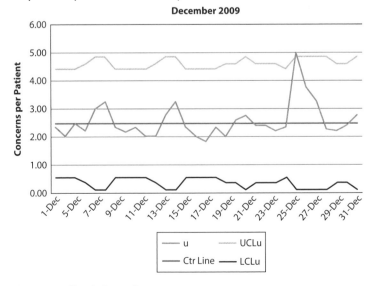

Figure 8.3 u Chart for Dietary Concerns

Step 5: Interpret Performance

The number of concerns stays between the established control limits all month except on December 25 (Christmas), when 5.00 concerns per patient were recorded and the UCL was exceeded. The effect of patient census is easy to see: when census is down and the number of patients surveyed is low, the control limits expand due to the lower accuracy of small samples.

Besides the breach in the upper control limit, a pattern also appears. When inpatient census is down on the weekends, days 5, 6, 12, 13, 19, 20, 26, and 27, the control limits expand and the number of complaints tends to be above the center line.

Step 6: Investigate Instability and Improve as Needed

The breach on December 25 could emanate from patient expectations (patients feel blue since they are hospitalized on Christmas Day, have higher expectations for a holiday meal and a desire for companionship on the holiday), labor (reduced staffing), supplies (since food deliveries do not occur on Christmas Day, perhaps food was stockpiled and spoiled), equipment failure, or an environmental issue.

The higher number of concerns reported on the weekends may emanate from the same factors that caused the higher complaints around Christmas. The recurring nature of a high number of concerns on the weekends presents a more pressing problem as well as an opportunity to identify the cause of the complaints. A once-a-year occurrence or an infrequent problem is by its nature difficult to diagnosis and correct. What set of conditions gave rise to the problem? Additionally, when a solution is formulated and implemented, it could take months or a year to determine if the change was successful. One can think of an infrequent breach of a control limit as a check-engine light that sporadically illuminates but goes off before the car is taken to a mechanic for service.

Weekly occurrences provide the opportunity to identify frequently recurring events and compare a process that meets expectations (meal delivery Monday through Friday) with one that does not meet expectations (meal delivery on Saturday and Sunday). Each week provides a case study to theorize why the two processes are achieving different levels of performance. In addition, corrections can be tested rapidly to determine whether the solution reduced the number of concerns reported or was ineffectual. Recurring events provide the opportunity to fully implement the PDCA cycle and continuous quality improvement.

The medical records and dietary examples have taken the reader through the SPC process. There are two important points to note: one, the process of establishing control limits and tracking performance is straightforward and strictly defined, steps 1 through 4; and two, the output of the defined portion provides direction only to the more challenging part of the process. Steps 1 through 4 provide definitive answers: What is performance, within what limits should a stable system operate, and is there a limit breach, trend, pattern, or series? While definitive numbers can be produced, we cannot conclude based on the numbers alone whether a system is operating at an acceptable level.

Step 5, interpret performance, and step 6, investigate and improve as needed, move the user from science and mathematics into art and insight. Where SPC provides clear signals of instability, investigation and improvement require insight into the goals sought and the behavior of people and systems. In the real world, managers must deal with conflicting goals and deviant behavior that is frequently removed from theoretical models of how systems should operate. In the dietary example, the breach of the control limit was clear, but as discussed in Chapter Seven identifying trends and patterns requires understanding the data and the process. After identifying a breach of the UCL and a pattern of higher concerns on the weekends, the manager must determine whether this indicates subpar performance or higher patient expectations on the weekend. Imagination is needed in interpreting performance and identifying the potential causes of unstable performance, while fixing problems requires the ability to motivate and direct groups of people toward a goal.

Is the breach on Christmas Day or the higher concerns reported on weekends remediable? Does it reflect a food service issue or another issue? If it is a food service issue, what will be required to improve service? Is it a matter of ensuring that weekday procedures are followed on the weekends, or are additional resources needed on weekends? If additional resources are needed, is the organization willing to commit more resources? If corrections are needed, how will they be implemented, what controls will be introduced to ensure procedures are followed, and what incentives will employees have for incorporating the new routines into their work?

Medicare Hospital Quality Initiative Example

The two previous examples dealt with relatively homogenous events, but c and u charts can also be used to monitor dissimilar activities. Clinical practice guidelines specify a wide range of activity, ranging from observation to surgery to discharge instructions. What providers need to know is how closely these guidelines are being followed. Defining and tracking the dozens or hundreds of activities specified in a guideline would be an arduous task. The Medicare Hospital Quality Initiative provides an opportunity to use c and u charts to monitor the delivery of a variety of medical activities.

The Medicare Hospital Quality Initiative prescribes nine measures for treating acute myocardial infarction (AMI): aspirin at arrival, aspirin prescribed at discharge, ACE inhibitor for left ventricular systolic dysfunction, smoking cessation, beta blocker at arrival, beta blocker prescribed at discharge, fibrinolytic therapy within 30 minutes of arrival, PCI within 90 minutes of arrival, and 30-day mortality. All of these measures can be monitored using p or np charts to determine whether the treatment was delivered or the patient survived. Those whose effectiveness depend on timeliness of delivery, aspirin at arrival, beta blocker at arrival, fibrinolytic therapy and PCI, can be monitored using $\bar{X}$ and R charts. However, to obtain an overview of AMI treatment, a c chart or u chart could be used. Data on all nine measures could be collected, and a c chart on the first eight process measures created. The mortality rate (a dichotomous outcome measure) is best monitored using p or np chart and should not be incorporated into a c chart or u chart that tracks process measures.

Step 1: Collect Data

The first step in monitoring AMI treatment would be to create a check sheet based on the Medicare measures. The check sheet is an easy-to-use tool to record whether treatment was received within the prescribed time period. Second, three decisions must be made: the number of patients to review (five randomly selected patients), the frequency with which reviews will be conducted (monthly), and the personnel responsible for data collection. The last step is to collect and record the data (Figure 8.4 and Table 8.4).

Step 2: Calculate Descriptive Statistics

The check sheet in Figure 8.4 provides a wealth of information. Summing the check marks indicates that on average 6.2 or 77.5% (31/40) of the recommended eight treatments were provided. Summing the individual rows shows that the hospital consistently delivered aspirin prescriptions at discharge, ACE inhibitors for left ventricular systolic dysfunction, beta blockers at arrival, beta blocker prescriptions at discharge, and PCI within 90 minutes of arrival; all five patients received each treatment. The obvious problems are the lack of timely delivery of fibrinolytic therapy (only one patient received) and smoking cessation counseling (only two received).

Summing the individual columns shows that patient #1 received all eight of the recommended treatments whereas the other four patients received between five and six of the recommend treatments. The recognition that certain patients received all the recommended care provides a starting point for exploring why others, such as patient #4, did not receive a significant amount of care. Are the differences in the delivery of care due to the patient care team, the condition of the patient, their arrival time for treatment, or other factors?

Sample 1, Date: MM/DD/YYYY

Process Measure:	Pat #1	Pat #2	Pat #3	Pat #4	Pat #5	Total
1. Aspirin at arrival	√		√		√	3
2. Aspirin prescribed at discharge	√	√	√	√	√	5
3. ACE inhibitor for left ventricular sys. dys.	√	√	√	√	√	5
4. Smoking cessation	√	√				2
5. Beta blocker at arrival	√	√	√	√	√	5
6. Beta blocker prescribed at discharge	√	√	√	√	√	5
7. Fibrinolytic therapy within 30 min. of arrival	√					1
8. PCI within 90 minutes of arrival	√	√	√	√	√	5
Total	**8**	**6**	**6**	**5**	**6**	**31**

√: delivered, not required (e.g. nonsmoker), or contraindicated

Outcome Measure:	Pat #1	Pat #2	Pat #3	Pat #4	Pat #5	Total
30-day mortality	√	√	√	√	√	5

√ : survived.

Figure 8.4 Check Sheet for AMI Treatment

Step 3: Calculate Control Limits

The calculated center line across samples shows that the hospital, on average, delivers 90% of the recommended Medicare treatments, or an average of four treatments are missed for every 40 recommended interventions. The formulas for the control limits, $4 \pm 3 \times \sqrt{4}$, show that acceptable variation will be six treatments above or below the average number of missed treatments. The lower limit $(4 - 6)$ is set to zero, while the "acceptable" number of missed treatments is ten $(4 + 6)$. The c chart will conclude that the system is stable if missed treatments amount to 25% or less of the recommended treatments when the mean number of nonconformities equals 10%.

Step 4: Graph Actual and Expected Performance

Table 8.4 records the number of nonconformities and the calculated center line and control limits from which the control chart is created.

Table 8.4 AMI Treatment, January 2011–August 2012

Sample	Conformities	Nonconformities (c)	Center Line	UCL$_c$	LCL$_c$
Jan 2011	31	9	4	10	0
Feb	39	1	4	10	0
Mar	37	3	4	10	0
Apr	33	7	4	10	0
May	35	5	4	10	0
Jun	35	5	4	10	0
Jul	34	6	4	10	0
Aug	37	3	4	10	0
Sep	39	1	4	10	0
Oct	35	5	4	10	0
Nov	38	2	4	10	0
Dec	34	6	4	10	0
Jan 2012	36	4	4	10	0
Feb	36	4	4	10	0
Mar	38	2	4	10	0
Apr	34	6	4	10	0
May	35	5	4	10	0
Jun	39	1	4	10	0
Jul	38	2	4	10	0
Aug	37	3	4	10	0
Average	36	4			

Step 5: Interpret Performance

The c chart in Figure 8.5 demonstrates that the system is stable. None of the data points exceeds the UCL. They lie around the center line, and no trend, pattern, or series is evident.

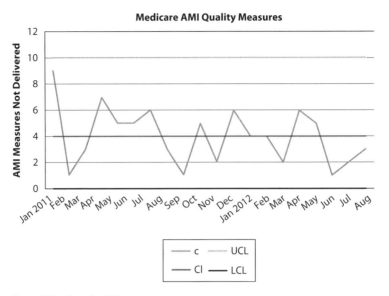

Figure 8.5 c Chart for AMI Treatment

Step 6: Investigate Instability and Improve as Needed

No investigation is needed, but the control chart and the check sheet together are powerful tools for assessing performance. First, the control chart provides an early warning system to identify significant changes in performance to allow rapid investigation of potentially unstable and undesirable situations. Second, as demonstrated in step 2 (calculate descriptive statistics), if an unstable situation is identified, the potential causes of the situation can be traced back to a specific period, a treatment, or a patient by using the check sheets. The user can determine if an undesirable situation is driven by a single cause or an across-the-board failure.

SPC combined with check sheets allow users to determine if unstable performance is due to sporadic delivery of care across all recommended interventions, systematic failure for one or more interventions, or systematic failure for one or more patients. The ability to track nonconformities back to patients provides the ability to determine if extraordinary circumstances surrounding one or more patients produced a breach of a control limit. In the hypothesized example, if a single patient did not receive any of the eight recommended treatments, the organization is 80% of the way to breaching the upper control limit (since only ten missed treatments are necessary to reach the upper limit).

Tracking nonconformities back to specific interventions allows the user to pinpoint where correction is made. Based on sample 1, the employees and process for delivering fibrinolytic therapy and smoking cessation counseling must be examined. The ability to pinpoint correction will simplify and facilitate change because the entire process and all involved employees will not require attention.

Perhaps the most difficult case for correction is when there is no pattern to the nonconformities. If no specific intervention is consistently missed and nondelivery cannot be traced to a specific patient, sample, or group of care givers, the quality improvement team must examine the entire process to determine where attention must be given to improve care.

The goal of using a c chart or a u chart to track the performance of a treatment process encompassing various activities is to establish a holistic monitoring system. This system may not generate intense opposition since it is a composite of various activities. No single employee or group of employees should feel they have been singled out for unwarranted attention. The control chart will provide an overview to all employees involved in care, may focus their attention on the measured activities, and allow them to instigate changes when they see opportunities for improvement. Finally, if the control chart identifies declining performance, other quality tools can be implemented and the justification for enhanced monitoring will be clear.

Cases and Applications

SPC and MRSA: Application 1

Curran et al. (2008) sought to determine if introducing SPC feedback and other diagnostic tools to nursing units could reduce the methicillin-resistant *Staphylococcus aureus* (MRSA) infection rate. They studied 75 wards at 24 hospitals in the United Kingdom over 49 months: 25 months prior to introduction of SPC feedback and 24 months after introduction. A prior article documented that MRSA infections had increased from fewer than 100 cases in 1992 to almost 900 in 1999 at four Glasgow hospitals (Curran, Benneyan, and Hood 2002). The introduction of an SPC feedback program coincided with a 50% reduction in the MRSA infection rate. The 75 studied wards were divided into three groups. One group received SPC charts documenting the MRSA infection rate and diagnostic tools including cause and effect diagrams and Pareto charts. The second group received only SPC charts, and the third received no new information.

C charts were used to record the number of MRSA infections per ward per month, which were subsequently distributed monthly to each unit. At the end of the study, the MRSA infection rate had fallen by 19.6% in the SPC-plus-tools wards, 32.3% in the SPC group, and 23.1% in the control group. Figure 8.6 records performance for one ward that received SPC charts and diagnostic tools. There was no statistically significant difference in the reduction of infection rates between experimental and control groups. The wards receiving only SPC feedback had greater reductions in their infection rates than the group receiving the greatest support, SPC plus diagnostic tools.

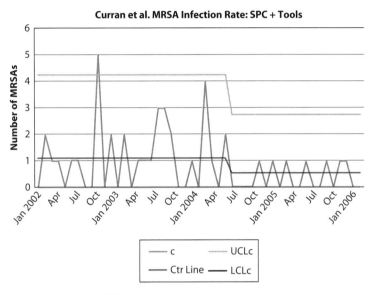

Figure 8.6 Curran et al. SPC Chart

Although there was no significant difference in the rate of reduction between wards, there was a significant reduction in infection rates in all groups. As seen in Figure 8.6, the reductions were large enough to require recalculation of the control limits in each group. As noted in Chapter Seven, a change in a process can be assumed when a series of points falls below the center line; the majority of postfeedback infection counts in Figure 8.6 fell below the preintervention center line. Given the lack of difference in the rate of MRSA infection reductions across units, the authors suggest that the reductions may have occurred due to "unprecedented government and media focus on healthcare-associated infections" that occurred while the study was taking place. A Hawthorne effect was also predicted, but the researchers deemed it unlikely to be sustained over a two-year period. A third possibility is that simple feedback was sufficient to drive the reductions. While the reduction in infection rates in the control units clearly clouds the relationship between the use of SPC and the lower infection rates, health care providers should embrace the fact that infections rates declined by 19.6% to 32.3% while control charts were in use.

SPC and a Public Health Outbreak: Application 2

Walberg, Frøslie, and Røislien (2008) were concerned by the slow reaction of Norwegian public health officials to an outbreak of *Pseudomonas aeruginosa* in 2001–2002. Their goal was to determine whether control charts could have led to more rapid detection of the outbreak. The c chart in Figure 8.7 was constructed using the number of infected patients per month for Asker and Baerum Hospital, and it showed a breach of the upper control limit in January 2002, signaling a significant change in the rate of infection.

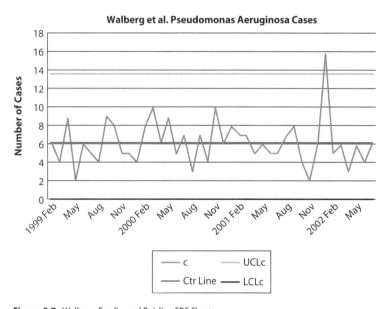

Figure 8.7 Walberg, Frøslie, and Røislien SPC Chart

The Norwegian National Public Health Institute did not declare the outbreak until mid-March 2002. Early detection combined with rapid and effective correction may have saved some of the 71 patients who died out of the 231 infected during the outbreak. The cause of the outbreak was eventually traced to contaminated mouth swabs, in April 2002. While a c chart would have identified the outbreak five weeks earlier than the official warning, the authors demonstrated that use of a g chart, examining days between event (not discussed in this text), would have identified the outbreak nine weeks earlier than when it was officially declared. For rare events, the g chart measures the time between one occurrence and the next, and if special cause variation has entered a system, the time between events will significantly increase or decrease. The bottom line from this study is either a c chart or a g chart would have reduced the time necessary to identify the outbreak and may have reduced the number of infections and deaths that arose from the outbreak.

SPC and Volume of Surgical Procedures: Application 3

Pollard and Garnerin (1999) used c charts to determine whether a shift in surgery from inpatient to outpatient would change the number of surgical procedures performed or the quality of care. A c chart utilizing control limits and warning limits (UWLc and LWLc) documented that the total number of procedures did not breach the upper control limit, indicating that the total number of procedures performed did not significantly increase as a result of the change in surgical setting (see Figure 8.8). A second c chart documented that there was a substantial shift in the distribution of surgeries, with outpatient surgery increasing from 24.7% to 45.4% of total surgeries performed.

Quality of care was measured by the number of complications or deaths occurring within 30 days of the procedure. Pollard and Garnerin were concerned that the shift to outpatient surgery could increase the number of complications or postoperative deaths. They found no significant increase in deaths in either setting and no increase in complications

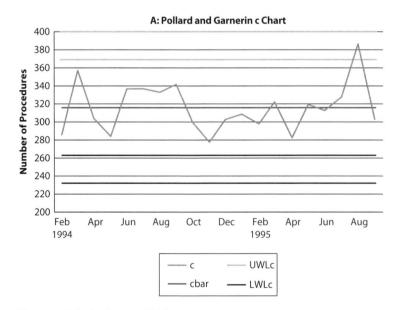

Figure 8.8 Pollard and Garnerin SPC Charts

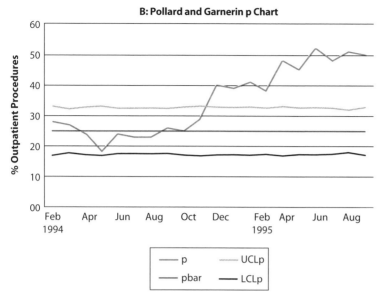

B: Pollard and Garnerin p Chart

Legend:
p, UCLp, pbar, LCLp

Figure 8.8 Continued

in the outpatient setting. There was a significant increase in inpatient complications from 2.31% to 3.50% (p < 5.0%) after the shift to outpatient surgery. The increase in inpatient complications was attributed to an increase in the average age of the inpatients and percentage of patients with severe systemic disease. In this study, the control charts were used to evaluate whether health care outcomes would be affected by a change in practice setting. This study demonstrates again the usefulness of control charts to determine whether a stable system would be affected by a change in clinical operations.

Selecting a Control Chart

Six control charts have been introduced in the last three chapters, and more charts are available. How does a potential user identify the right chart for the process she wishes to monitor and control? The first question is: What is the purpose of the analysis? Is it to determine how a task was performed (for example, timeliness, duration, dose) or whether a task or event occurred? The purpose of the analysis will often dictate the type of data required and the appropriate control chart. Questions about how a task was performed typically require that the variable of interest be measured on a continuous scale, indicating the use of $\bar{X}$ and R (or s) charts. Users must generate both charts for each variable to determine whether average performance and the variability of performance are acceptable.

If the data is discrete (that is, it cannot be measured on a continuous scale) and the user is attempting to determine whether something occurred, the user must select one of four charts. To narrow the choice, the user must determine the number of nonconformities that could arise per observation. If only one nonconformity can arise, then the user must select a p chart or an np chart. If more than one nonconformity per unit is possible, a c chart or a u chart must be created.

A final question must be answered: Is the sample size constant? If sample size is not constant and only one nonconformity per observation can occur, either a p chart or an np chart can be created, but if sample size is not constant, an np chart must be used. When more than one nonconformity can arise per observation and the sample size is constant, either a c chart or u chart can be created, but if sample size varies, a u chart is required. The advantage of np and c charts over p and u charts is that they do not require the user to calculate or interpret percentages.

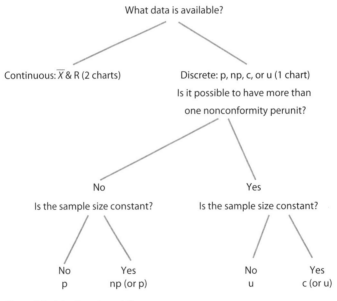

Figure 8.9 Selecting a Control Chart

Figure 8.9 provides an easy-to-use diagram that users can reference to determine which type of chart should be used. The six charts for continuous, binomial, and count data provide users with the ability to monitor a vast array of medical activity and distinguish between natural and special cause variation. SPC, when applied correctly, allows users to maximize their managerial effectiveness by focusing attention on only those areas that require investigation.

Benefits of SPC

SPC provides five distinct benefits to health care organizations; these benefits are part and parcel to the process of SPC. First, SPC is designed to identify areas in need of improvement. Organizations that undertake the effort to collect and analyze their operating processes and outcomes will know how their systems are operating and recognize changes in performance. Is average performance different from its historical performance? Is it above or below the organization's goals and the performance of competitors? Additionally, organizations will be able to monitor the variability of processes and outcomes by the width of control limits (wide limits indicate large variability) and how each sample compares to the limits. Do samples routinely approach or break the upper and lower limits (versus clustering around the center line)? Are there large differences in samples collected within short periods of time? The mere act of data collection will focus the organization and its employees on what is being measured.

Second, SPC is designed to separate normal and special cause variation. All systems are subject to variation, so the ability to identify unexpected, special cause variation is required for effective control. SPC sends clear signals when systems operate outside their historical experience. These signals provide early warnings that investigation is needed. The timeliness of the signal should increase the ability of employees to identify the cause and implement corrective action to minimize the duration of suboptimal performance. Equally important is the knowledge that nothing needs to be done. SPC provides the information necessary so managers can feel comfortable allowing processes to run without modification.

Third, SPC provides a wealth of information to diagnose and correct problems that may be difficult or impossible to recognize from individual customer complaints. Relying on individual customers to report problems falls short because some customers do not complain, complaints may be made only after a prolonged delay, or customers may complain to different employees and the complaints may never be collected; thus the magnitude of a problem and when it arose may never be clear. By introducing sampling to a process, SPC provides timely and accurate information on production problems, allowing employees to correct problems quickly and reduce the cost of poor performance.

When special cause variation is identified, SPC supports rapid and informed decision making and corrective action. In the case of breaches of control limits, SPC can identify production problems within minutes of when a problem arises. The timeliness of the signal will depend on how often samples are collected. Recognition of trends or patterns may take at least six periods to identify the problem due to the need to collect enough data points to establish a series.

Fourth, after corrections are implemented, SPC can be used to assess their impact. Was the correction effective, partially effective, or ineffective? If the correction was effective, continual monitoring is essential to ensure that hard-won gains are not subsequently lost. When implementing CQI initiatives, that is, modifications to stable systems, SPC can be used to determine whether performance or outcomes have improved. If improvements have been effective, an SPC chart should be able to document reduced error rates or higher compliance (the mean) or lower variability, or both. If improvement cannot be documented, employees know they must explore other avenues to improve performance.

The four preceding benefits arise from working through the SPC process and learning how a system operates. SPC outputs also afford a fifth substantial benefit, that of an effective communication tool (see Table 8.5). SPC charts display performance over time and can be used to define organizational goals and document progress. SPC goals are clear and unambiguous. SPC charts do not implore workers to "improve quality" but rather define specific tasks, define performance, and point employees in the direction of improvement. Interpreting an SPC chart requires little more than recognizing the goal and the direction of performance: is performance stable, increasing, or decreasing? Is it moving toward or away from the organization's goal? If the process of monitoring and controlling performance is left to the personnel operating the system, one would hope that employees would take ownership and implement corrections and improvements on their own initiative. This outcome is the one envisioned by Shewhart: employees would be free from oversight as long as output was maintained within control limits.

Table 8.5 Benefits of SPC

1.	Measure performance and outcomes
2.	Identify natural and special cause variation
3.	Support rapid and informed decision-making and action
4.	Assess effectiveness of improvements implemented
5.	Communicate with employees, customers, and regulators

SPC is more than a tool; it is a way of thought and action. Users must not only understand what SPC is and what the signals mean but they must also know their roles, responsibilities, and authority within the system. It is unlikely that simple graphing of performance and control limits will improve work processes or patient outcomes if the user does not understand the science and the art of SPC or lacks the authority to implement timely corrective action.

Inhibitors of the Use of SPC

The last three chapters devoted a significant amount of time to the discussion of how SPC could be used in health care and reviewed multiple cases in which SPC was used to improve health care delivery. Other industries make extensive use of SPC, but its use in health care remains unfortunately limited. At least seven factors account for its limited application in health care.

Several of the largest factors preventing more widespread usage are cultural. First, health care remains an industry controlled by individuals. The production process is determined by autonomous physicians, and practice patterns are widely divergent. Physicians are entrusted with the responsibility of defining and monitoring quality, and external accountability has been limited. Unlike other industries, where quality is everyone's job, the authority structure in health care organizations does not encourage lower-level employees to question the decisions of physicians. Health care will have to become more team-oriented, incorporating patients, other health care workers, and payers, before widespread use of SPC occurs.

Second, individual physicians do not have the time, incentive, or sufficient data to undertake SPC. The primary job of physicians is to deliver care to patients. Analyzing outcomes does not increase revenue or decrease cost, so time away from medical practice may reduce their incomes. In addition, individual physicians are dealing with relatively small groups of patients for any particular medical condition so the occurrence of adverse events may be extremely rare. The rarity of adverse outcomes observed by individual providers may suggest to them that analysis is not needed, but the frequency of adverse events at the system level cries out for attention. In large production systems, such as automobile manufacturing, an organization can devote significant resources to quality management and spread the cost over thousands, if not millions, of units. When total outputs can be measured in the dozens or hundreds, the costs of administering an SPC system may be unrecoverable.

Third, physicians are trained to deal with the needs of individual patients, and medical education does not devote enough time to evaluating group outcomes. An individual case approach to outcomes and the rarity of failure among small groups make it easy for physicians to attribute failure to the particular characteristics of patients as opposed to shortcomings in the health care decision-making or delivery process. SPC represents a sea change in the way physicians are taught to think. Physicians and other health care workers need to start identifying common failures and documenting the conditions present when the failure occurred.

A fourth factor is the greater variation in health care. A prime difference between health care and other industries is that other industries exercise greater control over inputs to the production system and are less dependent on people. Patients and their behaviors and conditions are a major complicating factor in the health care process. Patient factors (inputs) combined with the unpredictability of labor (throughput) result in health care providers facing much higher levels of variability than other industries. When building automobiles, manufacturers evaluate inputs before they enter the production system, and inputs likely to produce defective output can be screened out. Health care providers must treat all patients, and their medical and behavioral issues may complicate the care process and reduce the probability of successful treatment. Other industries rely more heavily on capital than on labor; in addition, machinery is often more consistent than human performance. Automated processes are less susceptible to variation than are processes carried out by workers who experience fatigue, stress, boredom, and other emotions and factors that affect human performance.

Fifth, another cultural factor that inhibits the use of SPC is the fact that health care workers do not receive extensive training in statistics or quality management. Although cognizant of what quality health care is, health care workers may be unable to operationalize their conception. The goal of this text is to introduce to health care workers the tools and techniques necessary to define, measure, and control performance. The dearth of quality training in health care programs is often reinforced by the widely held fear of, or desire to avoid, statistics and the idea common among health care workers that quality management techniques used in other industries are not applicable to health care.

A sixth barrier is the failure to understand the total production process. Workers in many organizations are only familiar with their part of a production process and cannot make the connection between their jobs and the final outcome sought. Health care, with its proliferation of medical specialties, division of labor, and rapid increase in medical knowledge, suffers from the same weaknesses. SPC requires knowledge of the entire production process to understand the objective of the system, identify what should be monitored and where monitoring occurs, and when corrective action should be initiated. The fragmentation of health care systems and increased emphasis on driving large numbers of patients through these systems has reduced focus on outcomes (total process) and increased attention to tests, procedures, and therapies (outputs).

Finally, there is the question of data collection. Data collection is a time-consuming and costly process. Once data has been collected, it is relatively easy to create control charts and understand what the information can tell us about the performance of a system. The hard part is getting the data. Health care information systems to date are still focused on individual patients and do not produce enough easily accessible information to evaluate system performance. The goal of this book is to demonstrate that the time and cost associated with data collection and analysis will be more than offset by the value that control charts can add to patient care.

While there are many benefits to the use of SPC, many barriers must be overcome to ensure better outcomes for patients (see Table 8.6). Without data, we can comfort ourselves with the idea we are doing all we can for our patients, but in the absence of information we can never be sure we are producing the best possible outcomes. The goal of this text is that, given knowledge of SPC and a vision of possible health care improvement, readers will be motivated to challenge these barriers and institute multiple SPC programs.

Table 8.6 Barriers to the Use of SPC

1.	Physician-driven production system
2.	Insufficient medical training on group outcomes
3.	Small production lots
4.	More sources of variation than other industries
5.	Insufficient understanding of the total production process
6.	Insufficient training in statistics and quality management
7.	Cost of data collection

Final Thoughts on SPC

In a typical day, a provider may engage in dozens, if not hundreds, of tasks. The job of SPC is not to create more work but rather to improve patient care by monitoring a small number of critical processes. The critical processes that should be monitored are ones in which poor performance or the failure to perform will have a substantial negative impact on the outcomes sought. Control charts should be created for processes that are important to outcomes; they are not required for every task. The second criterion required to justify ongoing control charting is that the process must be in need of improvement. Processes requiring improvement are those performing at a low level or having large variation in performance that could harm patients. Finally, attention should be targeted on processes where there is reasonable hope the process can be improved. All tasks do not require control charts. Charts should only be created for critical processes with unacceptable performance that can be changed.

In determining when to create a control chart, a critical factor is performance. But how are goals and targets selected? Process **capability** asks the question of what level of performance is achievable. This is a difficult question because health care providers have historically not collected sufficient data to understand outcomes across groups of patients. Chapters

capability
the level of performance a process can achieve versus what it does achieve

Six through Eight used a historical approach to answer the question "How do you establish targets?" The process documented prior performance and asked: How does current performance compare with prior outcomes? Is performance similar to past performance, or is it improving or declining? If performance is declining, it raises the question of why current results have fallen below what was previously achieved. While this approach is useful in controlling deterioration of performance, it does not address the more fundamental question of whether the process is operating at its potential.

A second way of establishing performance targets would be to research industry outcomes. What performance is achieved on average by the industry, or what is the performance of the industry leader? Improvement is possible if the organization's performance is less than average or less than that of the industry leader. The key issue, however, is by how much does the performance of two organizations differ, or by how much do the performance of the organization and the industry average differ? Is the difference large enough to seek improvement, or will managerial and employee efforts bear more fruit if applied to other areas?

A third method would be to survey patients or physicians to understand their expectations. Setting targets based on expectations would provide an organization with a minimum standard; the goal of an organization should be to exceed expectations. Surveying customers or benchmarking against the industry leader comes closest to the idea of process capability.

The goal of SPC is process improvement, and this requires changing the mean or reducing variation (or both). Changing the mean requires reducing the average rate of error or increasing compliance with generally accepted standards of practice. Reducing variation requires achieving more consistent performance. The purpose of both goals is to make a process more effective and predictable; that is, the system should produce the expected outcome more often and consistently. Process improvement requires more than SPC; it also requires understanding how process analysis tools (Chapter Four) determine what processes should be monitored, documentation of processes, and discovering the causes of problems.

Unintended consequences always arise from any initiative that attempts to alter human behavior, and SPC is no exception. When job performance is based on quantifiable measures, there will be an incentive for individuals to attempt to alter the data to cast themselves in the best light. Managers must recognize this incentive and periodically audit SPC data to ensure that the reported data accurately reflects job performance or the outcomes produced.

What gets measured gets attention. This idea is emphasized in this text, because it is common for employees to put more attention on the tasks they know are being monitored. Added attention to one task, however, may come at the expense of other duties. In the process of improvement, managers and employees must be sure that improvements in one area are not offset by decline or deterioration in other areas.

Summary

This chapter has reviewed how to create control charts for monitoring events that can have multiple nonconformities. Chapters Six, Seven, and Eight demonstrated how to monitor single events, but health care is a multifaceted product often encompassing dozens, if not hundreds, of activities. Busy providers do not have the time to create and review dozens or hundreds of control charts, but they still need to know how their overall process is performing. As demonstrated in this chapter, if health care providers can identify a set of critical activities, a c chart or u chart can provide a necessary overview of the delivery process. Only when the overview indicates a problem will providers have to disaggregate the data to discover the cause of the problem.

The cases and applications demonstrate that c charts have been successfully applied to a variety of health care situations. Even though SPC's applicability in health care is extensive, it remains underused, a situation that, if reversed, would provide benefits in the future.

One of the problems affecting potential users of SPC is determining which control chart is appropriate for the process they want to monitor. The prime determinants are: What is the goal, what do we wish to control, and how is it measured? Is the data continuous, binomial, or countable? Can the variable of interest be measured on a numeric scale, does it meet a standard, or can multiple nonconformities arise for a single observation? The second consideration is whether the sample size is constant or variable. Constant sample sizes provide the opportunity to track the number of nonconformities while variable size samples require rates be monitored.

Many of the primary benefits of SPC spring from the need to thoroughly understand and collect data on a process before creating control charts. Process understanding requires users to identify critical processes and goals and explicitly define them. Simply obtaining the agreement of users regarding what to monitor may be a substantial step toward improving the delivery of care. The second primary benefit of SPC is the ability to use the data after it is collected. Control charts are easy to interpret, and employees can readily see whether performance is improving or declining and whether it meets a target. Real-time identification of unstable performance facilitates the search for the causes of the variation and reduces the length of time an unsafe situation is allowed to continue.

There are many barriers to the use of SPC in health care, as seen by the limited effect SPC has had on health care processes. Many of the barriers arise from the nature and culture of health care. Health care has historically been a production process characterized by individualism and has not adapted the controls routinely used in other industries. The product of health care is often unique because of patients and their specific conditions, and because the way care is delivered is often determined by a single physician and his or her practice style. Medical education is built around treating individual patients, and insufficient training is given to evaluating outcomes across patients. Reinforcing this orientation is a reimbursement system that rewards individuals and organizations for what they do rather than what they achieve.

KEY TERMS

c chart   Nonconformities

Capability   u chart

REVIEW QUESTIONS

1. When can a c chart rather than a u chart be used to monitor system performance? What are the advantages of a c chart over a u chart?

2. What are the three questions that determine the type of control chart that should be used to monitor a process?

3. What are the primary benefits of implementing SPC?

4. What are the primary barriers to the use of SPC?

5. What is the difference between stability and capability?

6. Which processes should SPC be applied to?

PROBLEMS

1. A hospital introduced hip protectors to reduce the frequency of injury-producing patient falls. The hip protectors were introduced in July. The following table records the number of injury-producing falls from January through December. Create and interpret a c chart for patient falls. Were the hip protectors effective in reducing injury-producing patient falls?

Month	Falls	Month	Falls
Jan	5	Jul	3
Feb	5	Aug	3
Mar	3	Sep	2
Apr	4	Oct	2
May	2	Nov	3
Jun	2	Dec	3

2. The director of medical records conducts a monthly audit of 50 medical records to iden-tify coding errors. The Chapter 08.xls, Problem 08–02 tab records the data. National sta-tistics indicate that approximately 15% of medical records contain errors, and in the past the director has found multiple errors in a single record. Create a c chart to analyze perfor-mance. Interpret the department's performance based on your control chart and identify any issues that should be investigated. Is the department doing a good job?

3. The chief medical officer is concerned that the long lengths of stay at her hospital may be the result of missed oxygen treatments. She has enacted a program to reduce the number of missed treatments. The Chapter08.xls, Problem 08–03 tab, records the number of missed oxygen treatments over the last 40 weeks. The improvement program was introduced in week 20. Was the program effective?

4. Implementing regular nursing rounds has been demonstrated to increase patient satisfac-tion and reduce patient falls. A hospital has collected data on ten patients per month over the past 24 months. The first twelve months the hospital did not have a formal rounding system. During the second period nurses were required to make rounds on an hourly basis from 8:00 AM through 8:00 PM and every two hours from 8:00 PM to 8:00 AM. The Chapter 08.xls, Problem 08–04 tab displays the number of call lights received per day for the ten-patient sample. Create a c chart to determine the effect of the rounding system on the use of call lights. Did the rounding program reduce patients' use of call lights? Are there any issues that should be investigated?

5. To supplement their patient satisfaction survey, End Result Hospital conducts in-depth tele-phone interviews of past patients. The interviews are based on a 1% sample of the completed surveys from the prior month. The sample varies widely due to differences in monthly admis-sions, the rate at which surveys are completed, and the willingness of patients to participate in the telephone interview. The Chapter 08.xls, Problem 08–05 tab records the total number of the patients' concerns noted by the interviewers. These concerns range from the effective-ness of medical treatment to the cleanliness and comfort of the patient room and ease of parking. The interviewer addresses the same items found on the patient satisfaction survey, solicits additional information for any item on which the patient indicated performance was less than "Good" or "Very Good," and provides the patient with the opportunity to voice any other concerns. Create a control chart to summarize the results. Are patient concerns stable?

References

Curran E, Benneyan J, and Hood J, 2002, Controlling Meticillin-Resistant *Staphylococcus aureus*: A Feedback Approach using Annotated Statistical Process Control Charts, *Infection Control and Hospital Epidemiology* 23 (1): 13–18.

Curran E, Harper P, Loveday H, Gilmour H, Jones S, Benneyan J, Hood J, and Pratt R, 2008, Results of Multicentre Randomised Controlled Trial of Statistical Process Control Charts and Structured Diagnostic Tools to Reduce Ward-Acquired Meticillin-Resistant *Staphylococcus aureus*: The CHART Process, *Journal of Hospital Infection* 70 (2): 127–135.

J.D. Power and Associates, n.d., J.D. Power and Associates 2008 Initial Quality Study, http://www.autoblog.com/2008/06/04/j-dd-power-releases-2008 -initial-quality-study/.

Juran JM and Godfrey AB, 1999, *Juran's Quality Handbook*, 5th ed., McGraw-Hill, New York, NY.

Pollard JB and Garnerin P, 1999, Outpatient Preoperative Evaluation Clinic Can Lead to a Rapid Shift from Inpatient to Outpatient Surgery: A Retrospective Review of Perioperative Setting and Outcome, *Journal of Clinical Anesthesia* 11: 39–45.

Walberg M, Frøslie KF, and Røislien J, 2008, Local Hospital Perspective on a Nationwide Outbreak of Pseudomonas aeruginosa Infection in Norway, *Infection Control and Hospital Epidemiology* 29 (7): 635–641.

CHAPTER 9

EXPLORING QUALITY ISSUES WITH STATISTICAL TOOLS

Introduction

Chapter Nine places a more rigorous statistical foundation under the quality management approach given in prior chapters. Chapter Four gave four reasons to analyze data: to identify problems, to determine their potential causes, to propose possible solutions, and to monitor implemented solutions to determine if they achieve what was intended. Chapters Six through Eight introduced statistical process control (SPC) to determine whether a system was stable and capable. Determining stability is vital to improvement; in unstable systems individual elements can be identified and altered to improve performance. In stable processes that are not meeting expected performance, a total system review must be conducted. Improvements to underperforming but stable processes require changing the system rather than "tweaking" to produce better results. Improving human performance requires better designed processes, education and training, and better materials and equipment.

Process analysis tools and SPC focus on identifying problems and changes in systems and their effect on output. Once a correction or an enhancement is implemented, the same tools can be used to determine whether the changes improved performance. Table 9.1 links chi-square, **analysis of variance** (ANOVA), **analysis of means** (ANOM), and **regression** to problem identification (where do significant variations arise?), cause identification (what factors are related to problems?), and monitoring outcomes (is there a difference in outcome after an intervention or correction is made?). Ishikawa

analysis of variance
a test to determine if a continuous variable is independent of a categorical variable that can assume two or more values; that is, are group means significantly different

analysis of means
a test to determine if the mean for one or more groups is significantly different than the mean for all groups

regression
a test to determine the relationship between a dependent continuous variable and one or more independent continuous or categorical variables

statistical significance
the probability that a finding is due to chance; that is, when p is 5% or less the probability that the result is due to chance is less than 5% or conversely there is 95% or more probability that the result is not due to chance

noted that "quality control which cannot show results is not quality control" (Ishikawa 1985, 13), which points out that quality management, to be worthy of its name, must demonstrate predictable outputs that meet or exceed expectations. The bottom line is that decisions and actions must be data-driven.

Statistical tests that employ Donabedian's structure-process-outcome paradigm can be used to determine whether changes in resources and organization, or in diagnosis and treatment, improve outcomes (see Table 9.1). Statistical tests do not prove one variable *causes* a change in another variable; statistics only demonstrate whether two variables are correlated. It is important to understand how correlation and statistical significance are determined in statistics; that it, how to determine whether two variables are correlated or whether a statistically significant relationship exists between two variables. The standard rule for **statistical significance** is 5.0%. That is, based on the changes observed in the magnitudes of two variables, is there a 5.0% or less chance that the change in one is not related to the change in the other?

Table 9.1 Uses of Statistical Tests

1.	Identify problems—ANOM + chi-square and ANOVA
2.	Identify the causes of problems—regression
3.	Identify potential solutions and select a solution
4.	Monitor change—chi-square and ANOVA

While we know that all processes are subject to natural variation, the challenge is to institute improvements that not only demonstrate better performance but performance that is significantly better. The size of the improvement must render it unlikely to have occurred by chance: there must be less than a 5.0% chance that an observed change is due to random fluctuation in performance. The goal of this chapter is to explore the quality issues to which chi-square, ANOVA, analysis of means, and regression can be applied and to demonstrate their use in Excel. The chapter highlights the overlap between quality management and research (see Figure 9.1).

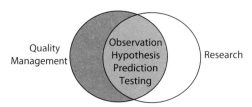

Figure 9.1 Quality Management and Research

Quality management is applied research. Basic research grounded on the scientific method—observation, hypothesis, prediction, and the testing of predictions—aims at the creation of knowledge. Quality management uses the same tools to study and improve existing practice. Statistics is not only a tool to improve operations; it is also the language to document and communicate improvements to patients and providers. This chapter does not provide exhaustive coverage of statistical tools; statistical references are provided at the end of the chapter for readers interested in expanding their knowledge of these statistical methods.

Chi-Square Analysis

Chi-square analysis is used to determine whether there is a statistical relationship between two categorical variables. Chi-square can be used to identify problems, potential causes, and whether interventions were effective. A **categorical variable** takes on one of two or more possible values, and these values are labels rather than numbers. For example, a categorical structure variable would be whether a physician is board certified. A categorical process variable would be whether a recommended drug was delivered at the appropriate time. And categorical outcome variables could be whether the patient improved, lived, or developed an infection. Each of these variables would be measured as yes or no. Chi-square analysis can also be used when a variable takes on more than two possibilities, such as an outcome variable measuring mobility after treatment classified as improved, no change, or diminished.

Before testing statistical significance, there is the question of data collection. Since we are concerned with the relationship between two variables, we must be able to obtain the counts of each set of variables. This could be a time-consuming process with a data set containing hundreds, if not thousands, of observations. Excel has functions that count numbers (**=Count**), events meeting a criterion (**=Countif**), and events meeting multiple criteria (**=Countifs**). The more powerful function, **=Frequency**, allows users to establish bins and count the number of occurrences within a range. Excel's PivotTable function provides another method to extract information from a data set.

PivotTable allows a data analyst to construct a contingency table, or cross tabulation, between two sets of variables. The variables can be either numeric or nonnumeric. The PivotTable function allows users to see the joint distribution of two variables; that is, to count the number of occurrences of each set of combinations of two variables. Live births and gender provide an example. Both variables are categorical and a 2 × 2 table could be

chi-square analysis
a test to determine if a categorical variable is independent of another categorical variable

categorical variable
a variable that can take on one of two or more possibilities that denote group membership rather than a numerical relationship

PivotTable
a table that counts the number of times (or the sum, average. . .) of the various combinations of two variables; also known as cross tabulation or a contingency table

produced with male and female and the whether they were live or stillborn. If a difference between the survival rates is observed in the PivotTable, chi-square can determine whether the difference is large enough to conclude that the probability of live birth and gender are not independent, that is, that gender predicts the probability of live birth.

For quality management, chi-square allows us to explore the potential relationship between two or more categorical variables. One example using a structure-process-outcome approach might be: Do board-certified physicians have lower readmissions than doctors that are not board certified? Board certification, a structure variable, would be the **independent variable** (IV), that is, the variable expected to predict or "cause" a change in another variable. Readmission, an outcome, would be the **dependent variable** (DV), which we may predict would be lower for board-certified physicians.

Chi-square analysis can also explore whether changes in process affect outcomes, for example, whether following a recommended treatment protocol reduces mortality. The common assumption in statistics, the **null hypothesis**, is that a change in an IV will have no impact on the DV. The **alternative hypothesis**, the idea researchers attempt to support, is that a change in the IV is related to changes in the DV. Chi-square analysis asks the question: Is there enough difference between what is observed between two groups (different levels of training or experience, or before and after a process change) and what we expect to observe (no difference) to conclude that the variables are dependent, that is, correlated?

Assume a hospital has instituted a hand-washing program (IV) to reduce the incidence of hospital-acquired infection (DV). Chi-square analysis will examine the actual number of infections before and after implementation of the program to determine whether infections have declined significantly after the program was initiated. The formula is:

9.1

$$\chi^2 = \sum (O_i - E_i)^2 / E_i$$

Where:

O_i: observed infections before and after the hand-washing program was implemented

E_i: expected infections assuming the hand-washing program was ineffective

The hospital has collected the following data, available online in Chapter09.xls, in the Tables 09–02–05 tab:

independent variable
the variable expected to predict a change in another variable

dependent variable
the variable that is expected to change with changes in the independent variable

null hypothesis
the assumption of no difference, that is, changes in the dependent variable are unrelated to changes in the independent variables; any change observed is due to chance

alternative hypothesis
what a researcher believes is true and is tested; that is, changes in the dependent variables are related to changes in one or more independent variables

Table 9.2 demonstrates that postimplementation infections have been reduced, but is the amount of change sufficient to conclude there is a statistically significant relationship between the hand-washing program and the infection rate? Prior to the program the infection rate was 5.13% (14/273). After the program was implemented, the rate fell to 2.65% (8/302). Is the difference of 2.48% (a reduction of 48.3%) in the infection rate sufficient to conclude that hand washing is related to the decline?

Table 9.2 Observed Infections, January–April 2012

	Infection	No Infection	Total
Preimplementation: Jan–Feb	14	259	273
Postimplementation: Mar–Apr	8	294	302
Total	22	553	575

The overall infection rate is 3.826% based on 22 infections among 575 patients; three decimal places were used to ensure the accuracy of subsequent calculations. The overall rate of infection is used to calculate the number of expected infections in the pre- and postimplementation groups based on the number of patients in each group. The assumption is if the program was not effective, the pre- and postimplementation groups should have roughly a 3.826% infection rate. The preimplementation group is expected to have 10.45 infections (3.826% * 273) and the postimplementation group should have 11.55 (3.826% * 302). Table 9.3 shows the expected occurrences in each group.

Table 9.3 Expected Infections, January–April 2012

	Infection	No Infection	Total
Preimplementation: Jan–Feb	10.45	262.55	273
Post-implementation: Mar–Apr	11.55	290.45	302
Total	22	553	575

The row and column totals are the same in Tables 9.2 and 9.3. Chi-square analysis calculates the squared difference between the observed values and the expected values to determine whether the difference is large enough to be statistically significant given the degrees of freedom: ((number of rows − 1)* (number of columns − 1)).

The χ^2 calculation for this example is:

$$(14 - 10.45)^2/10.45 + (259 - 262.55)^2/262.55 + (8 - 11.55)^2 /11.55$$
$$+ (294 - 290.45)^2/290.45 =$$

$$12.64/10.45 + 12.64/262.55 + 12.64/11.55 + 12.64/290.45 =$$
$$1.21 + 0.05 + 1.09 + 0.04 = 2.39$$

degree of freedom

the number of values in a statistic that are free to vary; in a sample of ten with a given mean only nine values can vary ($n - 1$) because the value of the tenth is determined by the sample average and values of the nine known values

critical value

a measure of the difference between observed and expected values that must be exceeded to establish statistical significance

test statistic

a measure of the actual difference between observed and expected values

χ^2, 2.39, is the calculated difference between the observed and expected values. Is the difference between the pre- and postimplementation infections large enough to conclude that the hand-washing program is related to the lower rate of infection? The amount of change required to conclude there is a statistical difference is determined by the degrees of freedom, the significance level (or the desired confidence level), and the chi-square distribution. Using a 5.0% significance level and a two-by-two matrix with a **degree of freedom** of 1, $(2 - 1)*(2 - 1)$, the chi-square distribution requires the difference to exceed 3.84, the **critical value**, to be significant.

The **test statistic**, χ^2, is less than the critical value of 3.84, so the null hypothesis of no difference between groups would be accepted. From a statistical perspective, the result indicates that the hand-washing program had no significant impact on the number of infections. That is, there is a greater than 5% probability that the reduction in the number of infections could have occurred without the hand-washing program.

Excel does not calculate the expected values (Table 9.3) or the test statistic, $\chi 2$, but it provides two formulas to calculate the probability of finding the difference between (1) the observed and expected values given that the null hypothesis is true and (2) the test statistic, χ^2, and critical value that must be exceeded to be significant. To access the chi-square functions, select **Formulas** from the main tool bar, **Insert Function**, and then type "chi" into the Search for a function field, as shown in Figure 9.2.

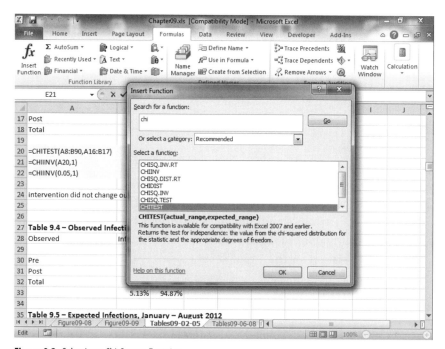

Figure 9.2 Selecting a Chi-Square Function

=CHITEST(*actual_values,expected_values*) returns the probability of finding χ^2 this large when the null hypothesis is true (no difference or variables are independent). When the observed and expected values are entered, =CHITEST(B6:C7, B14:C15), the function returns 0.1217. There is a 12.17% probability that the reduction in infections is random variation.

The second function is =CHIINV(*probability,d.f.*), and it returns the test statistic χ^2 calculation, $\Sigma(O_i\text{-}E_i)^2/E_i$, or the critical value that must be exceeded to establish statistical significance. The test statistic is calculated based on the value generated by =CHITEST. When the analyst enters =CHIINV(0.1217,1), the function returns 2.39. The critical value is calculated by replacing the 0.1217 with the desired level of confidence, typically 5.0%. Entering =CHIINV(0.05,1) returns 3.84.

Anytime =CHITEST produces a value greater than 0.05 (as it did in this case, returning 0.1217), the null hypothesis of no significance must be accepted. The test statistic and critical values of χ^2 show that the null hypothesis must be accepted because the test statistic of 2.39, =CHIINV(0.1217,1), is less than the 3.84 threshold, =CHIINV(0.05,1), required to conclude that the hand-washing program was related to the reductions in infections. That is, the reduction in the rate of infection is within the range we would expect infections to vary, thus we cannot conclude the hand-washing program improved the system.

Although the difference in infection rates may be statistically insignificant, from a quality improvement standpoint there has been a reduction in infection rates. Before the program, the rate was 5.13%, and after the program began, the rate declined to 2.65%. Assume the hospital continues to track infection rates for another four months (effectively tripling the size of the postimplementation sample) and the lower infection rate is maintained. Will there now be a significant difference between the observed and expected rates, in Tables 9.4 and 9.5, to change the conclusion?

Table 9.4 Observed Infections, January–August 2012

	Infection	No Infection	Total
Preimplementation: Jan–Feb	14	259	273
Postimplementation: Mar–Aug	24	882	906
Total	38	1141	1179

Table 9.5 Expected Infections, January–August 2012

	Infection	No Infection	Total
Preimplementation: Jan–Feb	8.80	264.20	273
Postimplementation: Mar–Aug	29.20	876.80	906
Total	38	1141	1179

=CHITEST returns a probability of 4.2%, which is now less than 5.0%. This probability indicates that the reduction in infections is related to the hand-washing program. The difference of 2.48% (5.13% − 2.65%) between the original pre- and postimplementation groups was not significant, but the same difference is significant when the size of the postimplementation group increased. This result highlights an attribute of statistics: as sample size increases, smaller differences become statistically significant. In terms of quality management, it highlights the fact that although differences among small groups may not be significant, if the difference is maintained over time it may demonstrate the effectiveness of a change.

Let's return to the impact of board certification. A hospital wants to compare mortality rates between board-certified and non-board-certified surgeons. The hospital has chronologically recorded all surgical patients (n = 18,742), the certification status of the surgeon (1 = board certified, 0 = not board certified), and whether the patient survived (1 = died, 0 = survived). Table 9.6 shows a portion of the data file from the Chapter09.xls file in the Tables 09–06–08 tab. Patient 652 was treated by a board-certified physician and survived, while patient 653 was also treated by a board-certified physician but died. The first thing an analyst must do is summarize the data set using PivotTable to count the number of patients in each of the four possible groups.

Table 9.6 Board Certification and Mortality Data

Patient #	Board	Died
652	1	0
653	1	1
654	1	0
655	0	0
656	1	0
657	1	0
658	1	0
659	1	0
660	1	0
661	1	0
662	0	0
663	0	1
664	0	0

To use the PivotTable function, select **Insert** and then **PivotTable**. The input screen shown in Figure 9.3 will appear. Enter the range, including the column headings into the Table/Range field, for example, A7 through C18749, and specify placement—new or existing worksheet.

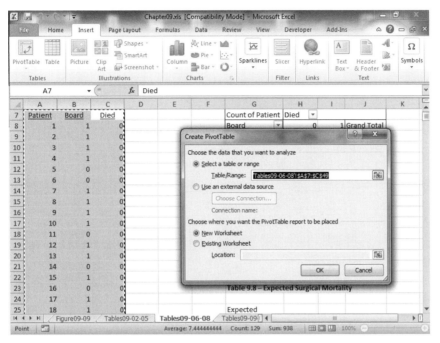

Figure 9.3   Create PivotTable

After the range and placement, G7 in the existing worksheet, are specified and accepted (by clicking the OK button), the screen in Figure 9.4 is generated. Next, drag and drop the column headings from the PivotTable Field List to the columns, rows, and body of the table: drag **Board** to the rows G8, **Died** to the columns H8, and **Patient** to the body H9 or anywhere from H9 through I11; this will produce a PivotTable that displays the sum of patients. To obtain the count of patients, as displayed in Figure 9.4, left click on the downward arrow following Sum of Patient in the bottom right of the screen, left click on Value Field Setting . . . and select Count from pop-up screen.

Table 9.7 has rearranged the PivotTable and replaced the 1s and 0s with titles to improve readability. Table 9.7 reveals that the average mortality rate is 0.91238% (171/18,742; rate is calculated to five decimal places to ensure subsequent calculations do not have rounding errors) and non-board-certified surgeons have higher mortality rates: 1.39% (39/2,800) versus 0.83% (132/15,942) for board-certified physicians. Is this difference large enough to conclude that there are different outcomes between the two groups?

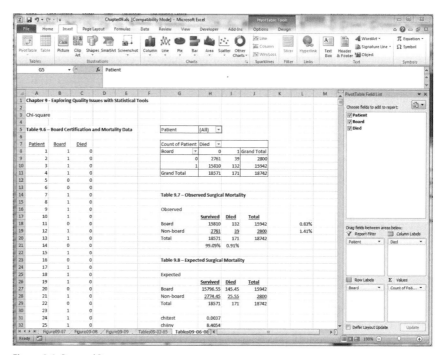

Figure 9.4 Drag and Drop

Table 9.7 Observed Surgical Mortality

	Survived	Died	Total
Board Certified	15,810	132	15,942
Not Board Certified	2,761	39	2,800
Total	18,571	171	18,742

Table 9.8 is created using the overall mortality rate to calculate the expected deaths for each group of physicians. Assuming no difference between the two groups, non-board-certified surgeons should have 25.48 fatalities (0.91% * 2,800), approximately 13 fewer fatalities, and board-certified physicians should have 13 more.

Table 9.8 Expected Surgical Mortality

	Survived	Died	Total
Board Certified	15,796.55	145.45	15,942
Not Board Certified	2774.45	25.55	2,800
Total	18,571	171	18,742

Based on the observed and expected deaths, chi-square analysis produces a test statistic of 8.45 and a threshold of 3.84. The probability of observing this amount of difference between the two groups is 0.37%, below the 5.0% required to be statistically significant. The higher mortality rate among non-board-certified surgeons appears to be due to something other than chance.

Based on the higher mortality rate for non-board-certified physicians, the hospital must determine why this is true. Is it due to lower ability among non-board-certified physicians? If so, can the gap between board-certified and non-board-certified physicians be narrowed by education and training? A second possibility is that there is a difference in the type of patients treated by each group. The group treating the sicker patients should have lower outcomes; can these patient factors be identified and accounted for? Do non-board-certified physicians treat sicker patients? Using this finding, the hospital should identify the potential causes to the different mortality rates and determine what actions should be taken. If action is taken, follow-up is essential to determine whether there is any convergence of the mortality rates across the two groups.

Applications of Chi-Square Analysis

Chi-square analysis is a widely used tool in quality management. Armola and Topp (2001) studied the variables related to LOS and readmission for heart failure patients. They found that angiotensin converting enzyme (ACE) therapy, physician type, and heart failure education were not related to either LOS or readmission. A prime objective of their study was to determine the effect of a case manager and discharge plan on their two outcome variables. The presence of a case manager was associated with a longer LOS but was unrelated to readmission. Discharge plans were unrelated to LOS but were associated with lower readmissions. The finding that the presence of a case planner was related to higher LOS was unexpected; the researchers expected that case managers would reduce LOS, consistent with prior research. Armola and Topp attribute the higher LOS to the way the case managers work, which Armola and Topp describe as a discharge planning function, and the possibility that patients assigned case management had a higher severity of illness.

A study by Harrison et al. (2010) examined the relationship between inattention in elderly patients and impulsivity-related falls (IRF). Research was required because IRFs comprise 28% of all falls, two-thirds of patient falls involve people over the age of 64, and because of the effect of falls on patients' health and the cost of hospitalization. Inattention was measured using the short form Confusion Assessment Method. They found that 79% of falls in inattentive patients were related to impulsivity, while only 18% of attentive patients suffered an IRF. Chi-square analysis produced a test statistic of 45.5 with a probability of 0.00%, supporting their hypothesis that patient inattention is related to IRFs. Further analysis dismissed gender and age as explanatory variables. The authors conclude that their results emphasize the need for nursing staff to identify inattention in patients and implement additional precautions for inattentive patients to prevent falls.

Analysis of Variance

continuous variable
a variable that can assume any numeric value

Analysis of variance (ANOVA) is used to determine if there is a statistical relationship between a categorical variable (typically the IV) and a **continuous variable** (the DV). ANOVA, like chi-square, is commonly used to identify problems, potential causes, and whether interventions were effective. The continuous variable measures phenomena on a numeric scale, and the categorical variable divides the observations into groups based on some ordering scheme. The ordering scheme may indicate that the variable was measured before or after a system change, care was delivered by different providers, or different treatment protocols were used. ANOVA determines whether there is sufficient difference in the numeric scores between groups to conclude that group membership is related to different outcomes.

ANOVA could examine if physicians or groups of physicians have significantly different outcomes in measures such as LOS, A1c levels, systolic blood pressure, or cholesterol levels. ANOVA differs from chi-square analysis in that the dependent variable is no longer placed into two or more categories but could take on any numeric value, and statistical significance is based on assessing the difference in group means. Is there a large enough difference in group means to conclude that group membership is correlated with outcomes?

The null hypothesis is that there should be minimal difference in individual or group scores. That is, if a test is conducted between pre- and post-implementation groups, providers, or treatment protocols, the difference in their numeric scores will be insufficient to conclude that a change in the IV had any impact on the DV. If there are large differences in group means, we accept the alternative hypothesis: the DV and IV are correlated.

Assume a hospital has instituted a pain management education program for staff and patients. The hospital forms four groups to determine the effectiveness of the program. In group 1 no one receives education (the control group); in group 2 only staff are trained; in group 3 only patients are educated; and in group 4 staff and patients receive training and education. The dependent variable is the reported level of pain based on the 11-point American Pain Society Patient Outcome Questionnaire (APS-POQ), where 0.0 indicates no pain and 10.0 the "worst pain possible." ANOVA examines if the average level of reported pain was significantly different in any group. The formula is:

$$x_{ij} = \mu + \tau_j + e_{ij}$$

9.2

where:

x_{ij} is value of a single observation; x_{ij} in this example represents the pain reported by patient i in group j.

μ is the grand mean or sum of the pain scores divided by the number of observations.

τ_j is the difference between group j's mean and the grand mean. This coefficient measures the change in pain scores predicted by group membership or the treatment effect.

e_{ij} is the unexplained difference between an observation and its group mean or the **error term**. The error term in this example demonstrates the difference in pain scores reported by a patient and what is expected based on his or her group.

error term
the unexplained difference between an observation and its expected value

Reviewing the means for each group in Table 9.9 shows that reported pain levels were less in the groups receiving education. Is the difference in reported pain between groups large enough to conclude the difference is related to the intervention?

Table 9.9 Patient-Reported Pain

Patient #	Control	Staff	Patient	Staff and Patient
1	5	3	6	6
2	8	5	9	7
3	6	5	5	2
4	4	8	8	3
5	7	8	9	5
6	10	4	4	5
7	6	9	9	2
8	7	4	4	7
9	7	6	5	2
10	8	7	7	3
Mean	6.8	5.9	6.6	4.2

To run an ANOVA, the analyst selects **Data** from main toolbar. After Data is selected, a second toolbar pops up and the user selects **Data Analysis**. Data Analysis is not included in the standard Excel setup so the analyst must add in this feature through Excel Options.

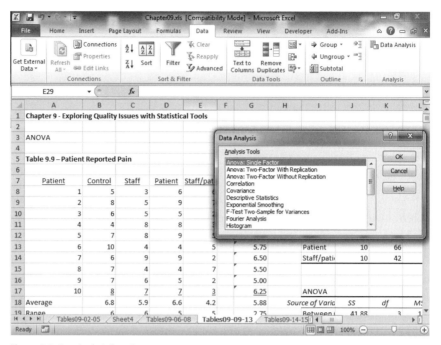

Figure 9.5 Data Analysis Functions

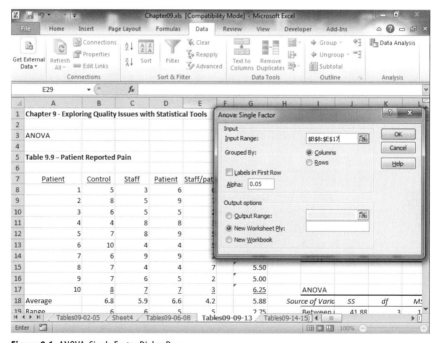

Figure 9.6 ANOVA: Single Factor Dialog Box

Input Range: The data range entered must be at least two columns (or rows), with each column (or row) representing a different group.

Grouped By: The default is Columns. Change if groups are recorded in rows.

Labels in first row. Check this box. Data files should be created such that the first row of each column contains the name of the group; thus output will name specific variables. If unchecked, output will report "Column 1, Column 2. . ."

Alpha: The default is 0.05 for the level of statistical significance. Adjust downward (upward) if higher (lower) level of confidence is desired.

Output options: The ANOVA results can be placed in the current worksheet, in a new worksheet, or in a separate workbook.

Clicking the OK button produces output shown in Table 9.10

Table 9.10 Excel ANOVA Output

ANOVA: SINGLE FACTOR				
SUMMARY				
Groups	**Count**	**Sum**	**Average**	**Variance**
Control	10	68	6.8	2.84
Staff	10	59	5.9	4.10
Patient	10	66	6.6	4.27
Staff-and-patient	10	42	4.2	4.18

ANOVA						
Source of Variation	**SS**	**df**	**MS**	**F**	**P-value**	**F crit**
Between Groups	41.88	3	13.96	3.63	0.0219	2.87
Within Groups	138.50	36	3.85			
Total	180.38	39				

The ANOVA output summary shows the number of observations in each group (*Count*), the reported pain levels (*Sum*), the group mean (*Average*), and *Variance*. Variance is the sum of the squared differences of each observation from its group mean divided by n-1, $\sum(x_{ij} - \overline{X}_j)/(n - 1)$. The bottom half of Table 9.10 reports whether the null hypothesis should be accepted or rejected. Statistical significance is determined by the **p-value**. The p-value indicates that the probability of observing the test statistic when the null hypothesis (no change or independence) is true. The p-value of 0.0219 indicates the probability that this amount of difference between group means, F = 3.63, would be observed if there were no relationship between the education and training program and reported pain levels. Given that the probability of observing this amount of difference is 2.19% and statistical significance requires a probability of 5.0% or less, we can conclude that group membership is related to pain levels.

p-value
the probability of obtaining a result as extreme as the one observed when the null hypothesis, no relationship, is true

Statistical significance can also be assessed using the F and F $crit$ values. When F (the test statistic) exceeds F $crit$ (the critical value), the null hypothesis of no relationship can be rejected. Since F, 3.63, exceeds F $crit$, 2.87, we can conclude that there is a difference among the four group means. ANOVA does not identify which group means are different, only that one or more groups has a mean that differs substantially from the other groups. For medical management, we do not know which programs work, that is, whether everybody, only staff, or only patients should be trained. All we know is that reported pain levels for at least one of the groups is significantly different from the others.

We can assume that there is significant difference between the control group, which has the highest average level of reported pain, 6.8, and the staff-and-patient group, which has the lowest at 4.2. We can also assume that there is probably no difference between the control and the patient-only group due to the small difference between the two groups, 6.8 versus 6.6, so designing an education program solely for patients will not achieve the desired goal of reducing patient pain levels.

The easiest way to determine whether reported pain is different between groups is to run an ANOVA on groups of two. For example, comparing the control group to the staff-and-patient group produces Table 9.11. There would be no need to run pairwise comparisons if the four-group ANOVA had found no statistical difference.

Table 9.11 Excel ANOVA Pairwise Output, Control vs. Staff-and-Patient

ANOVA: SINGLE FACTOR				
SUMMARY				
Groups	**Count**	**Sum**	**Average**	**Variance**
Control	10	68	6.8	2.84
Staff-and-patient	10	42	4.2	4.18

ANOVA					
Source of Variation	**SS**	**df**	**MS**	**F**	**P-value**	**F crit**
Between Groups	33.8	1	33.80	9.63	0.0061	4.41
Within Groups	63.2	18	3.51			
Total	97.0	19				

Table 9.11 confirms our assumption that training of both staff and patients produces a statistically significant reduction in reported pain levels compared to a group receiving no training. The p-value indicates that the difference between group means, 6.8 versus 4.2, would be observed only 0.6% of the time if there were no relationship between the reported pain levels (DV) and group membership (IV).

The reported pain levels were the extreme values. Would a staff-only education program reduce reported pain? To answer this question, a third ANOVA must be run, comparing the control group to the staff-only group. The output is shown in Table 9.12. One advantage of a staff-only program is that fewer people would be trained, so the training may be easier to manage.

Table 9.12 Excel ANOVA Pairwise Output, Control vs. Staff Only

ANOVA: SINGLE FACTOR				
SUMMARY				
Groups	**Count**	**Sum**	**Average**	**Variance**
Control	10	68	6.8	2.84
Staff	10	59	5.9	4.10

ANOVA						
Source of Variation	**SS**	**df**	**MS**	**F**	**P-value**	**F crit**
Between Groups	4.05	1	4.05	1.17	0.2944	4.41
Within Groups	62.50	18	3.47			
Total	66.55	19				

The results indicate that there is no statistical difference in the reported pain levels between the control (6.8) and staff-only group (5.9). The p-value indicates that we would expect to see this amount of difference, 0.9, between the group means 29.4% of the time if there were no relationship between the education program and reported pain levels. Consequently, we conclude that there is no statistical difference between the two groups: a staff-only education program is as ineffective as providing no training. Let's explore the difference between the staff-only group and the staff-and-patient group, which was previously shown to be effective. Table 9.13 displays the results.

Table 9.13 Excel ANOVA Pairwise Output, Staff Only vs. Staff-and-Patient

ANOVA: SINGLE FACTOR				
SUMMARY				
Groups	**Count**	**Sum**	**Average**	**Variance**
Staff	10	59	5.9	4.10
Staff-and-patient	10	42	4.2	4.18

ANOVA						
Source of Variation	**SS**	**df**	**MS**	**F**	**P-value**	**F crit**
Between Groups	14.45	1	14.45	3.49	0.0781	4.41
Within Groups	74.50	18	4.14			
Total	88.95	19				

The results indicate that there is no significant difference in reported pain levels between the staff-only group, 5.9, and the staff-and-patient group, 4.2. The p-value indicates that we would expect to see a difference of 1.7 in group means 7.8% of the time if there were no relationship between the education program and reported pain levels.

The seeming paradox is that the effectiveness of the staff-only training in reducing reported pain levels was shown to be equivalent to the control group but was also shown to be equivalent to the significantly lower pain levels reported in the staff-and-patient group. This paradox is based on the amount of difference between the group means and the sample sizes. The reported pain levels in the staff-only group were not sufficiently different from either group to be statistically significant. In samples of greater than ten, a difference of 1.7 may be statistically significant. From a managerial standpoint, the conclusion should be that training must include staff and patients to achieve lower reported pain levels.

Applications of ANOVA

Shaw et al. (2010) wanted to assess whether accreditation or ISO (International Standards Organization) certification were related to quality management measures in Europe. The sample, n = 71, contained 34 accredited hospitals, 10 hospitals with ISO certification, and 27 which were neither accredited nor certified. A four-point scale was used to evaluate 229 criteria, which were summarized in six categories: management, patient rights, patient safety, clinical organization, clinical practice, and environment. Certified and unaccredited hospitals had the lowest scores, and ANOVA found that these hospitals had significantly lower scores than the accredited hospitals in every category except patient rights. Accredited hospitals had significantly higher scores than ISO-certified hospitals in management, patient safety, and clinical practice. This study used ANOVA effectively to determine whether quality management processes differed systematically across three distinct groups.

Analysis of Means

Analysis of means (ANOM) is used to determine whether individual or group performance, measured by the number of events, is significantly different from the average. This determination is based on comparing individual or group means against a grand mean calculated for all individuals or groups. ANOM can be used to identify potential problems and their causes.

ANOM is similar to SPC and ANOVA. Like c charts, ANOM creates control limits but rather than asking whether the process stable, the question in ANOM is: Do any individuals or groups differ from the grand mean? Unlike SPC, ANOM is not time-dependent but rather assesses individual or group performance across multiple time periods, accounts for the number of observations in each group, and assumes that the system is stable. ANOM uses a single rule to determine excessive variation: Is a control limit broken? ANOM can be used to measure compliance with treatment recommendations (process) or outcomes.

$$\text{Mean} = \sum \text{Observed events of interest/Total opportunites (N), also know as the grand mean} \tag{9.3}$$

$$\text{UCL}_i = \text{mean} + 3 \times \sqrt{\text{Mean} \times (1 - \text{mean})/n_i}, \text{ upper control limit for group i} \tag{9.4}$$

$$\text{LCL}_i = \text{mean} - 3 \times \sqrt{\text{Mean} \times (1 - \text{mean})/n_i}, \text{ lower control limit for group i} \tag{9.5}$$

n_i = group i sample size

p_i = observed events$_i$/n_i – group i mean

In the United States in 2000, approximately one in eight children were prescribed Ritalin for treatment of attention deficit hyperactivity disorder. A managed care company wants to analyze physician prescription rates to determine if over- or underuse is occurring.

Table 9.14 Ritalin Prescription Rates

MD	On Ritalin	Patients	Percent
1	12	103	11.65
2	8	54	14.81
3	24	98	24.49
4	14	200	7.00
5	10	75	13.33
6	11	93	11.83
7	4	66	6.06
8	35	255	13.73
	118	944	

In many cases a column chart would be created using only the number of patients prescribed Ritalin and would ignore a physician's case load. Figure 9.7 demonstrates if only raw counts are graphed attention is immediately drawn to the highest prescriber, physician 8, but should this doctor be the focus of attention? When case load is incorporated into the analysis, as shown in the last column of Table 9.14, prescription rates vary from 6.06% to

24.49%, indicating that concern should be based on the rate of prescription (observed events of interest/sample size) rather than on the total number of prescriptions. Over- and underprescription may be a problem; does a low rate indicate unmet patient needs, or do high rates indicate overprescribing?

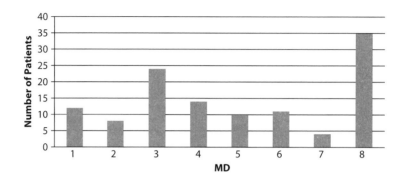

Figure 9.7 Number of Patients Prescribed Ritalin

ANOM asks: Is any physician's prescription rate too high or low? An average, p_i, must be calculated for all eight physicians, and control limits need to calculated for each physician based on the size of their specific patient population. The calculations below are for physician 1.

$$\text{Mean (center line)} = 118/944 = 0.1250$$

$$UCL_1 = 0.1250 + 3 \times \text{square root } (0.1250 \times (1 - 0.1250/103))$$

$$= 0.1250 + 3 \times 0.326$$

$$= 0.1250 + 0.0978 = 0.2228$$

$$LCL_1 = 0.1250 - 3 \times \text{square root } (0.1250 \times (1 - 0.1250) / 103)$$

$$= 0.1250 - 0.0978 = 0.272$$

As long as physician 1's prescription rate remains between 2.72% and 22.28%, her prescription practices do not require investigation. Investigation will be necessary to determine if patient needs are being unmet if her rate falls below 2.72%. If her prescription rate rises above 22.28%, investigation will be required to ensure that she is not overprescribing Ritalin.

Calculating the control limits for MD 1 in Excel requires the following calculations:

$$\text{Mean: } = B32/C32$$

$$UCL_1 := D\$16 + 3 \times SQRT (D\$16 \times (1 - D\$16)/C8)$$

$$LCL_1 := D\$16 - 3 \times SQRT (D\$16 \times (1 - D\$16)/C8)$$

Note that the $ proceeding row number 16 indicates that the function will always reference the grand mean, and C8 references the physician-specific patient population, so these formulas can be copied down the spreadsheet for physicians 2 through 8. Table 9.15 shows the results of these calculations, and Figure 9.8 is the result of inserting a line chart referencing the following columns: %, Mean, UCL, and LCL (B through E).

Table 9.15 Upper and Lower Control Limits for Ritalin Prescription Rates

Physician	%	Mean	UCL	LCL	
1	11.65%	12.50%	22.28%	2.72%	
2	14.81%	12.50%	26.00%	0.00%	* increased from −1.00%
3	24.49%	12.50%	22.52%	2.48%	
4	7.00%	12.50%	19.52%	5.48%	
5	13.33%	12.50%	23.96%	1.04%	
6	11.83%	12.50%	22.79%	2.21%	
7	6.06%	12.50%	24.71%	0.29%	
8	13.73%	12.50%	18.71%	6.29%	

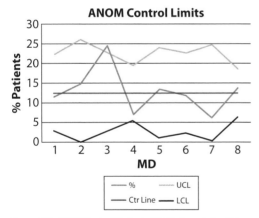

Figure 9.8 ANOM Control Limits for Ritalin Prescription Rates

Figure 9.8 shows that the range of acceptable performance varies inversely with the size of a physician's patient population: as the number of patients increases, less variation is expected and tighter control limits are established (MD 4). Conversely, as the patient population shrinks, more variation is expected and looser limits are created (MDs 2 and 7). MD 2's lower limit was increased from −1.00% since negative prescription rates are not possible. The UCL and LCL are symmetrical around the mean; that is, the UCL and LCL for each physician is an equal but opposite distance from the center line. The control limits are mirror images.

Physician 3's prescription rate of 24.49% requires investigation since it exceeds the expected UCL of 22.52% based on a population of 98 patients. The examination of MD 3's prescribing patterns will conclude either that the rate is appropriate given the physician's patient population (he may be a specialist and be referred the most difficult patients) or that the rate is inappropriate (overprescribing of medication is occurring and the physician needs education and training on prescribing practice).

Applications of ANOM

Karen Homa (2007) used ANOM to examine referral patterns. The goal of her study was to determine whether there were any significant differences in referral rates across providers for patients with low mental health scores or other patient characteristics. She found an overall referral rate of 38%, with a range of 18% to 74%. Three providers' referral rates were significantly above the average, and three significantly lower.

Further investigation found that other patient characteristics explained the different referral rates; higher rates were documented for patients who rated their health as poor, those that had prior surgery, and those between the ages of 30 and 39. Referral rates were significantly lower for patients over 60 years of age. As with the stratification charts introduced in Chapter Four, Homa demonstrated how data could be sliced at various levels to identify providers with significant variation in referral patterns and track these differences to other patient characteristics. This tracking ability greatly enhances an analyst's understanding of variations and ability to assess whether differences are justified.

Homa concluded that a stable system of behavioral medicine referral does not seem to exist, given the vastly different provider-referral rates. This type of analysis provides the starting point—ascertaining where referral differences exist—for a discussion with providers and patients into why differences exist and the ramifications of these differences.

Regression Analysis

Regression is used to determine whether there is a statistical relationship between two continuous variables; that is, does a change in an IV predict a change, whether positive or negative, in a DV? This tool can be used to identify the potential causes of a quality issue, that is, to identify what factors are significantly related to disease and outcome.

A scatter diagram can be used to graphically document the relationship between two variables. In Chapter Four, a scatter plot was created documenting the inverse relationship between LOS and the number of DRG 143 cases a hospital handles. Figure 4.20 demonstrated that an increase in the number of cases performed was correlated with a decrease in LOS. When a linear trend line was inserted into the scatter diagram, it plotted the best fitting line. While the relationship between the two variables was clearly demonstrated, it did not tell us how much we can expect LOS to decrease for each case performed or if the relationship was statistically significant.

Using the same data set, Chapter09.xls, Table 09–16 tab, we will plot the number of cases and average charge. In a two-variable regression, the tool estimates the **intercept** (the value of the DV when the IV equals zero) and the coefficient (the expected change in the DV for a one-unit increase in the IV). The question is: Do more cases lead to lower charges (through greater efficiency), or do more cases drive charges upward (through diseconomies of scale)? An additional feature of regression is that it can estimate the percentage of the change in the DV explained by changes in the IV.

intercept
the predicted value of the dependent variable when all the independent variables are zero

The formula for the best fitting (regression) line is:

$$Y = a + bX + e$$

9.6

Where:

Y is the dependent variable

X is the independent or explanatory variable

a is the intercept, the value of the DV when the IV is zero

b is the slope of the best fitting line and describes the change in the DV for every one-unit increase in the IV

e is the error term, the unexplained change in the DV

Figure 9.9 shows a positive relationship between cases and average charge, but the issue is how much can we predict charges to increase for each additional case a hospital performs?

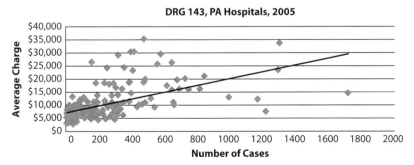

Figure 9.9 Scatter Diagram of Average Charge and Case Volume

To produce the regression, select **Data** from the Excel main menu, select **Data Analysis**, and then select **Regression** from the Data Analysis menu.

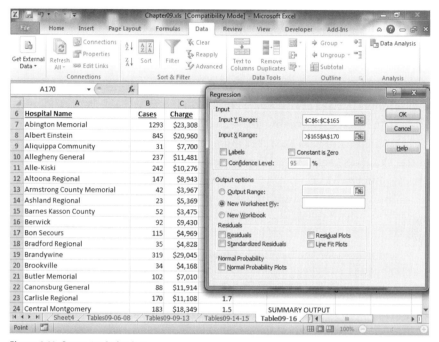

Figure 9.10 Regression Dialog Box

Input <u>Y</u> Range: enter the DV range

Input <u>X</u> Range: enter the IV range

Labels: Check <u>L</u>abels if data columns have headings describing the data. Labels are highly recommended to ensure that the output is easy to interpret. If labels are not checked, the regression output will list independent variables as: X Variable 1, X Variable 2. . .

Con<u>f</u>idence Level: Adjust confidence level if necessary; default = 95% <u>O</u>utput options: may select <u>O</u>utput Range and enter a cell to display the regression output in the current worksheet, New Workbook <u>P</u>ly, and designate a name to create a new worksheet within the existing file, or New <u>W</u>orkbook, to create a new file

coefficient of determination

the amount of change in the dependent variable that is explained by changes in the independent variables

Clicking the OK button produces the output shown in Table 9.16.

The **coefficient of determination**, *R square* or R^2, provides the amount of change in the DV explained by changes in the IV. In this example, $R^2 = 0.3087$, which indicates that 30.87% of the change in the average charge for DRG 143 is explained by changes in the number of cases a hospital handles. Conversely, this means that 69.13% of the variation in average charge

Table 9.16 Excel Regression Output

SUMMARY OUTPUT	
Regression Statistics	
Multiple R	0.5556
R Square	0.3087
Adjusted R Square	0.3043
Standard Error	5586.53
Observations	159.00

ANOVA					
	Df	**SS**	**MS**	**F**	**Significance F**
Regression	1	2.19E+09	2.19E+09	70.12	2.92E-14
Residual	157	4.9E+09	31209279		
Total	158	7.09E+09			

	Coefficients	**Standard Error**	**t Stat**	**p-value**	**Lower 95%**	**Upper 95%**
Intercept	7159.06	596.79	12.00	6.06E-24	5980.29	8337.83
Cases	13.10	1.56	8.37	2.92E-14	10.01	16.19

is explained by other variables. The maximum value for R^2 is 1.0; that is, 100% of the variation in the DV is explained by changes in the IV. On the other hand, 0.0 is the minimum value, indicating that none of the variation is explained by changes in the IV.

The intercept and slope (*Coefficients*), 7159.06 and 13.10, show that when cases are zero, the expected charge would be $7,159.06 and that the average charge increases by $13.10 for each case performed. The *p-value* column records statistical significance. The p-value for the intercept of 6.06E-24 is in scientific notation, with 24 zeros after the decimal point, showing that the probability that this value would be observed by chance is below 5.0%. Similarly, the p-value for the **slope coefficient** is 2.92E-14, and it is also significant. The *Lower 95%* and *Upper 95%* demonstrate the possible range of the effect of the IV. For each case handled, there is a 95% chance that the average charge per case will increase from $10.01 to $16.19.

The regression results can be used to predict charges. If a hospital produces 100 cases per year, their predicted average charge would be:

$$\$7,159.06 + (\$13.10 \times 100) = \$8,469.06$$

A hospital producing 1,000 cases would be:

$$\$7,159.06 + (\$13.10 \times 1000) = \$20,259.06$$

slope coefficient
the change in the dependent variable that is predicted by a one-unit increase in an independent variable

If we can identify a variable that has a documented statistical relationship with a desired outcome variable, then we can use this information to predict and possibly control the DV. That is, we can change the IV to attempt to increase or decrease the DV to improve outcome. Regression does not prove that the number of cases causes a change in average charge, and as stated earlier, only 30.13% of the change in average charge was explained by changes in the number of cases. Researchers should identify other factors that may explain changes in charges, such as patient age, existence of other medical factors, cost of living in the area in which the provider is located, and so on.

Multiple Regression

Multiple regression uses more than one IV to determine the impact of multiple factors, including various patient and clinical factors, on health outcomes. Assume a physician wants to determine which patient behaviors may have the greatest impact on cholesterol levels, and he collects data from 15 patients to determine the potential causes of high cholesterol (see Table 9.17).

Table 9.17 Cholesterol Data Set

	Y	X_1	X_2	X_3	X_4	X_5	X_6
Patient	Total Cholesterol	Weight	Exercise (Days/ Week)	Diet (Saturated Fat)	Smoking	Rx	Pulse
1	240	203	0	120	0	1	68
2	180	165	4	80	0	0	66
3	196	182	1	95	1	0	60
4	221	196	1	100	0	0	66
5	279	254	0	150	1	0	78
6	233	221	0	110	0	0	82
7	165	168	7	70	0	1	87
8	245	212	0	125	0	1	81
9	193	180	3	90	0	0	69
10	302	274	0	150	1	0	72
11	251	238	0	125	1	0	68
12	188	163	3	80	0	0	76
13	146	158	5	120	0	0	60
14	265	278	0	170	1	0	73
15	213	194	0	105	0	0	75

Where

Total cholesterol is measured as mg/dL. Over 240 indicates high cholesterol, between 200 and 240 is borderline high, and under 200 is desirable.

Weight: measured in pounds

Exercise: recorded as number of 20-minute-or-more episodes per week

Diet: measured as percentage of daily recommended saturated fat consumption

Smoking: 1 = smoker, 0 = nonsmoker

Rx: 1 = prescribed diuretic, 0 = no medication

Pulse: measured as beats per minute

Note that the variables Smoking and Rx are categorical IVs, which highlight the fact that regression can be used to determine the relationship between a numeric DV and a categorical IV as well as numeric IVs. Regression quantifies the size (how much the DV changes with a one-unit increase in the IV) and strength (how much of the change in the DV is explained by changes in the IV) of the relationship.

Formula:

$$Y = a + b_1X_1 + b_2X_2 + \ldots + b_nX_n + e$$

Where

b_n is the coefficient of the nth variable and describes the expected change in the dependent variable for every one-unit increase in the nth variable when all other independent variables are constant.

The cholesterol example recognizes that typically more than one IV is related to a DV. The typical regression model includes multiple IVs and calculates a slope coefficient and p-value for each IV. The analyst selects **Data, Data Analysis**, and **Regression** as before. The only change from the two-variable regression is the inclusion of more than one column in Input X Range; that is, more than one IV will be used to predict changes in the DV.

R^2 shows 95.1% of the variation in total cholesterol is explained by changes in the six IVs. *Adjusted R Square* considers the number of IVs used and recognizes that as more variables are added to the regression equation, the explanatory power will increase even if poorly chosen variables are used. Adjusted R^2 penalizes a researcher for using an excessive number of IVs by reducing the estimate of the change explained by the IVs; in this case explanatory power is reduced by 3.7% to 91.4%.

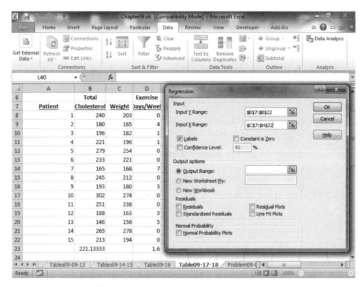

Figure 9.11 Multiple Regression Dialog Box

Table 9.18 Excel Multiple Regression Output

SUMMARY OUTPUT	
Regression Statistics	
Multiple R	0.9751
R Square	0.9509
Adjusted R Square	0.9140
Standard Error	12.84
Observations	15

ANOVA					
	Df	**SS**	**MS**	**F**	**Significance F**
Regression	6	25526.61	4254.43	25.80	8.07E-05
Residual	8	1319.13	164.89		
Total	14	26845.73			

	Coefficients	**Standard Error**	**t Stat**	**p-value**	**Lower95%**	**Upper 95%**
Intercept	63.97	40.06	1.60	0.1490	−28.41	156.35
Weight	1.08	0.32	3.32	0.0106	0.33	1.82
Exercise (Days/Week)	−6.02	2.39	−2.51	0.0361	−11.54	−0.50
Diet (Saturated Fat)	−0.36	0.30	−1.19	0.2679	−1.06	0.34
Smoking	−3.35	12.85	−0.26	0.8010	−32.98	26.29
Rx	12.14	9.92	1.22	0.2558	−10.73	35.02
Pulse	−0.21	0.69	−0.30	0.7682	−1.80	1.38

F, shown in the ANOVA section of the regression output, records whether the group of IVs as a whole is significant in explaining the change in the DV. In a two-variable regression, the significance of the F stat is equal to the p-value of the sole IV. When more than one IV is used, the group of IVs as a set may be significant while the individual variables are insignificant. *Significant F*, 8.07E-05, in the regression output shows that the probability of observing this relationship between the DV and the IVs is below 5% and the set of IVs is significantly related to cholesterol levels.

From a medical management perspective, the provider wants to understand which IVs may have the largest effect on cholesterol and which should be focused on to improve cholesterol levels. *Coefficients* shows the calculated change in the DV from a one-unit change in an IV when the other IVs are held constant, and the *p-value* indicates whether the relationship is statistically significant. Significance is determined if the p-value is equal to or less than 0.05 (5.0%).

The only variables that are significantly related to cholesterol are weight and exercise. The regression equation indicates that total cholesterol increases by 1.07 units for every one pound increase in weight. The p-value for weight indicates that there is a 1.1% probability that this increase would be observed if there was no relationship between cholesterol and weight. Since the p-value is less than 5.0%, we reject the null hypothesis, no relationship between weight and cholesterol, and conclude that cholesterol increases with weight. The coefficient for exercise indicates that for every episode of exercise per week cholesterol will decrease by 6.02 units. The p-value for exercise indicates that there is a 3.6% chance an effect of this size would be observed if there were no relationship between cholesterol and weight.

Statisticians hesitate to describe these relationships as cause and effect, instead relying on the term **correlation**. Correlation does not assume causation; in the extreme case a researcher could reverse cause and effect—total cholesterol causes exercise—and the coefficients, significance, and explanatory power would be the same. Based on existing medical knowledge, we can describe the relationships between weight and exercise and total cholesterol level as cause and effect. The remaining IVs—diet, smoking, Rx, and pulse—were not statistically significant as their p-values exceeded 5.0%.

correlation documents the percentage of time that two variables move together; the movement of the two variables may be may be direct or inverse

For management purposes, identifying the cause of a problem or selecting a solution, we would focus on weight and exercise. The cause of high cholesterol is excess weight and lack of exercise; to reduce cholesterol levels a physician should recommend losing weight and increasing exercise. Given the statistically insignificant results for the remaining four issues, no change in cholesterol level is expected if diet, smoking, pharmaceutical use, or pulse change.

Applications of Regression Analysis

Damberg et al. (2010) explored the factors associated with better medical performance, given the demands that providers face to improve care and the scarcity of evidence on what to implement. They identified three dependent variables: diabetes management, processes of care, and intermediate outcomes (LDL and HbA1c control). Their independent variables were the use of care management processes (CMP) and electronic medical records (EMR) and participation in quality improvement (QI) initiatives. Their results showed higher use of CMPs were associated with improvements in diabetes management ($p = 0.001$) and intermediate outcomes ($p < 0.001$). CMP was measured as an index of six distinct processes: electronic patient lists, guideline-based reminders, physician feedback, patient reminders, patient education, and case managers, where each one-unit change in the index increased diabetes management performance by 3.2 points on a 100-point scale and intermediate performance by 0.6 points. EMR use was not associated with any change in the three dependent variables. Participation in QI initiatives was associated with a positive change only in care processes ($p = 0.02$). Their regression models produced adjusted R^2 between 0.17 and 0.30. Based on their findings, the best use for scarce resources would be investing in CMP, but the authors advise that their findings do not distinguish which of the six CMP processes produced the greatest improvement in care.

David Becker (2007) used regression to study a provocative question: Is quality of care lower in hospitals on weekends? We assume that quality should be the same regardless of what day a patient is hospitalized, but is this assumption valid? If the quality of care varies by day of admission, this knowledge can be used to improve care. Becker's study examined Medicare patients admitted for acute myocardial infarction and found that patients admitted on the weekend were significantly less likely to receive timely cardiac catheterization, angioplasty, and bypass surgery. Weekend patients also had lower overall expenditures; they consumed less care and had higher one-year mortality rates. Becker calculates that weekend patients' mortality risk increased by 0.38%, which translated into a 67.9% to 87.5% increase in expected mortality. This study provides evidence that quality in hospitals varies by the day of admission and suggests a clear path to improve care.

Quality Improvement and Research

Quality management is applied research; taking what is known about best practice and determining if it is followed in practice and whether it produces better patient outcomes. Quality management is based on the scientific method and begins with identifying a potential for improved outcomes. Once a perceived performance gap is identified, the quality improvement team considers how outcomes can be improved. The team should review the literature to determine whether other organizations have achieved superior outcomes and, if so, how they produced better results. After identifying better methods, the quality management team seeks to implement these methods and monitor practice to ensure that better results are realized.

The literature review marks one distinction between quality management and basic research. Basic research seeks to discover "new" knowledge or new ways of doing things, while quality management seeks better use of existing knowledge. In practice the principal differences between quality management and research lie in the study population and goal. Quality management projects lack the rigorous study design of research. In quality management, the study population may be based on convenience rather than **randomization**. A **convenience sample** is drawn from a population that is easily accessible and the sample may not reflect the general population. Randomization in clinical research seeks to ensure that every member of a population has an equal chance of being assigned to experimental or control groups, and as Guyatt, Sackett, and Cook (1993) note, randomization ensures that known and unknown factors that could affect outcomes are equally distributed among the two groups.

Quality management runs a greater risk of **selection bias**; that is, the patients and providers in the experimental group may be more motivated to participate, and their motivation, more than the intervention, may explain any results produced. Selection bias and lack of randomization may lead to profound differences between experimental and control groups. Thus authors of basic research studies control **confounders** by excluding participants based on specified criteria. Medical practice must treat all patients, so quality management projects must identify and quantify confounders to the extent possible.

Research also attempts to limit variation in treatment through the use of rigorous treatment protocols to ensure that any outcome can be attributed to the intervention and not to changes in other variables. Similar to the situations in which all patients are accepted, quality management attempts to assess the effect of one intervention across multiple providers without establishing a strict treatment standard. The rigorous specification of research studies—who is treated, how they are treated, and by whom—is designed to increase the generalizability of the findings, so that the same intervention will produce the same result at other sites. Guyatt, Sackett, and Cook (1993) note that when using observational studies, the user should determine whether the groups were randomized, all subjects are accounted

randomization
assignment of an individual to a control or experimental group by chance; in a random sample every individual has an equal probability of being assigned to either group

convenience sample
the selection of test subjects based above ease of access; unlike samples chosen randomly, the results of studies using convenience samples are less generalizable to other groups

selection bias
patients and providers in experimental groups may be more motivated to participate, and their motivation, more than the intervention, may explain the results produced

confounders
variables other than the independent variable(s) included in a study that are correlated with the dependent and independent variables

for at the end of the study, selection bias was controlled (and if so, how), and whether groups were equally treated. The extent of differences between groups (confounders) should also be determined.

Of course, medical practice does not operate according to strict research standards. There are wide variations in treatment, and this raises the question of whether quality management or research is more useful to everyday medical practice. Research establishes efficacy, the power to produce an effect, but does it establish effectiveness, the ability to produce a result in practice? Naylor and Guyatt (1996) remind users of observation studies to recognize that differences in outcomes may arise from what services are provided, as well as who, where, and when the services were provided.

Tunis, Stryer, and Clancy (2003) note that the advantage of quality management studies versus randomized clinical trials is the range and distribution of patients seen in practice. Besides variations in treatment, practice must deal with patient diversity, including patient compliance, and with an array of complications and comorbidities. The rigorous design of research bestows an often unwarranted superiority of research (more valid

generalizable
the extent to which the results of a study can be expected to be reproduced in another group

and **generalizable**) over quality management, but quality management may have greater applicability to the medical system, where patients and providers interact on a daily basis. The fallibility of research was documented by Ioannidis (2005), who found that one-third of reports published in highly rated medical journals turned out to be ineffective or produced opposite results from those originally cited.

A key distinction between research and quality management is **institu-**

institutional review board
a committee assembled to review, approve, and monitor research studies involving humans to protect test subjects

tional review board (IRB) approval. The goal of IRB approval is to prevent harm to patients. IRB approval is mandatory for research because research creates new knowledge and the impact of an innovation may be unknown, but the risk of harm is typically lower in quality improvement projects. Quality management often utilizes common medical interventions and standardizes care, neither of which carries the risk of implementing a new treatment process; thus IRB approval is not mandatory.

Information sharing is another factor that should be considered in determining whether an IRB is required. Many hold that any intent to publish requires IRB approval (Cepero 2011; Kemper, Denne, and Miles 2011; Ramachandran and Kheterpal 2011). In reality, every patient encounter is a clinical trial; physicians and patients choose treatment, observe results, and adjust their actions based on outcomes achieved and on their goals. Requiring an IRB for every improvement project will ensure that fewer projects are undertaken and less information is shared. Ellwood (1988) notes that outcomes management, the explicit recording of interventions used and outcomes in practice, could be a "clinical trial machine" where medical science could be constantly assessed and subject to revision.

Another primary difference is that research is defined and discrete. It addresses a single issue, whereas quality management is built on continuous quality improvement, the PDCA cycle, and the idea that "good enough is never good enough." Quality management continually assesses the system and performance and makes changes as necessary. Such "on-the-fly" adaptations are not allowed in research. Similarly, the results of research may take years to enter practice, but quality management discoveries may have immediate, if limited, impact. One can think back to Semmelweis's procedure of washing in chlorinated lime in 1847 and Lister's germ theory discovery in 1867. Semmelweis's discovery immediately improved the health of his patients and was an input to Lister's discovery. Lister's work ranks as one of the world's great discoveries. It explained why Semmelweis's procedure was effective, and it led to widespread, if belated, acceptance of antisepsis practices.

While research is the pursuit of new knowledge and is an input to quality management, quality management pursues the larger goal of ensuring the best use of existing knowledge. In ensuring and promoting this goal, quality management should use the same tools as research to show that quality initiatives are producing the intended results. Ellwood (1988) notes that the health care system "is unstable, confused, and desperately in need of a central nervous system that can help it cope with the complexities of modern medicine." Research and quality management are two tools to build an effective information system to ensure that one-on-one patient-physician encounters are creating the maximum benefit for patients and society. In Wernher von Braun's words: "We can lick gravity, but sometimes the paperwork is overwhelming." It would be unfortunate if we let the paperwork deny us the benefits of widespread application of quality management tools and distribution of their findings.

Summary

This chapter introduced additional statistical tools that can be used to explore quality issues. Chi-square is used to identify relationships between two nonnumeric variables, while ANOVA explores the relationship between a categorical DV and a numeric IV. Both tools can be used to identify differences in outcomes between groups and identify problems or causes and monitor improvement efforts.

ANOM is used for numeric data and identifies excess variation between groups. ANOM can be used to identify problems and causes; for example, does one or more groups have substandard outcomes or vary significantly in their care process? Regression also explores the relationship between numeric variables, in this case to determine whether two variables are related and, if so, how much the DV is expected to change with a one-unit increase in the IV. Unlike chi-square, ANOVA, and ANOM, regression can be used to predict the amount of improvement we can expect to achieve by altering an IV; for example, do more frequent physician visits improve A1c levels and by how much?

Quality management requires providers to understand how to evaluate care, whether measured as given/not given, acceptable/unacceptable, or along a continuous scale. A review of medical literature reveals that statistical tools are routinely employed to evaluate the effectiveness of medical interventions. In addition to process analysis tools and SPC, quality management can use the tools of research to explore medical issues and document improved patient outcomes. Like research, quality management projects should not be the proprietary information of a single institution but should be distributed as widely as possible to ensure that all patients in all institutions receive the best possible care.

KEY TERMS

Alternative hypothesis	Generalizable
Analysis of means (ANOM)	Independent variable
Analysis of variance (ANOVA)	Institutional review board (IRB)
Categorical variable	Intercept
Chi-square analysis	Null hypothesis
Coefficient of determination (R-square)	p-value
	PivotTable (contingency table or cross tabulation)
Confounders	
Continuous variable	Randomization
Convenience sample	Regression
Correlation	Selection bias
Critical value	Slope coefficient
Degree of freedom	Statistical significance
Dependent variable	Test statistic
Error term	

REVIEW QUESTIONS

1. What are null and alternative hypotheses? Which hypothesis does a researcher test or attempt to support?

2. Explain statistical significance.

3. What is the difference between independent and dependent variables?

4. Describe the uses to which chi-square, ANOVA, ANOM, and regression can be applied.

5. Describe the similarities and differences between applied research as exemplified by quality management and basic research using random control trials.

PROBLEMS

1. End Result Hospital has implemented a program to reduce the incidence of pressure ulcers. The table below shows the number of pressure ulcers observed before and after the program was implemented. Was the program successful?

	Pressure Ulcer	No Pressure Ulcer	Total
Preimplementation	11	89	100
Postimplementation	3	97	100
Total	14	186	200

2. A second hospital has implemented the same pressure ulcer reduction program as End Result Hospital and observed the following results. Compare the two outcomes. If there are differences, what factors could explain the differences?

	Pressure Ulcer	No Pressure Ulcer	Total
Preimplementation	8	92	100
Postimplementation	6	94	100
Total	14	186	200

3. End Result Hospital is examining the effect of high- and low-intensity rehabilitation for hip replacement patients. Patient mobility postreplacement is based on patient self-reports and is categorized as improved, no change, or diminished. High-intensity rehabilitation is a ten-week regime; low-intensity is four weeks. Are outcomes different between the high- and low-intensity groups?

	Improved	No Change	Diminished	Total
Low-Intensity Rehab	121	22	12	155
High-Intensity Rehab	143	17	9	169
Total	264	39	21	324

4. End Result Hospital wants to assess the effectiveness of diabetes education through A1c levels. The hospital has created three groups. In the control group no instruction is provided, in group two instruction is provided by physicians, and in the third group RNs provide instruction. Are A1c levels different between groups?

Control	MD	RN
10	7	6
7	6	5
5	4	5
14	8	7
12	11	7
8	7	6
6	5	4
10	9	8
9	10	7
5	5	4

5. End Result Hospital wants to assess different approaches to the control of cholesterol. Fifty-three patients are randomly assigned to four groups: control, diet, exercise, and diet and exercise. Is there any difference between the four treatment options? What is your treatment recommendation?

Control	Diet	Exercise	Diet and Exercise
247.2	234.4	224.1	173.0
172.2	167.0	195.1	131.0
188.4	204.2	145.2	185.0
181.6	162.6	142.2	150.7
219.4	164.9	238.6	163.2
221.8	148.5	192.3	152.1
188.0	236.0	174.3	128.6
153.4	182.7	241.2	140.3

165.8	158.7	226.2	210.7
226.4	174.6	193.8	162.8
203.9	193.5	162.2	191.1
248.1	217.5	156.5	132.0
	161.5	220.6	192.8
	159.5	194.7	

6. The vice president of nursing services is concerned with the number of complaints her office has received concerning her nursing units. She has collected the following data. Do any of her departments have an excessive number of complaints?

Unit	Complaints	Patient Days
Medical	779	47250
Surgical	656	44550
Maternity	181	7650
Pediatrics	208	12825
ICU	396	19800
Psychiatric	375	18000

7. The director of surgical services has decided to study the number of post-op complications for general surgeons. Do any surgeons have an excessive number of complications?

MD	Complications	Patients
1	52	800
2	74	753
3	23	462
4	79	1125
5	68	1034
6	57	822
7	69	611
8	35	436
9	86	1348
10	52	1129
11	12	312

8. Using the Ch09Problems.xls file under the Problem 09–08 tab, run a regression on number of cases (IV) and LOS (DV). Interpret R^2, F, the IV coefficient and p-value, and the intercept. Describe the relationship between cases and LOS.

9. A physician wants to assess the potential causes of high cholesterol among her patients to tailor self-care instructions. She has collected data on total cholesterol, BMI, physical activity, age, gender, alcohol consumption, and stress. Use the Chapter09.xls file under the Problem 09–09 tab. Which variables have a statistically significant relationship with total cholesterol? If BMI can be reduced by two points, what is the expected impact on total cholesterol?

10. End Result Hospital is examining their LOS for coronary artery bypass surgery (CABG). Using past research, they collected data on LOS, patient age, smoking, BMI, comorbidities, and hospital-acquired infections, Using the Chapter09.xls file under the Problem 09–10 tab, interpret adjusted R^2, F, and the intercept. Which variables have a statistically significant relationship with LOS, and how do they affect LOS?

References

Armola R and Topp R, 2001, Variables that Discriminate Length of Stay and Readmission Within 30 Days for Heart Failure Patients, *Lippincott's Case Management* 6 (6): 246–255.

Becker D, 2007, Do Hospitals Provide Lower Quality Care on Weekends?, *Health Services Research* 42 (4): 1589–1612.

Cepero J, 2011, Differences Among Quality Improvement, Evidence-Based Practice, and Research, *Journal of Neuroscience Nursing* 43 (4): 230–232.

Damberg C, Shortell S, Raube K, Gillies R, Rittenhouse D, McCurdy R, Casalino L, and Adams J, 2010, Relationship Between Quality Improvement Processes and Clinical Performance, *American Journal of Managed Care* 16 (8): 601–606.

Daniel W, 1999, *Biostatistics: A Foundation for Analysis in the Health Sciences*, 7th ed., John Wiley and Sons, Inc., New York, NY.

Ellwood PM, 1988, Shattuck Lecture—Outcomes Management: A Technology of Patient Experience, *New England Journal of Medicine* 318 (23): 1549–1556.

Guyatt GH, Sackett DL, and Cook DJ, 1993, How to Use an Article about Therapy or Prevention: Are the Results of the Study Valid? *JAMA* 270 (21): 2598–2601.

Harrison B, Ferrari M, Campbell C, Maddens M, and Whall AL, 2010, Evaluating the Relationship Between Inattention and Impulsivity-Related Falls in Hospitalized Older Adults, *Geriatric Nursing* 31 (1): 8–16.

Homa K, 2007, Analysis of Means Used to Compare Providers' Referral Patterns, *Quality Management in Health Care* 16 (3): 256–264.

Ioannidis JP, 2005, Contradicted and Initially Stronger Effects in Highly Cited Clinical Research, *JAMA* 294 (2): 218–228.

Ishikawa K, 1985, *What Is Total Quality Control? The Japanese Way*, Prentice-Hall, Englewood, NJ.

Naylor CD, Guyatt GH, 1996, Users' Guides to the Medical Literature. X. How to Use an Article Reporting Variations in the Outcomes of Health Services, *JAMA* 275 (7): 554–558.

Kemper AR, Denne SC, and Miles PV, 2011, Publishing Quality Reports: Spreading Research and Innovation, *Pediatrics* 128 (3): e687–e688.

Ramachandran SK and Kheterpal S, 2011, Outcomes Research Using Quality Improvement Databases: Evolving Opportunities and Challenges, *Anesthesiology Clinics* 29, 71–81.

Shaw C, Groene O, Mora N, and Sunol R, 2010, Accreditation and ISO certification: Do They Explain Differences in Quality Management in European Hospitals? *International Journal of Quality in Health Care* 22 (6): 445–451.

Tunis SR, Stryer DB, and Clancy CM, 2003, Practical Clinical Trials: Increasing the Value of Clinical Research for Decision Making in Clinical and Health Policy, *JAMA* 290 (12): 1624–1632.

Veney JE, Kros JF, and Rosenthal DA, 2009, *Statistics for Health Care Professionals: Working with Excel*, 2nd ed., Jossey-Bass, San Francisco, CA.

CHAPTER 10

FAILURE MODE AND EFFECTS ANALYSIS

Introduction

This chapter shifts from a process view toward a holistic view of an organization's entire production system to emphasize the big picture. While previous chapters concentrated on tools that can be used to study parts of the health care delivery process to determine how they are functioning and whether improvements is needed, this chapter examines what the organization does, how it is structured, and what constitutes success. General system theory and the **value chain** emphasize the interrelationships between work performed within an organization and its effect on customers and employees. Activities that integrate seamlessly into the flow of work and facilitate the ultimate goal of a production process not only make customers happy but they increase job satisfaction of employees.

Failure mode and effects analysis (FMEA) examines how malfunctions can arise, their impact, and whether the malfunction can be detected and their consequences minimized. FMEA is not implemented after an error has arisen but is a prospective system review designed to identify system weaknesses and institute preventative changes before error occurs. FMEA recognizes that all errors are not created equal and generates a prioritized work list to correct the most serious system deficiencies before lesser weaknesses are tackled.

Once a system weakness is identified, effort shifts to deciding if it can be fixed. **Reengineering** is a methodology to improve the effectiveness, efficiency, quality, and customer responsiveness of operations by examining workflows. Failure is often reduced and effectiveness and

LEARNING OBJECTIVES

1. Understand general system theory
2. Apply the value chain perspective to health care
3. Apply failure mode and effects analysis
4. Understand reengineering concepts and design better systems

efficiency increased through simplifying processes, resequencing of activities, and automation.

General System Theory

Many believe that the production of health care is fundamentally different from producing other goods and services and that health care is immune from the laws that apply to the other production processes. This view obfuscates the examination of current processes and impedes the development of higher quality and safer processes. All production processes are systems designed to achieve a goal. Systems are sets of interrelated elements with definitive points at which inputs are applied and outputs produced.

Every system is perfectly constructed to produce the output it achieves. But is the output the best it could be? If the response is yes, no change is needed. If output is not the best it could be or often fails to produce the desired outcome, then a second question must be asked: Can improvement be successfully introduced to improve output? The structure of systems can be the result of conscious design or may be the result of evolution. That is, individuals working with a system adapt over time to challenges and the system is the result of action more than design. In either case, current output may be less than desired due to design errors or a design developed for an earlier time which has not been updated to incorporate changing consumer needs and desires or technological advances. On-the-fly evolutionary adaptations may have been undertaken without due consideration of their effects on other parts of the production process or may not be the best response to system challenges. System thinking allows one to visualize a process in order to simplify and understand it, monitor its performance, and identify corrective actions that could improve performance.

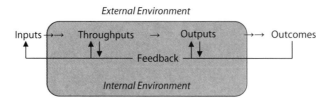

Figure 10.1　The System View

Figure 10.1, a simple model of a production system, reproduces Figure 1.4, and is repeated for the reader's convenience. The five major components are in place, and the system's dependence on the external environment for inputs and receptivity to its outputs is also shown. In the simple model the transformative process is represented as a single step, but in the real world production requires multiple transformations and hand-offs of work before a final product is produced. Figure 10.2 presents a more complex model without the feedback loop to recognize the multiple hand-offs that occur within an organization.

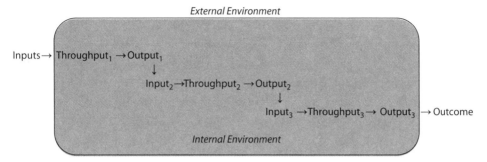

External Environment

Inputs→ Throughput$_1$ →Output$_1$
↓
Input$_2$→Throughput$_2$ →Output$_2$
↓
Input$_3$ →Throughput$_3$→ Output$_3$ → Outcome

Internal Environment

Figure 10.2 A Production Process

Most production processes are a series of input-output chains: one process produces an output that becomes the input to another process and so on. Hand-off of care is a frequent occurrence in health care; patients receive a multitude of tests and treatments from a wide array of providers. To ensure quality, the ability to measure system performance should be embedded at each step of a process and in the transitions from one subsystem to another. Failure at any point complicates later work and jeopardizes the desired outcome.

The system view emphasizes the primacy of the outcome over output. It highlights the desirability of evaluating inputs before they enter the production process, measuring the efficacy of the work performed in the transformation process, and documenting the attributes of the output produced at each step. Few people relish the opportunity to clean up problems created by others, and Figure 10.2 recognizes the interrelationship between employees and the need to produce outputs that facilitate, rather than impede, the work of coworkers. Ishikawa noted "the next process is your customer," emphasizing that the people who should evaluate intermediate outputs are those who must use them in subsequent operations (Ishikawa 1985, 104). A well-designed system should evaluate intermediate outputs of subsystems to be sure they are fit for subsequent processes; does output$_1$ meet the standards necessary to be input$_2$?

If the final output has been produced, it should be evaluated to determine how well it fulfills the goals for which the system exists. Will output$_3$ produce the desired effect or outcome? Work can and often is performed without these checks, but more effective and efficient processes determine as early as possible if preceding elements facilitate or hamper later efforts and lead to the desired outcome. If preceding elements are acceptable, producers continue to the next step in the process. If incoming elements are unacceptable, then producers should undertake the necessary steps to correct the situation before additional work is performed and institute changes to ensure that the same deficiencies do not reoccur.

The primary advantages of the system view are that it builds understanding of processes, specifies the desired level of performance, and facilitates monitoring of output through the explicit recognition of performance standards and desired outcomes. Acceptable outputs can then be passed to the next step in a system or released to the external environment. Identified substandard outputs should be corrected or discarded and redone to ensure that the desired outcome is produced. The desired output at each point in the health care process is often not explicitly defined. Health care processes suffer from the fact that they often have no definitive beginning or end point, few quality measures or measurement systems, and minimal feedback. Communication deficiencies plague interactions between physicians and patients and between health workers.

Outcome

Outcome is the value of the good or service produced (the output) to the consumer. Focusing on outcome emphasizes that the mission of the organization is not the production of goods and services but rather the production of goods and services that are valued by consumers.

Outcome should be both the starting and ending points of a process. The desired outcome is the starting point that should dictate the design of the system. Systems exist to fulfill some human need or desire; that is, the outputs of systems are designed to produce a desired outcome. Satisfying patients requires that health care outputs fulfill their intended function (an objective standard) and meet consumers' perceptions and expectations (a subjective standard). The fact that placebos produce real health benefits is a prime example of a product that does not fulfill generally accepted scientific standards for effectiveness but that nevertheless produces real benefit for patients. On the other hand, history is replete with examples of goods that performed at a high level in terms of technical standards but were rejected by consumers.

Outcome is the final measure of the effectiveness of the system. Is the system operating as designed? Is the outcome satisfying patients? Outcomes, as shown in Figures 10.1 and 10.2, exist beyond the confines of the producing organization, emphasizing that the performance of products and services is ultimately outside the control of the producer. It is easier to produce a set of outputs (such as lab tests and procedures) than an outcome (such as improved health), since uncontrollable factors beyond the walls of the organization may ultimately determine the outcome.

Health care has relied on physicians to define outcomes. Physicians have developed a system strong in technical ability (production oriented), but they have often placed less emphasis on satisfying patients' psychological needs (consumer oriented). Consumerism is refocusing health care's orientation on the needs and desires of patients. Kizer (2001) states that consumerism is refocusing patients away from service quality and access and toward clinical performance data. Cleary and Edgman-Levitan (1997), however, note the extreme difficulties of creating measures that are important and useful to patients. They note that patients want reports from people like themselves, that is, those who have similar demographic backgrounds and medical conditions, rather than Likert scale ratings of satisfaction or excellence. Patients with complicated conditions do not evaluate care on an encounter-by-encounter basis but rather as a single episode of care. A problem experienced in an initial encounter may sour a patient's perception of the entire episode of care despite exemplary care in all subsequent encounters.

Those in the health care industry must recognize that the goal is the creation of a sense of health, well-being, and respect rather than a hospital day, a **CBC**, or a **CABG**. The demand for a sense of health, well-being, and respect places a significant burden on providers to communicate clearly what the probable, not the best possible, outcome of treatment will be. Unrealistic expectations (built on prior medical miracles) are a major cause of dissatisfaction with health outcomes.

CBC
complete blood count

CABG
coronary artery bypass graft

Health care providers do not control the final outcome of care, which lies outside the contained and controlled clinical environment. Outcomes depend heavily on the patient's behavior, and this behavior is largely outside the view and control of providers. In the Coronary Drug Project, no significant difference in mortality was discovered between the treatment group and a placebo group. High adherers in both groups had significantly lower mortality than low adherers (Coronary Drug Project Research Group 1980). This study demonstrates the effect of nonmedical factors in determining outcomes. Self-selection is at work. The high-adherence groups were more willing to change their lifestyle to improve their health. In this study, adherence was more important in determining outcome than was treatment. Providers, when setting outcome standards, need to differentiate between effectiveness—the benefits obtained in a *practice*, or clinical, setting—and efficacy—the benefits obtained in an *ideal* setting (IOM 2001b).

Providers need to develop additional ways of measuring outcomes to supplement patient satisfaction. Patient satisfaction surveys focus on short-term and highly subjective criteria. Improvement in quality will depend on lengthening the measurement period. Codman noted in 1914 that health is not a short-term phenomenon and pointed out the need to develop objective measures. Clinicians are rightly reluctant to equate clinical quality with patient satisfaction scores, but in the absence of better measurement systems, patient satisfaction will continue to be used (both rightly and wrongly) for assessing medical care.

Changing provider perspectives and processes is the crucial task facing the health care industry, and change will occur only if providers are given valid and reliable outcome data. Outcome data must be more than subjective assessments of satisfaction in order to change provider behavior. Wennberg (1984) showed that physicians, when given credible data on use of medical procedures, would explore the reasons for these differences and change their practice patterns.

On the other hand, providers must be responsive to subjective assessments if they affect patient behavior after patients leave the control of the provider. Noncompliance for chronic disease has been estimated to average about 50% (Eraker, Kirscht, and Becker, 1984). Studies show that patient compliance is correlated with the quality, duration, and frequency of interaction between the patient and physician. Compliance also depends on the physician's attitude toward the patient, ability to convey information, and belief in the efficacy of treatment (Griffith 1990).

A final concern is simply the mechanics of establishing a long-term patient monitoring system. Outcomes depend on the patient's ability to manage his or her condition, but how often will behavior be measured, and who will track it? Where will the funds come from to monitor patients' behavior after they are released from care? How should patients pay for and how should providers be paid to ensure good outcomes? Outcomes must be emphasized more than outputs to ensure that providers, insurers, and patients have appropriate incentives to produce health rather than health care.

Output

Output is the end result of the transformation process on the inputs. The outputs of health care include checkups, treatments, procedures, tests, and bundles of individual items such as a physician visits or admissions. Like health outcomes, health care outputs are unpredictable; health care goods and services can be applied identically to two similar patients and the results may be greatly different. The results of treatment are probabilistic;

that is, a range of outcomes can occur as a result of appropriate treatments delivered without error. Outputs could be produced proficiently without any knowledge-, rule-, or skill-based error, yet a patient outcome may be less than desired due to the patient's physiological or psychological reaction to treatment or environmental factors.

A patient's condition may be difficult to measure because it is unstable or not explicitly assessed against standards or because standards may be lacking. The seemingly infinite number of combinations and treatments has had a detrimental effect on the development of quality measurement systems. The difficulty of measuring inputs, throughputs, and outputs has eclipsed the fundamental need to measure. The gold standard is the randomized clinical trial, but this standard ignores the fact that in the uncontrolled environment, health outcomes are paramount. Clinical practice (with more than 33,000,000 hospital admissions in the United States every year) provides a wealth of information whose input, throughout, and output could be measured. The subjectivity of quality measures is often derided for being imperfect, and the entire quality management process viewed as an unnecessary drain of resources from the more important task of meeting patients' needs. To make matters worse, many reimbursement systems consider all hospital admissions or physician visits to be of equal worth, and they pay accordingly. Unfortunately these attitudes hamper efforts to develop quality measurement systems.

Throughput

Throughput is the transformation of inputs into outputs. Throughput describes the process by which labor, resources, energy, and information are combined to produce an output. Obviously, it is impossible to define the process of care for every patient, but it is possible to provide an outline for treatment of common medical conditions; Chapter Eleven will discuss clinical practice guidelines that attempt to place medicine on a more scientific and standardized footing.

Throughput is often described as a black box. The inputs that enter the black box and the outputs that emerge from the process are clear, but what occurs inside the box is less than clear. Part of the problem lies with the idea of **equifinality**; that is, objectives can be achieved with different amounts and types of inputs and methods.

Not only can health care outputs be produced in a multitude of ways but they are also heavily reliant on labor. Many industries are more dependent on raw materials and machines, which are easier to control than human behavior. Health systems are dependent on human variability, and output is directly affected by this variability in performance, unlike the more

equifinality
the ability to achieve an objective with different amounts and types of inputs and methods

consistent output of machines. Human variability emanates from differences in skills among employees doing the same job, illness or fatigue that impairs performance, and overreliance on memory to complete tasks.

Compounding the problem of human variability is the absence of a standardized process. Brent James (1993) reports that 80% to 90% of medical practice is based on medical tradition and experience rather than published scientific research. The lack of scientific grounding does not undermine the effectiveness of most treatments but it does inhibit us from determining best practice. The absence of a standardized process makes it difficult to monitor and control the process. Without clear treatment plans including what should be done, when care should be rendered, and how a patient should be responding, one cannot determine if a patient is making appropriate progress and whether correction is needed.

Input

Inputs are labor, resources, energies, and information that enter a system. Moving farther back through the production process (Figure 10.1) we again cross the boundary separating an organization from its external environment. The significance of this passage is that the organization has less control over what occurs in the external environment than what occurs within the organization. Control over inputs entering from outside the system is essential to what is produced (outputs) and achieved (outcomes).

Quality processes in other industries begin before inputs enter the production process. Manufacturers have the ability and incentive to inspect and reject substandard inputs before work is performed. Inspection assures the producer that the materials entering the system are of sufficient quality to fulfill the purpose for which they are intended. This type of inspection and evaluation is easier with raw materials and labor, where effort can be translated into outputs with easy-to-measure quantities and quality attributes.

Health care processes use two primary human inputs, the patient and the physician, and both introduce variation into the system. As we saw in Chapter Two, physician practice styles vary dramatically, and no two patients are identical. Patients introduce many sources of variation, including medical, demographic, economic, social, and psychological factors, into a system that already produces outputs that are unpredictable.

Health care providers cannot reject patients the way other industries can reject raw materials, but they should intensively screen patients. Attention must be given to identify and define risk factors, that is, factors the patient brings into the treatment process that can diminish the effectiveness of treatment. Differences in patients' health status, attitudes, and abilities necessitate different interventions to achieve desired outcomes; otherwise the same process will result in different outcomes due to differences in the input. The IOM (2001a) reports that 40% of people with chronic conditions have more than one chronic condition and that those with two or more conditions have per capita expenditures six times higher than acute patients. High-risk patients increase the likelihood of poor outputs and outcomes. Health care processes can and do change to handle higher-risk patients, but the problem is that these accommodations are not systematically determined. Each physician is allowed to alter his or her treatment plan implicitly, and the successes and failures of these accommodations are not widely shared so that other providers and patients can learn and benefit.

Systematic improvement in quality requires that accommodations be explicit and that planners identify and quantify why the accommodations are being made, for example, what incoming risk factors the patient presented with. This task may seem burdensome and nonproductive, but the system view demonstrates why this effort is necessary: different inputs require different processes to achieve the same outcomes. The high-risk designation may reduce the likelihood of a poor outcome. A side benefit may be reduced liability; if a patient is defined as high risk prior to beginning treatment, a poor outcome is more probable and can provide a defense against claims of negligence. The other primary labor input and health care decision-maker is the physician. Physician services account for roughly 25% of total health spending in the United States but are disproportionately instrumental in determining the use of inpatient, outpatient, and home care services, and pharmaceuticals (Feldstein 1999). As with patients, the physician input is not subject to a high degree of control. Physicians typically are not employees and are not subject to the same amount of supervision and control as other health care workers. Physicians and the hospitals they work in often seem to be partners with different objectives. Although both value the patient, the differences in incentives to use one process or another must be reconciled (while still meeting the patients' and the system's goals) if the health system is to function efficiently. For example, in the DRG system there is an incentive for hospitals to discharge patients expeditiously although continued hospitalization may increase inpatient consultations for independent physicians.

Feedback

Feedback is information on system performance that reenters the system to affect subsequent performance. Feedback can be collected at any point in the process. For example, it can be collected at input and be used to stop substandard input from entering the system or to correct deficient inputs before they enter the system. In either case, standards are required. Inspection could be performed by employees, or the organization could rely on self-policing by vendors and suppliers.

Health care providers cannot refuse emergency care to patients, so information collected prior to the delivery of care should be fed forward to change the throughput process. Access to the patient's medical history could be vital when rapid treatment is needed; this information might determine not only the outcome of care but also its cost. For example, one of the challenges to health care providers has been methicillin-resistant *Staphylococcus aureus* (MRSA) because of its resistance to antibiotics and its effect on treatment of other conditions. From 2005 through 2008, the United States saw a 28% decrease in hospital-onset MRSA infections and a 17% reduction in health care–associated community-onset infections (Kallen et al. 2010). Part of the decline in MRSA infections was due to individual hospitals' recognizing the threat that patients who carry the infection pose for their patients and operations. For example, Vidant Medical Center in Greenville, NC, screens all inpatients for the MRSA virus, and patients found to be carrying the virus are placed in isolation, instructed in hand hygiene, provided dedicated equipment, and given a decolonizing bath. Controlling the input, the patient, should dictate subsequent treatment processes. In the case of MRSA, the additional precautions may reduce the cost of treatment, prevent the spread of infection, and increase reimbursement—documenting the infection at admission is vital since Medicare will not pay for hospital-acquired infections.

Performance data can also be collected during the transformation process, at the point of output, or at the point of use (outcome) to improve system performance. During the transformation process, workers should note how inputs facilitate or impede the delivery of care and feed this information back to the intake process. If the patient, providers, supplies, or equipment impede care, these obstacles must be noted so future care can be more effectively delivered.

There are times when the effectiveness of care cannot be evaluated until a definitive output is created, such as a lab test or x-ray. The users of these outputs must report any deficiencies they observe so the causes can be rectified at the point of intake or during the transformation process. Ultimately, the measure of health care success is the patient outcome: did the patient recover or improve? The feedback link between outcome and the production process is the most vital and least controlled as it requires the cooperation of the patient and may require months or years to determine the effectiveness of treatment. Health care requires communication between health care workers and between patients and providers, but this area is where health care is often most deficient. Studies find that approximately 50% of patients and their physicians disagree on the reason for the visit (Rosenberg, Lussier, and Beaudoin 1997). The goal of this text is to improve the feedback of quantitative information between workers using data of various types—continuous (timeliness, completeness), binomial (success rates), and count (number of nonconformities)—as well as information that stretches beyond the confines of the organization (readmission rates and postdischarge mortality).

Other producers engage in continuous quality monitoring, involving all members of the production team and consumers. Health care providers tend to rely on isolated and retrospective review. Continuous quality monitoring is relatively easy when products or services can be defined throughout their production cycle to determine whether they meet standards and when each part of the system communicates effectively with the other parts. The health care industry is grappling with the questions of who should measure, when to measure, and what are acceptable variances. The challenges to greater feedback in health care include expanding the monitoring and evaluation function to incorporate workers other than physicians, dealing with potential liability issues surrounding the identification of health care problems, and the lack of financial incentive to undertake quality review.

General system theory presents a way of thinking about any type of system. System theory emphasizes the essential components of a process, its internal relationships, and the interaction between the system and its environment. The external factors, besides those already noted, that play large roles in determining the effectiveness of a system include economic, social, political, legal, and physical factors. The next section introduces the idea of a value chain to advance our understanding of production processes in general and health care processes and their desired outcomes in particular.

The Value Chain

The value chain is a means of identifying where and how value is created within an organization. A value chain describes graphically the relationships between different parts of an organization and what the organization as a whole produces and achieves. Like system theory, the value chain emphasizes activities and functions, outputs, and outcomes. Michael Porter popularized the idea and describes it as a means of identifying an organization's competitive advantage. Competitive advantage is that which an organization does better than its rivals.

Figure 10.3 demonstrates the two principal components of the value chain: the parts of the organization that interact with customers (primary activities) and those that provide service to the employees dealing directly with customers (support activities) (Curran and Ladd 2000). Primary activities occur at distinct points in time, while support activities, which serve other employees, are ever present. Support activities cut across primary activities and are the foundation for all work the organization performs. Both sets of activities should be designed to increase the value to customers of the goods and services produced by the organization and to increase profits.

Porter defines five primary activities: inbound logistics, operations, outbound logistics, marketing and sales, and service. Inbound logistics encompasses acquisition of resources, inventory control, and production scheduling. All of these functions occur prior to production. Operations describes an organization's throughput activities or how goods and services are produced. In a manufacturing organization this would include machining, assembling, and packaging. Outbound logistics is concerned with connecting the product to the consumer, including order processing and delivery. Before products can be sold, customers must be identified, which is the job of marketing and sales. Marketing and sales involves all presale (or preorder) activities, including advertising and promotion and price quoting. The final primary activity is service, which includes all activities after a good or service has been provided to a customer, for example, installation, training, and repair.

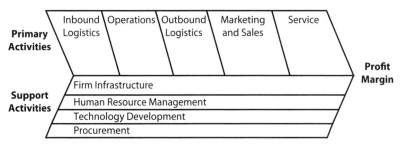

Figure 10.3 Porter's Value Chain

Support activities are designed to facilitate primary activities by ensuring that employees working with customers have the inputs (human, technology, informational, etc.) they need to quickly and effectively complete their jobs. Porter defines four support activities: procurement, technology development, human resource management, and firm infrastructure. Procurement, also known as materials management, is concerned with purchasing, inventory management, and distribution functions (Curran and Ladd 2000). Technology development is designed to ensure that employees have access to the tools that allow them to complete their tasks in the most effective and efficient manner. Technology development involves the evaluation and acquisition of technology. Human resource management involves hiring, compensation, training, evaluation, and disciplinary action. Firm infrastructure addresses the organization's structure, its decision-making process, and its culture, values, norms, and goals.

Swayne, Duncan, and Ginter (2008), in Figure 10.4, refined the value chain for health care by replacing profit maximization with patient satisfaction and focusing on primary activities that deal directly with patients at three distinct points; preservice, point of service, and after service. The three distinct service activities emphasize providing the right services (designing the care process to achieve the most desirable outcomes), delivering effective and patient-pleasing care at the point of service, and following up care to measure long-term effectiveness and identify opportunities to provide more services.

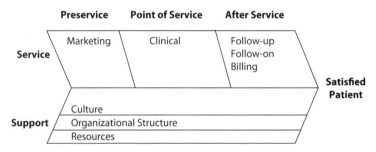

Figure 10.4 Health Care Value Chain

Source: LE Swayne, WJ Duncan, and PM Ginter, 2008, *Strategic Management of Health Care Organizations*, 6th ed., San Francisco: Jossey-Bass, 128.

Preservice activities can be viewed as the Four Ps of marketing: product, price, promotion, and physical distribution. Marketing is tasked with designing a product to meet patient needs, establishing a price patients are willing and able to pay, promoting the availability of the product, and determining where care will be provided. Point-of-service activities revolve around the patient-provider encounter and should ensure that patients receive prompt, courteous, and effective care. Swayne, Duncan, and Ginter include a product development function within point-of-service activities; that is, providers should identify unmet patient needs and desires and develop products and services to satisfy those needs. After-service activities encompass all activities occurring after a patient is released from care. Follow-up activities are designed to determine patient response to care and satisfaction with the care they received. When dissatisfaction is identified, it should be fed back into the system to improve future care. Follow-on activities are designed to identify other services patients could benefit from after they are released from care, for example, postdischarge rehabilitation or home health services. Finally, billing is recognized as a service activity because billing personnel interact directly with patients, and a pleasant and competent billing service can enhance the value of the health care experience. If billing personnel are rude, lack knowledge or skill, or produce incorrect billing statements, any goodwill created by point-of-service personnel can be destroyed. All service activities should be provided in a manner that enhances the value of the care provided in the eyes of the patient.

Support activities provide the foundation for effective and efficient service. Support activities should provide the culture, organizational structure, and required resources to employees who interact with patients to ensure they can complete their tasks as designed. If an organization believes that patients value prompt care and it wants to implement a rapid treatment system, support personnel should create an environment in which timeliness is valued and an organizational structure that facilitates rapid decision making, and provide the necessary resources to make rapid care achievable.

Figure 10.4 is deliberately drawn to emphasize patient satisfaction as the end point and purpose of the system. All activities should be designed to satisfy the patient and increase the probability of organizational success. Value chain thinking should be used to break down the silos that develop within organizations. Too often departments see themselves as the primary reason for the existence of the organization and think that other employees should modify their work to facilitate the goals of the department. The value chain makes explicit that the only reason for departments such as finance, human resources, and information technology is to facilitate the work of employees who have direct contact with patients. Similarly, the only reason for the frontline service activities is to produce satisfied patients.

The value chain examines the goal of the organization from the organizational level but emphasizes that value is added or reduced by the activities of departments. FMEA is a tool to proactively evaluate systems to identify weaknesses and strengthen processes to increase value.

Failure Mode and Effects Analysis

Failure mode and effects analysis (FMEA) is a systematic method of identifying and preventing product or process failures before they occur (Kaiser Permanente, 2002). Unlike concurrent system feedback, FMEA is a prospective approach to determine how and why a system could fail and to introduce design changes, safeguards and barriers, and monitoring and **mitigation** systems to eliminate or reduce the probability of failure and minimize the effects of failure should it occur. Ideally, FMEA is conducted before a system is constructed and put into operation; however, FMEA can also be applied to currently operating systems to improve their performance. The key to FMEA is the focus on possible system failures and **prevention** thereof versus on remediation of extant failures.

mitigation
action to make an event less severe or painful

Substantial insight into FMEA can be gained by examining the meaning of its components. *Failure* signifies any inability to function in a desired manner, including deficiency, defect, or nonperformance. *Failure mode* signifies all the ways a process can fail; that is, what can go wrong to prevent the system from working as designed or expected? FMEA recognizes that a single deficiency, defect, or nonperformance can arise from a multitude of factors. The third component, *effects*, is concerned with the consequences of each type of failure identified. The effects may range from the insignificant to the catastrophic. Finally, *analysis* indicates a systematic examination of a complex system or process based on generally recognized principles.

prevention
action to preclude an event from occurring

FMEA has risen in prominence in health care due to the mandate of the Joint Commission, which requires hospital leaders to conduct proactive risk assessment activities every 18 months (Joint Commission 2010, LD.04.04.05). This standard also requires annual reports to the hospital's governing body reporting on failures and corrective actions that have been taken proactively and in response to sentinel events.

The FMEA Process

A brief review of FMEA processes reveals that it is implemented differently by different users. There is no one right approach, so the focus should be on the overall goal and structure of the FMEA process rather than on seeking a definitive model. FMEA should be adapted based on system complexity and type of failure being examined. There are two primary approaches to FMEA. The first is the hardware (or bottom-up) approach. This approach is often used when failure can be traced to specific components. The hardware approach is used when failure can be traced to the malfunction or absence of a component and is used when the source of the problem can be localized. The second and more appropriate approach for health care is the functional approach. The functional approach is used for complex systems that are not well defined and where failure often cannot be traced to a single factor. One can discern eight essential steps in the FMEA process. The steps described in Table 10.1 are an amalgam of different approaches.

Table 10.1 FMEA Steps

1.	Define the failure and its boundaries
2.	Define the process
3.	Identify failure modes
4.	Identify potential causes of each failure mode
5.	Evaluate the potential effects of failure
6.	Identify corrective actions to reduce or eliminate failure
7.	Document the analysis and recalculate residual risk
8.	Monitor

Step 1: Define the Failure and Its Boundaries

The team preparing the FMEA (generally a multidisciplinary group encompassing suppliers, workers providing patient care, support personnel including management and quality management specialists, and patients) begins by defining the FMEA boundary, which requires defining the system or subsystem to be analyzed. Step 1 is an information-gathering phase during which the system's goals, standards, procedures, equipment utilized, floor plans, records of failure (if available), literature reviews and expert consultations are obtained and studied to provide the foundation for the FMEA. The boundaries should define and delimit; that is, the boundaries establish the problems to be addressed and recognize what will not be addressed.

Step 2: Define the Process

Step 1 took inventory of the available documentation on a system. In step 2 the goal is to document how the system operates, which may or may not agree with current documentation. As systems evolve, adaptation takes place to improve the process or make work easier for employees. The goal of step 2 is to document the current process, identify any adaptations, and determine if they improved performance. The problem with on-the-fly adaptations is they may improve one part of the process but have a detrimental effect on other parts of the process.

Flowcharts (Chapter Four) are designed to simplify and clarify complex processes to build comprehension. Flowcharts signify events, processes, information, and interfaces and define the level of analysis. A flowchart to document a complete system, such as all the activities that are comprised in a hospitalization, will require multiple pages. On the other hand, if the analysis is concerned only with a subsystem, such as anesthesia administration, the total process may be captured on a single page. Flowcharts are often used to resolve differences in how individuals believe a system operates and document the final consensus on how the system works. Upon completion of the FMEA, the flowchart can be used to document and communicate any changes made as a result of the analysis. In addition, the flowchart can specify operating and environmental conditions that affect performance.

Step 3: Identify Failure Modes

The task in step 3 is to determine all the ways a system could fail to perform in the expected manner. This is challenging, given the multitude of ways a system can fail to deliver a desired output, but the flowchart developed in step 2 should provide a guide. The FMEA team should be more capable of identifying potential failures when a process is divided into discrete, sequential steps. Each step can then be analyzed in terms of who and what is involved and when the activity should take place.

As shown in Table 10.2, types of failures can be identified by timing, including events occurring prematurely (too soon) or belatedly (too late). A second type of failure is simply the absence of performance, that is, a required step that is not undertaken. The third and fourth types of failure deal with incomplete performance, including intermittent performance or premature conclusion of a task. A fifth failure is excess performance, the continuation of a process that should be terminated. An example would be an IV pump that should infuse a set amount of medication in a defined time period but does not shut down when the defined dose is delivered. The sixth type of failure, degraded performance, may arise from underskilled labor (lack of experience, impaired, etc.) or miscalibrated or poorly maintained machinery. The task is complete but was performed in a manner that it does not fulfill the end for which it was produced. A seventh category, *other*, can be used for failures that do not fall into the preceding types (MIL-STD-1629A 1980).

Table 10.2 Types of Failures

1.	Premature operation (timing) + belated operation (timing)
2.	Failure to operate (absence)
3.	Intermittent operation (incomplete)
4.	Failure during operation (incomplete)
5.	Failure to cease operation (excess)
6.	Degraded performance (performance)
7.	Other

A Why-Why diagram is an appropriate tool to delineate possible failure modes. The Why-Why diagram starts with one failure and then subdivides the problem into major causes to demonstrate how different factors can produce the problem. As seen in Table 10.2, a single failure can arise from timing problems, incomplete or faulty performance, absence, or excess, and each of these general problems can be broken into a myriad of other factors; for example, what produced premature operation? The beauty of FMEA is its emphasis on identifying and developing safeguards for the most important types of failures.

Step 4: Identify Potential Causes for Each Failure Mode

Possibly the most intellectually challenging and time-consuming task is to determine all the potential causes for a system failure. Just as the idea of equifinality states that an end can be achieved in a multitude of ways, failure can be the result of an infinitesimal number of factors. Identifying causes is challenging, given the multitude of ways a system can fail to deliver a desired output. As seen with the cause and effect diagram (Chapter Four), the main categories of failure may be manpower/human error, machines/equipment failure, materials/supply failure, method/process, and mother nature/environment. In health care, given the probabilistic nature of disease and biological processes and the variation in patient compliance, one could never definitively catalog all the factors and combinations of factors that could produce an undesired outcome.

As seen in Table 10.2, error arises from timing issues emanating from convenience, lack of attention, or poor scheduling, and from the absence or omission of function, incomplete performance, excess or overperformance, or degraded performance. Error can also arise from poorly designed systems, machines, supplies, or the environment. A cause and effect diagram can be used to pinpoint the most likely causes of a problem and point the way to correction.

Step 5: Evaluate Potential Effects

The potential effect of failure commonly encompasses three areas and produces a priority rating to guide improvement efforts. The effects of a failure can be categorized by severity, probability of occurrence, and probability of **detection**. Prevention and improvement efforts should be directed toward the failures that cause the most harm, are most likely to occur, and cannot be detected or mitigated. The output of step 5 is a prioritized list of failures that should be worked sequentially from the most important failures to the least important.

Severity is concerned with the effect or damage of a failure. At one extreme, failure may occur without harming a patient; at the other extreme, failure may kill the patient. The following scale was used by the U.S. military to gauge weapon system failures (MIL-STD-1629A 1980):

detection
the ability to identify a failure after its occurrence

Category I—Catastrophic: a failure that may cause death or weapon system loss. Rank: 4

Category II—Critical: a failure that may cause severe injury, major property damage, or major system damage, which will result in mission loss. Rank: 3

Category III—Marginal: a failure that may cause minor injury, minor property damage, or minor system damage, which will result in delay or loss of availability or mission degradation. Rank: 2

Category IV—Minor: a failure not serious enough to cause injury, property damage, or system damage, but which will result in unscheduled maintenance or repair. Rank: 1

The military wants to allocate resources to prevent failures that could produce the greatest threat to human safety and equipment. Category IV, minor failures, though undesirable, do not warrant attention if more damaging failures are possible. The goal of FMEA is to reduce harm by systematically working on the most damaging types of error first, and when these systems have been made safer, devoting attention to less serious failures. The output of the FMEA analysis is a numeric score that ranks potential failures based on the mathematical product of severity, probability of occurrence, and detectability. Based on the rankings given by the military, failures are worked from the highest to the lowest scores (rank 4 is worked prior to lower-ranking failures). Unlike the military, Sematech, the semiconductor manufacturing technology consortium, categorizes severity of failure on a one-to-ten scale, with higher numbers indicating more severe failures (Villacourt 1992).

Rank	Description
1–2	Failure will probably not be detected by customers (internal or external).
3–5	Failure will result in slight customer annoyance or slight deterioration in system performance.
6–7	Failure will result in customer dissatisfaction and deterioration in system performance.
8–9	Failure will produce a high degree of customer dissatisfaction and cause system failure.
10	Failure will produce major customer dissatisfaction, cause system failure or noncompliance with government regulation.

These two classification schemes emphasize that FMEA teams design their own severity scales based on industry standards or on the particular needs of their organization. The relevant point is simply to list failures in order of their impact on people and system operation. Following is a possible severity scale for health care:

Rank	Description
1	Minor failure: no injury to patient; no additional care required.
2	Modest failure: no injury to patient, minor, short-term care required.
3	Moderate failure: short-term injury to patient, major, short-term care required.
4	Critical failure: long-term injury to patient, ongoing care required.
5	Catastrophic failure: patient dies.

Estimating the likelihood of a failure occurring is the next step in assessing the effect of failure. Similar to severity, the FMEA team should concentrate its efforts on failures that are likely to occur. In many cases, the ranking of likelihood is based on best guesses. The first three columns in Table 10.3 (Apkon et al. 2004) reflect the subjectivity of the process. For remote and low probabilities, reasonable people may differ greatly due to the rarity of these events. Documentation should be available and collected for moderate events. Obviously, rankings will be more supportable when the FMEA can point to objective evidence, such as the number of failures per total number of events, failures per hours of operation, and so on.

Table 10.3 Probability of Occurrence

Likelihood	Data	Score	Probability
Remote	No known occurrence	1	1/10,000
Low	Possible but no data	2–4	1/5,000
Moderate	Documented but infrequent	5–6	1/200
High	Documented and frequent	7–8	1/100
Very High	Documented, almost certain	9–10	1/20

Column four, probability, provides a more objective measure by quantifying occurrence rates. Probability requires a common denominator that can be used across various treatments (number of events, hours of operation). One criticism that can be levied against this scheme is the gaps in the probability scale; for example, how would a probability of 1 in 7,000 be classified since it falls between a score of 1 and 2?

To avoid the problem of falling between the gaps in an arbitrary ranking scheme (or drawing bright-line distinctions between groups), an FMEA team could forgo the rank score and use probabilities, bypassing the need to translate a probability into an ordinal rank and introducing a higher degree of accuracy into the risk score calculation. Of course, probabilities can be calculated only for systems that are currently operating and that have collected data on failure. As stated earlier, the FMEA risk score is the product of severity, probability of occurrence, and detectability. Using an ordinal score rather than a probability will produce larger scores, but regardless of how big or small the risk score is, the important point is to produce a list of potential failures that is worked from the most serious to the least serious.

The third step in assessing the potential impact of a failure is determining the probability of a failure being identified before damage occurs. A patient death is easy to identify, but at this point, remediation is impossible. The team is not concerned with the theoretical ability to detect failure but rather with how likely it is that the failure will be detected in practice. Detectability can also be thought of in terms of long-term and short-term identification. Will a failure result in an immediate, observable problem, or will the effect only be identifiable at a future point in time? The hope is that failures that are immediately identified can be quickly counteracted to reduce damage, as opposed to errors whose effects can be seen only after an extended period of time. Rapid recognition of problems prevents the completion of additional work that might have to be undone to correct the original failure. Consider a foreign item left in a patient during surgery; if detected before closing, the patient will not have to be reopened. If the object is belatedly detected by an x-ray, the patient must be returned to the OR, reopened, and closed again.

Sematech uses a detectability ranking scheme based on a ten-point scale, and again the scale descriptions can be criticized for lack of clarity. Their descriptions, unlike the probability of occurrence used by Apkon et al. (2004), do not include quantitative measures of what each ranking means. The idea of "very high," for example, may mean different things to different individuals. Replacement of these rankings with the documented operational probabilities of detection (if available) would improve the calculation.

Rank	Description
1–2	Very high probability of detection: verification or controls will almost certainly detect deficiency or defect.
3–4	High probability of detection: verification or controls have a good chance of detecting deficiency or defect.
5–6	Moderate probability of detection: verification or controls are likely to detect deficiency or defect.
7–8	Low probability of detection: verification or controls not likely to detect deficiency or defect.
9–10	Very low (or zero) probability of detection: verification or controls will not or cannot detect deficiency or defect.

The final operation in evaluating the potential effects of failure is to establish a priority list to direct action to strength the system. Most FMEA systems rank failure by the product of severity, probability of occurrence, and probability of detection and label it the risk priority number (RPN).

10.1 RPN = severity * probability of occurrences * probability of detection

Improvement priorities are based on the failures with the highest numbers receiving first attention. For example, the Sematech system ranks severity, probability of occurrence, and probability of detection on ten-point scales. The maximum score, and the failure that would receive the most attention, would be one that scored 1,000. This type of failure could produce catastrophic damage, be extremely likely to occur, and be impossible to detect after occurrence (10 * 10 * 10). A failure that could produce catastrophic damage but is extremely unlikely to occur and easy to detect and mitigate would produce a score of 10 (10 * 1 * 1). This type of failure will not receive any attention as long as other failures produce higher risk scores based on the product of the severity, occurrence, and detection scores.

Table 10.4 provides an example of the FMEA processes using common medical errors. The scales used to evaluate severity, probability of occurrence, and probability of detection are shown at the bottom of the table.

Table 10.4 Failure Priority Calculation

Failure	Severity	Occurrence	Detection	RPN
Wrong-site surgery	4	5	3	60
Op or post-op complication	3	5	3	45
Delay in treatment	2	4	4	32
Medication error	1	4	3	12
Patient fall	1	3	1	3
Unintended retention of foreign body	2	3	3	18
Perinatal death or loss of function	5	2	3	30
Restraint injury or death	2	2	2	8
Transfusion error	3	2	2	12
Infection	2	2	1	4
Anesthesia	3	2	4	24
Ventilator death or injury	4	1	2	8

Severity
5-Catastrophic; 4-Critical; 3-Moderate; 2-Modest; 1-Minor
Occurrence
5-Very High; 4-High; 3-Moderate; 2-Low; 1-Remote
Detection
5-Remote; 4-Low; 3-Moderate; 2-High; 1-Very High

Re-sorting by risk priority number (RPN) from highest to lowest produces the list in Table 10.5.

Table 10.5 Failure Priority Work List

Failure	RPN
Wrong-site surgery	60
Op or post-op complication	45
Delay in treatment	32
Perinatal death or loss of function	30
Anesthesia	24
Unintended retention of foreign body	18
Medication error	12
Transfusion error	12
Restraint injury or death	8
Ventilator death or injury	8
Infection	4
Patient fall	3

The top four candidates for attention are now clear: wrong-site surgery, surgical complications, treatment delays, and perinatal death or loss of function. Table 10.5 separates potential failures into three groups: high risk, RPNs of 30 or more; moderate risk, RPN between 12 and 24; and low risk, RPNs at 8 or below. Attention to low-risk groups such as patient falls and infections should be postponed until higher-priority failures have been minimized or eliminated.

Some FMEA processes focus on the product of severity and probability of occurrence and create a risk priority matrix. The risk priority matrix provides a visualization of the priority-setting process. In Table 10.6 severity is ranked on a four-point scale and probability of occurrence on a five-point scale, and each cell represents a different failure.

Table 10.6 Risk Priority Matrix

	PROBABILITY			
Severity	Catastrophic (4)	Critical (3)	Marginal (2)	Minor (1)
Very High (5)	20	15	10	5
High (4)	16	12	8	4
Moderate (3)	13	9	6	3
Low (2)	8	6	4	2
Remote (1)	4	3	2	1

The matrix highlights the potential failures that generate high scores, 12–20; these should receive immediate attention. Other potential failures, 8 to 10, will receive attention only if the probability of occurrence or severity of the highest rated failures can be reduced. Potential failures that have low or remote probability and marginal or minor effects (scores between 1 and 6) may never advance to the identification of corrective action in step 6.

As stated earlier, a desirable variation of the prioritizing system would be one that uses the typical severity ranking scheme but replaces the probability of occurrence and detection rankings with actual probabilities. If a four-point severity scale is used, the most severe failure would be 4.0, calculated as follows: 4.0 = 4 (catastrophic damage) * 100% probability of occurrence * 100% probability of nondetection. The least important failure would produce a score that approaches zero, 1 (minor damage) * 0.001 (occurs one time in a thousand) * 0.001 (failure detected 999 times in a thousand) = 0.000001.

Duwe, Fuchs, and Hansen-Flaschen (2005) identified high-risk medical processes as those combining two or more of the following characteristics: variability of patient condition and providers rendering care, complexity of treatment, lack of standardization, tight coupling of activities, dependence on human intervention, hierarchically structured delivery teams, and time constraints.

Step 6: Identify Corrective Actions to Reduce or Eliminate Failure

The quality improvement team should work on the most pressing issues first—those with highest severity, highest probability of occurrence, and lowest probability of detection before harm occurs—and prioritize countermeasures. The FMEA team is *not* attempting to immediately eliminate all failures but to systematically focus its efforts on minimizing the effects of failures. Interventions can be thought of in the same way that the risk score was calculated: how can severity be reduced, how can the probability of occurrence be lowered, and how can failures that arise be more easily identified? The team should rank and institute countermeasures based on those that have the greatest possibility of success. Once high-impact countermeasures have been successfully implemented, the team should sequentially adopt lower yield improvements.

Mitigation or compensating actions are undertaken to reduce the severity of injury after an error has been made. These actions can be thought of as recovery efforts and include second attempts, choosing alternative means to achieve the goal, and repair and restart. In medicine, mitigation techniques include recovery protocols and the stocking of reversal agents and crash carts. The Institute of Healthcare Improvement (2012) has developed a series of measures to reduce harm from high-alert medications that highlights the range of activities that can be taken for a single type of failure.

The best case would be to eliminate failure or reduce the probability of occurrence. A zero probability of failure is unlikely, but preventive measures, including standardized protocols, check sheets, order sheets, dose packaging of medications, and reminders, can be implemented to lower the likelihood of occurrence.

The third component of the RPN is detection. Methods to detect error or increase the visibility of failure include educating employees and patients to recognize signs of failure. Providers are of course trained to track vital signs, but the number of vital signs tracked should be expanded when the risk of failure increases. Etchells, O'Neill, and Bernstein (2003) claim that the best method for prospectively detecting errors includes attending clinical rounds, and undertaking daily chart reviews and interviews with care givers. Similarly, patients should be actively involved in the care process to provide another set of eyes to track their symptoms and progress. A third way to improve the detection of failure is the use of information technology, including electronic monitoring and automatic alerts when monitored vital signs move outside acceptable ranges.

Viewing health care as a system, the FMEA team must recognize that changes in one part of the system can affect performance in other areas, so foreseeable impacts must be identified. If the FMEA covers an entire system, the impact of change should be traceable. However, if only a subsystem is being examined, the team must recognize that the change could affect prior and later operations and should make personnel in these areas aware of the proposed change prior to implementation.

Step 7: Document the Analysis and Recalculate Residual Risk

Quality improvement is a continuous process, and it is unlikely that corrective action will entirely eliminate the possibility of failure or damage that could occur. Step 7 requires the FMEA team to document what was done—the actions that were taken to reduce the probability of occurrences, probability of detection, and the damage that will result if failure occurs. A primary concern is to document what could not be changed, to determine how risky the failure is after corrections are made.

The principal aim of this step is to reprioritize improvement activities. As high-priority failures are reduced or eliminated, lower-priority failures should be thrust to the top of the work list. It is possible that the corrections may not sufficiently reduce the failure risk and so the failure remains the number-one improvement priority. Following the intent of the PDCA cycle, the team would reexamine the failure to implement further improvement, or, if they conclude no further improvement is possible, proceed to the next item on their priority list.

Assume the FMEA team has enacted procedures that reduce the frequency of wrong-site surgery, the highest RPN in Table 10.5, from very high (5) to moderate (3) and has improved detection systems so the probability of detection is increased from moderate (3) to high (2). Given no change in severity (4), the recalculated RPN is 24 ($4 * 3 * 2$). These clinical changes place wrong-site surgery into the moderate risk category and elevate surgical complications to the top of the improvement work list. In this case, wrong-site surgery would not be reevaluated until surgical complications, delays in treatment, and perinatal death or loss of function RPNs were reduced to 24 or less.

Step 8: Monitor

One of the primary reasons for failure of quality improvement initiatives is the failure to follow up on recommended changes. Were changes implemented, implemented properly, and continued? Did the changes lower or eliminate the probability of failure, reduce its severity, or increase the ability to detect and mitigate harm?

Since FMEA is a prospective approach, FMEA teams often report on what expected risk was before and after modifications are identified. For a system or process that has never been put into operation, this is the limit of what can be done. For systems in the design stage, the team should document the expected RPNs before and after the proposed corrections. Once the system moves into operation, the team should determine whether the expected results are achieved.

The team should document the expected reduction in risk for systems that are operating and compare the frequency of occurrence, amount of damage sustained (severity), and the number of failures detected before and after changes were implemented. While review of performance may not document significant change in the rate or severity of wrong-site surgery, given the infrequency of these errors, tracking more common problems, such as patient falls, should document reductions in the rate and severity of falls if interventions are effective.

A plan is simply a plan if it is not implemented. If it is implemented, we cannot assume its effectiveness. Long-term quantification of results is vital to quality improvement.

Designing Better Systems

Nolan (2000) presents three general strategies for reducing the effects of failure. The first and perhaps most desirable strategy focuses on preventing errors. Prevention of error eliminates harm and negates the need to build detection and recovery systems and meets the quality objective of "do it right the first time." When elimination is not achievable, improvement efforts should strive to reduce the probability of occurrence.

Despite efforts to build the perfect system, errors will always occur. Recognizing the inevitability of error, Nolan presents two other strategies. The first attempts to make errors more visible (increase the possibility of detection), and the second focuses on mitigating the effects of errors (reducing severity). Detecting errors may involve instituting inspections after activities that are known to produce error and before costly activities, activities that will conceal defects, and irreversible activities. Mitigation of harm requires the anticipation of possible failures and the development of skills and processes to rapidly minimize or prevent injury.

In the discipline of business engineering, Curran and Ladd (2000) recommend the following methods for the examination and alteration of business processes: reexamination, simplification, reorganization, integration, communication, automation, and adaptation. The fundamental goal of reengineering is to improve the effectiveness, efficiency, quality, and customer responsiveness of operations.

Reexamination involves the fundamental rethinking and possible restructuring of processes, which requires a willingness to challenge long-held beliefs and methods and could lead to dramatic changes in how an organization is structured and the goals it pursues. **Simplification** is designed to make an organization more efficient and reduce production costs by eliminating redundancies and unnecessary or low-value-adding activities. **Reorganization** introduces new work flows in response to specific failures or lower than desired performance. Unlike reexamination, which is required when an organization faces significant problems that affect the entire organization, reorganization is appropriate when failures are localized to a department or single process. **Integration** recognizes the interdependencies between departments and functions and requires the organization to unify their processes so all employees pursue organizational goals and are cognizant of the impact of their actions (or inaction) on other departments. A simple example shows how two seemingly unrelated departments, food service and the operating room, must coordinate their actions. If patients eat before surgery, surgery should be cancelled; if the error is not detected, a patient may aspirate during surgery.

Improved communication seeks to ensure that all employees use the same terminology, understand each other and organizational goals, and are aware of their responsibilities to patients and other employees. **Automation** seeks to implement optimal use of technology. Automation is not simply

reexamination
the fundamental rethinking and possible restructuring of processes

simplification
the elimination redundancies and unnecessary or low-value-adding activities

reorganization
introduction of new work flows in response to specific failures or lower than desired performance

integration
unification of organizational processes so all employees pursue the same goals and are aware of the impact of their work on coworkers and other departments

automation
the substitution of technology for human effort

replacing human functions with machinery and technology but fundamentally asking whether a process should continue to be performed as it has in the past and whether technology can improve on human performance. Finally, **adaptation** is necessary for organizations in a changing environment. Patient needs and desires are constantly changing, so organizations must continually review their products and services and methods of production to ensure they provide the greatest value to their customers.

adaptation

the alteration of production processes and products in response to changing technology and consumer preferences

Table 10.7 fleshes out these broad strategies into implementable actions and demonstrates the gains that can be achieved. The primary goal of quality management is to improve patient care by reducing error. Table 10.7 shows that the expected result of elimination of steps, changes in hand-offs, and automation of steps is lower error. The rationale for fewer steps (simplification) is that more complicated processes have a higher probability of error. Similarly, the more times work is handed off, the more opportunity there is for miscommunication, duplication of already completed activities, or missing steps. Automation attempts to replace variable human performance with the consistency of machine processes. The other system changes target different aspects of quality valued by customers, such as timeliness and costs.

Table 10.7 Commonly Implemented System Changes

System Changes	Potential Impact
Elimination of steps	Fewer people, lower costs, fewer errors
Different sequence or hand-offs	Better work flow, reduced cycle time, fewer errors
Redesign	Better asset utilization, lower costs, fewer errors
Automation	Increased productivity, reduced variability, fewer errors
Outsourcing	Access to specialized skills, lower costs, fewer errors

Source: RC Camp and IJ DeToro, 1999, Benchmarking, in *Juran's Quality Handbook,* 5th ed., edited by JM Juran and AB Godfrey, McGraw-Hill, New York, NY, 12.11.

In moving from broad strategies to specific tactics to deal with failure, it is helpful to understand human error rates. Nolan (2000) provides insight, outlined in Table 10.8, which demonstrates that humans will do things wrong approximately three times in every 1,000 opportunities. Clearly, attempting to prevent general errors of commission is on par with attempting to change human nature. However, an examination of errors of *omission* can tell us how human error rates can be reduced. Humans fail to do something roughly once in every one hundred opportunities. Systems can be redesigned so the desired action is embedded into a sequence of steps. When actions are embedded into a series of steps, the failure-to-perform rate falls to three in 1,000 (one in 333), roughly one-third the nonembedded rate.

Given the one-in-ten probability that employees will fail to check equipment during shift change, the desirability of standardized processes at the start of duty is apparent. A perfect example of this is the preflight checklist reviewed by pilots prior to takeoff to ensure that their aircraft is ready for flight. These checklists require pilots to check their instrumentation, fuel status, route, and weather conditions, among other factors. The preflight checklist is designed to ensure airworthiness and reduce the need for information gathering once in flight, allowing pilots to focus their attention on flying the plane. The use of surgical checklists, such as the one provided by the World Health Organization, is a prime example of the health care industry's adaptation of the tools used in other industries to the needs of the medical field (see http://www.who.int/patientsafety/safesurgery/ tools_resources/SSSL_Checklist_finalJun08.pdf). Table 10.8 demonstrates that relying on inspection in a process will continue to allow failures to go undetected because only nine in ten errors are caught by inspection.

Table 10.8 Human Error Rates

General error of commission	0.003
General error of omission	0.01
General error of omission when embedded	0.003
Simple arithmetic with self-checking	0.03
Failure of inspection to detect error	0.10
Failure to check equipment at shift change	0.10
General error rate—high stress and dangerous activity	0.25

Source: TA Nolan, System Changes to Improve Patient Safety, *BMJ* 320: 773.

These statistics demonstrate that reengineering processes may be the best way to improve system performance. Reengineering typically pursues five types of changes. The first is to reduce complexity. If the number of steps and opportunities for error can be reduced, the number of errors can also be reduced. The second is to optimize information processing. Information problems contribute to failure in two ways: unnecessary activity occurs, or necessary activity does not occur. Either result can be produced by an absence of required information or the existence of incorrect information. Two of the fundamental rules of information processing are to capture data once (eliminating the possibility of conflicting information) and to disseminate information to all necessary parties in a timely manner. Health care providers have generally not been able to prevent multiple capture of the same data or guarantee that medical information will be available to providers on a timely basis.

The third type of change is to automate wisely. Wise automation means that what needs to be done and can be done more effectively by technology should be performed by technology. One common automation error is the attempt to automate all the steps in a manual process. Reengineering emphasizes simplification, so before automating a process the improvement teams should ask: Does the task, activity, or function need to be performed? If continued performance is necessary to produce the desired outcome, the next question is: Is automation more effective than human performance? Automation should be pursued if the team believes the task can be handled more effectively and efficiently by machines. The goal of automation should be the elimination of human error, for example, the 3% error rate for mathematical calculations noted by Nolan in Table 10.8.

Use constraints and forcing functions are a fourth set of interventions to reduce failure by restricting actions. As stated in Chapter Five, physical safeguards such as dedicated plugs and connectors prevent employees from connecting gas lines to inappropriate sources. Similarly, procedural safeguards such as order forms and formularies make it impossible to order incorrect medications. Two additional examples of forcing function come from the automobile industry. First, autos cannot be started if the vehicle is in gear and the operator's foot is not on the brake. Second, legislation is being considered to make it impossible to operate cell phones or other electronic devices, which can distract the driver, while the vehicle is in motion. Cohen (2007) provides a list of forcing functions for high-risk medications, including flow control IV pumps, epidural tubing without side ports, and oral syringes that cannot be connected to IV tubing. Similarly, she lists seven use constraints, including storage of medications, unit dose packaging, formularies, and rapid switching from IV to oral medications.

The final set of interventions focuses on mitigation of harm. Harm reduction requires employees to recognize the early warnings signs of failure and know what actions to implement to neutralize the effects of failure. Mitigation requires employee training and the incorporation of monitoring into standard work processes. Once a failure is identified, employees must have access to the personnel (rapid response teams) and materials (crash carts, antidotes, etc.) to ensure that effective mitigation can be initiated.

Reengineering is a commonly used term, but in practice how successful has reengineering been? Curran and Ladd (2000) report that its success rate is marginal, with 32% of reengineering initiatives rated as very successful, 45% somewhat successful, and 23% unsuccessful.

Where reengineering has succeeded, the organization undertook action for compelling reasons. Successful organizations responded to significant problems that, if left unresolved, could threaten the existence of the organization; "the need to improve" was not a compelling reason. Second, successful organizations employ qualified project leaders. Qualified leaders are not simply successful individuals within the organization but people who have mastered quality management tools and can manage people. The third requirement is frequent communication. Employees must be informed of the need for change, the goal of change, the desired improvements, and progress. Finally, successful organizations found new and innovative uses of technology (Curran and Ladd 2000).

Organizations in which reengineering has been unsuccessful demonstrate little knowledge of current processes. As the text emphasizes, the first step in the improvement process is to document what is being done and the results of these activities. Quantification is essential in deciding what needs to be done and whether improvements are successful. Second, reengineering often fails when information technology is not an integral part of the improvement process, that is, when information technology is seen as a tool to be called upon rather than a means to integrate operations and pursue organizational goals. Finally, failure is more likely when reengineering is employed to fix problems rather than redesign systems (Curran and Ladd 2000).

Summary

This chapter has reemphasized the need to think of processes as a system. We should avoid focusing on discrete processes but instead recognize that subsystems are integral parts of a larger system and that their performance, however remote from the ultimate outcome, affects organizational goals. If a system is to achieve its potential, all parts of the production process must be controlled and the hand-offs monitored.

The value chain reminds us that the goal of a health care system is to produce a satisfied patient and that satisfaction is determined by the medical services delivered and the manner in which they are provided. Employees who work directly with patients know how their actions add or reduce value; the value chain emphasizes the fact that employees who do not interact with patients have an equally vital function. Support personnel are tasked with providing service personnel with the tools and operating conditions to effectively and efficiently complete patient care. The value chain also demonstrates that latent errors, such as a non-patient-oriented culture, untimely or inaccurate information, or poorly maintained equipment, may make it impossible for frontline personnel to provide outstanding medical care.

Determining how a medical process can fail is the goal of FMEA. FMEA assesses risk according to the harm a failure could produce, the likelihood of failure, and the ability to detect and correct failure when it arises. FMEA creates a prioritized work list of the highest-risk activities and, following the structure of FMEA, points us toward improvement: to prevent, detect, and mitigate failure.

The chapter concluded by examining reengineering. The fundamental goal of reengineering is to improve the effectiveness, efficiency, quality, and customer responsiveness of operations through the fundamental redesign of operations. Redesign often takes the form of simplifying processes, resequencing of activities, and automation.

KEY TERMS

Adaptation	Mitigation
Automation	Prevention
CABG	Reengineering
CBC	Reexamination
Equifinality	Reorganization
Failure mode and effects analysis (FMEA)	Simplification
	Value chain
Integration	

REVIEW QUESTIONS

1. Describe the six components of a system, including the external environment, and how they contribute to achieving the goal of a system.

2. Describe how service and support personnel can increase patient satisfaction according to Swayne, Duncan, and Ginter's value chain.

3. How is the risk priority number (RPN) calculated, and what actions can an organization take to reduce the risk of failure?

4. What are the differences among reexamination, simplification, reorganization, and integration?

5. What benefits can be achieved through reducing the number of steps in a process?

PROBLEMS

1. An FMEA will be performed on postoperative infections. Data is available by surgery type on the frequency, severity, and detectability of these infections. The director of quality improvement wants you to prepare a priority list giving the order in which the various surgeries should be examined, to produce the greatest potential benefit for the organization. Severity is ranked from most severe (4) to least severe (1), and detectability is ranked from difficult to detect (4) to easy to detect (1). Calculate a frequency ranking from very high (5) to very low (1) based on the number of infections and cases shown in the following and the RPNs for each type of surgery. Which surgery should be examined first? Which surgery should be examined last? What is the maximum possible risk score for this analysis?

Surgery Types	Number of Infections	Number of Cases	Frequency	Severity of Infections	Detectability	Risk Priority Number
Thoracic	5	200		3	3	
Neuro	1	100		4	3	
Orthopedic	50	2,000		2	2	
Plastic	32	800		1	2	
Oral	25	500		1	1	
General	100	5,000		2	1	

2. Instead of the ordinal ranking of frequency, 1 to 5, used in problem 10.1, the director of quality improvement has collected data on the number of cases for each type of surgery and the number of patients that contracted a postoperative infection. The director wants you to recalculate the RPN using the actual incidence rates of infection. Infection severity and detectability are ranked the same as in problem 10.1. Compare your new RPNs with those calculated in 10.1. How does the use of the incidence rate change the improvement work list? Which surgery should be examined last? What is the maximum possible risk score for this analysis?

Surgery Types	Number of Cases	Number of Infections	Rate of Infection	Severity of Infections	Detectability	Risk Priority Number
Thoracic	200	5		3	3	
Neuro	100	1		4	3	
Orthopedic	2,000	50		2	2	
Plastic	800	32		1	2	
Oral	500	25		1	1	
General	5,000	100		2	1	

3. Assume that in problem 10.2 strict adherence to antibiotic administration one hour prior to thoracic surgery has reduced the rate of infection to 1.0% and severity to 2.0. How did this improvement affect the priority list? Which surgery should be the primary target for improvement?

4. A hospital is setting its quality improvement agenda for the upcoming year and will perform an FMEA in one area. The hospital has rated sentinel events for severity, probability, and detectability on the following scale: very high, high, moderate, low, very low. Calculate the risk priority number for each type of event. Which sentinel event should be the focus of the hospital's FMEA effort?

Event	Severity	Probability	Detectability
Hospital-acquired Infection	High	Moderate	High
Medication Error	Moderate	High	Moderate
Patient Fall	Low	High	Very high
Pressure Ulcer	Low	High	Very high
Treatment Delay	Low	High	High

References

Apkon M, Leonard J, Probst L, DeLizio L, and Vitale R, 2004, Design of a Safer Approach to Intravenous Drug Infusions: Failure Mode Effects Analysis, *Quality and Safety in Health Care* 13 (4): 265–271.

Camp RC and DeToro IJ, 1999, Benchmarking, in *Juran's Quality Handbook*, 5th ed., edited by JM Juran and AB Godfrey, McGraw-Hill, New York, NY, 12.1–12.20.

Cleary P and Edgman-Levitan S, 1997, Health Care Quality: Incorporating Consumer Perspectives, *JAMA* 278 (19): 1608–1612.

Cohen H, 2007, Protecting Patients from Harm: Reduce the Risk of High-Alert Drugs, *Nursing* (September 2007): 49–54.

Coronary Drug Project Research Group, 1980, Influence of Adherence to Treatment and Response of Cholesterol on Mortality in the Coronary Drug Project, *New England Journal of Medicine* 303 (18): 1038–1041.

Curran TA and Ladd A, 2000, *SAP R/3 Business Blueprint*, Prentice Hall PTR, Upper Saddle River, NJ.

DeToro IJ, 1995, *Business Process Benchmarking Workshop*, The Quality Network Inc., Rochester, NY.

Duwe B, Fuchs B, and Hansen-Flaschen, J, 2005, Failure Mode and Effects Analysis Application to Critical Care Medicine, *Critical Care Clinics* 21 (1): 21–30.

Eraker S, Kirscht J, and Becker M, 1984, Understanding and Improving Patient Compliance, *Annals of Internal Medicine* 100 (2): 258–268.

Etchells E, O'Neill C, and Bernstein M, 2003, Patient Safety in Surgery: Error Detection and Prevention, *World Journal of Surgery* 27: 936–942.

Feldstein PJ, 1999, *Health Policy*, 2nd ed., Health Administration Press, Chicago, IL.

Griffith S, 1990, A Review of the Factors Associated with Patient Compliance and the Taking of Prescribed Medicines, *British Journal of General Practice* 40 (332): 114–116.

Institute of Healthcare Improvement, 2012, How-to Guide: Prevent Harm from High-Alert Medications, http://www.ihi.org/knowledge/Pages/Tools/ HowtoGuidePreventHarmfromHighAlertMedications.aspx.

Institute of Medicine, 2001a, *Crossing the Quality Chasm*, National Academy Press, Washington, DC.

Institute of Medicine, 2001b, *Envisioning the National Health Care Quality Report*, National Academy Press, Washington, DC.

Ishikawa K, 1985, *What Is Total Quality Control? The Japanese Way*, Prentice-Hall, Englewood, NJ.

James BC, 1993, Implementing Practice Guidelines through Clinical Quality Improvement, *Frontiers of Health Service Management* 10 (1): 3–37.

Joint Commission, 2010, *Comprehensive Accreditation Manual for Hospitals*, Oakbrook Terrace, IL.

Kaiser Permanente, 2002, Failure Mode and Effects Analysis (FMEA) Team Instruction Guide, March 2002.

Kallen AJ, Mu Y, Bulens S, Reingold A, Petit S, Gershman K, Ray SM, Harrison LH, Lynfield R, Dumyati G, Townes JM, Schaffner W, Patel PR, and Fridkin SK, 2010, Health Care-Associated Invasive MRSA Infections, 2005–2008, *JAMA* 304 (6): 641–648.

Kizer K, 2001, Establishing Health Care Performance Standards in an Era of Consumerism, *JAMA* 286 (10): 1213–1217.

MIL-STD-1629A, 1980, Task 101, Procedures for Performing a Failure Mode, Effects and Criticality Analysis, November 24, 1980.

Nolan TWA, 2000, System Changes to Improve Patient Safety, *BMJ* 320: 771–773.

Rosenberg EE, Lussier MT, and Beaudoin C, 1997, Lessons for Clinicians from Physician-Patient Communication Literature, *Archives of Family Medicine* 6 (3): 279–283.

Swayne LE, Duncan WJ, and Ginter PM, 2008, *Strategic Management of Health Care Organizations*, 6th ed., Jossey-Bass, San Francisco, CA.

Villacourt M, 1992, Failure Mode and Effects Analysis (FMEA): A Guide for Continuous Improvement in the Semiconductor Equipment Industry, Sematech Technology Transfer #92020963B-ENG, September 30, 1992.

Wennberg JE, 1984, Dealing with Medical Practice Variations: A Proposal for Action, *Health Affairs* 3 (2): 6–32.

PART 3

MEDICAL PRACTICE MANAGEMENT

We have covered how to assess system performance and determine whether improvement is needed. Part Three focuses on how we can move toward improving patient health. What proven tools have been effective in altering medical practice and improving patient outcomes? Chapter Eleven discusses practice policies that seek to standardize treatment to the extent possible, to reduce variation and improve patient outcomes. It is essential that computer support supplement human efforts given the myriad of activities involved in a medical case. Research on practice policies shows mixed results. Some authors have found policies led to greater consistency in care processes and improvements in outcomes while others documented no significant change in either.

Chapter Twelve reviews case, disease, and outcomes management. All attempt to improve patient outcomes through assessment, planning, education, coordination, monitoring, and evaluation of treatment and outcomes. The difference between these medical practice tools lies in their orientation; case management focuses on individual high-risk patients, disease management focuses on high-cost medical conditions, and outcome management focuses on the results of care rather than on the processes of care. All three systems emphasize standardization to reduce variation while recognizing the need for rapid modification of care due to the unique circumstances of individual patients.

"The worst form of inequality is to try to make unequal things equal." Aristotle's quote encapsulates the challenge of physician profiling. Tracking of performance and comparison of results are essential to quality management, yet comparisons must be valid. Chapter Thirteen introduces the reader to measures that could be used as valid and reliable indicators of physician performance while pointing out that comparisons must recognize differences in patients or random events that affect outcomes. Although comparison of performance will always be a sensitive topic, the need for improvement must drive the use of cross-provider assessments; the sensitivity of providers should be addressed through reserve in judgment.

Chapter Fourteen introduces benchmarking and expands on the idea of comparison introduced in Chapter Thirteen. Benchmarking is used to compare one organization with another, with the goal of ensuring that best practices are employed across an industry. Balanced scorecards and dashboards are introduced to facilitate the achievement of an organization's goals by communicating targets to employees and providing the plans and tools needed for success. The chapter concludes by examining implementation strategies. Because planning is easy, but achieving employee buy-in is more difficult, the chapter reviews approaches that increase and decrease the probability of successful implementation and achieving one's goals.

Chapter Fifteen recaps the text. The goal of quality management is to improve patient outcomes, but this goal cannot be achieved if essential elements are not in place. The first element is a foundation of statistics, human behavior, and continuous quality improvement. These fields provide a knowledge base and define what can be accomplished. The second element, tools, provides techniques to measure and evaluate a system and determine if improvement is needed or desirable. The third element, goals, sets out how less-than-desirable processes can be improved to achieve desired ends. Mastering evaluation skills, evaluating performance, and correcting systems will improve patient outcomes, thus closing the circle. Quality management is not about assigning blame to individuals but a more comprehensive effort to improve systems.

CHAPTER 11

PRACTICE POLICIES

Introduction

Variability is a documented fact in medical practice, and often variability is good for patients. Physicians deal with uncertainty on a daily basis and must adapt treatments to the unique characteristics of their patients, but variability can injure when patients are subjected to procedures or pharmaceuticals that provide little or no benefit or that cause harm.

In one of the first definitive statements on evidence-based medicine (EBM), the Evidence-Based Working Group (1992) described traditional medical practice as relying on unsystematic observations based on a provider's experience built on his or her understanding of disease processes and pathophysiological principles. Traditional clinical practice relies on medical training, clinical experience, and common sense. Evidence-based practice accepts these premises but recognizes that systematic recording of outcomes across providers will increase an individual clinician's confidence in his or her treatment choices. Clinicians pursuing EBM practice must develop literature-searching skills (see Chapter Twelve) and the ability to evaluate evidence to "interpret literature on causation, prognosis, diagnostic tests, and treatment strategy" (Evidence-Based Working Group 1992, 2421).

The EBM approach does not eliminate physician authority in favor of documented evidence of effectiveness but rather seeks a balance between these two approaches to patient care. In addition to traditional problem-defining skills, EBM challenges physicians to search, evaluate, and apply the findings of clinical studies and meta-analyses when treating patients (Evidence-Based Working Group 1992).

LEARNING OBJECTIVES

1. Understand the idea of evidence-based medicine

2. Describe the idealized clinical decision-making process

3. Understand the goals, structure, and implementation of practice policies

4. Recognize the role of information technology for support of practice policies

5. Review the effect of practice policies

Practice policies
recommendations on treatment with applicability determined by the level of information known about the medical condition and patient preferences

Practice policies are one result of providers, insurers, and government recognizing the inherent uncertainty and variability of medical practice. Practice policies focus on the process of care: defined steps in treating a patient, providers understanding their role in the process, and deciding when action should occur. The goal of practice policies is to provide better patient care through effective and efficient medical practice. Widespread adoption of practice policies has been slow due to the passive manner in which they have been disseminated, the proliferation of competing guidelines, and the opposition of physicians to what is often perceived as "cookbook" medicine.

It is natural that physicians who have historically had almost complete latitude in making decisions would be hesitant to accept any encroachment on their area of authority. The explosive growth in medical literature has, however, made it impossible for any person to stay abreast of the progress in medical knowledge. Physicians need tools to assist them in keeping up with advances in medical knowledge while maintaining their practice. Innovations in information technology offer tools that providers have yet to fully capitalize on to improve patient care.

The demand for greater clarity in medical decisions can be attributed to multiple factors. The first two are the recognition of the inherent limitations of the human mind and the ability of computers to track information and assist decision making. Technology is expanding the opportunities in which information systems can assist providers by tracking and analyzing data and locating pertinent research. Providers should not have to rely on human memory to ensure that necessary treatments occur at the appropriate times in an era of fast computers and increasingly interwoven databases.

Third, there is a substantial literature documenting differences in practice patterns (Wennberg, as discussed in Chapter Two), patients receiving unnecessary treatments, and patients not receiving needed care (McGlynn, as discussed in Chapter Two). A fourth concern is the continuing growth in health care expenditures. It is hoped that practice policies will lower costs by eliminating unnecessary care and by ensuring that early and appropriate care is delivered, which will reduce the need for later, more expensive care. Fifth, there is the natural growth in demand for higher-quality goods and services as societies become wealthier. Finally, there is growing skepticism among the public toward professionals, a loss of respect that extends to medicine. Patients want to be increasingly involved in medical decisions, often arrive at the physician's office with research in hand, and demand fuller explanations from their physicians. The increased concern for quality and the mistrust of professionals is contributing to the demand for greater accountability in health care.

Providers must be able to respond to questions about what they are producing, beyond simplistic answers of tests and procedures. Providers need to address concerns over potential effects on lifestyle: Did the treatment improve a patient's life, or simply alleviate a health problem? Was the benefit of treatment greater than the cost? The threat to providers is that unless they can successfully answer the public's concern over medical practice, they may find that practice policies will be dictated by third-party payers or the government.

It is important to recognize that specific solutions are required for specific problems when studying practice policies. A chapter on practice policies runs the risk of wallowing in generalities that may not be particularly insightful or useful when confronted with a specific problem. The chapter will attempt to avoid overgeneralizations while providing broad parameters on what policies should include and on how information systems can assist in improving patient care by monitoring treatment and recognizing deviations from recommended care. The chapter ends with a review of cases in which specific problems were addressed and in which the success of the practice policies can be assessed.

Practice Policies

Before discussing the types of practice policies, a review of medical decision making is needed. As introduced in Chapter Two, Eddy (1990a) summarized the key issues and developed a well-known schematic diagram of the medical decision-making process, shown in Figure 11.1. This model, reproduced here for ease of reference, shows that the quality of health care treatment, like any other good or service, is determined by the decisions made regarding what actions should be undertaken, the treatment plan, and the skill with which it is executed (Reason). Determining if the appropriate treatments were provided should be based on the benefits and harms of treatment, the expected outcomes and costs, and opportunity costs. The benefits, harms, and expected outcomes of treatment are standard inputs into a medical decision,

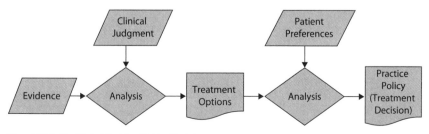

Figure 11.1 The Clinical Decision-Making Model

but U.S. health care providers have not had to deal with larger societal issues such as the crowding out of non–health care spending at the state and national level and reduced global competitiveness. As private insurance and government health programs face increasing financial pressure, the issue of limited resources and what will be sacrificed to fund health care will produce greater public scrutiny of medical cost and performance.

Understanding Eddy's clinical decision-making framework is essential for anyone concerned with individual patient care decisions or health policy.

The treatment selection, a practice policy, is the outcome of process, with six steps involving physicians and their patients. The treatment selection process starts with the existing evidence concerning a disease or injury. Evidence should be the product of rigorous testing across multiple providers and patients and not simply the outcomes observed by a single physician or small group of providers handling a small number of cases. The second input is the clinical judgment of the provider. In many cases, the evidence base may not address the particular circumstances of a patient, so the physician must consider how the patient's age, comorbid conditions, and other factors that may affect potential treatments. The physician's knowledge of the specific characteristics and behavior of the patient may shift the clinical decision from medical to surgical intervention or vice versa, or may favor one surgical or pharmaceutical approach over others. The job of the physician is to access patients, identify and utilize the existing medical evidence on their condition, and determine the appropriate treatments and potential outcomes including benefits and harms. The result of the analysis is a set of potential treatments and outcomes.

Once a set of treatments is determined, a second evaluation process begins by adding patient preferences. As part of this process, the physician explains the possible treatments and their expected outcomes, with risks and benefits, to the patient, and the patient and physician determine which course of treatment to pursue. The driving factor in this evaluation process is the preference of the patient since he or she will be the one that will live with the consequences of the clinical choice. The outcome of this evaluation is a practice policy—the treatment that will be pursued.

While this process is the optimal way to arrive at clinical decisions, the process cannot be economically implemented for every case, because it is extremely time consuming. First, there is often an extensive amount of evidence to consider. The Evidence-Based Medicine Working Group in 1992 reported that it took a resident 30 minutes to research an issue and cost $2.68 to conduct a computer search and print research. The major cost of the literature review was not the computer-related expenses or the cost of producing hard copies of articles but rather the half hour of provider time. When we add the time necessary to describe potential treatments and hammer out a clinical choice with the patient, it is clear that this method of medical practice cannot be widely implemented. Ioannidis (2005) documents a second major problem: published evidence is often contradictory, so literature searches may fail to limit treatment choices.

The arduous tasks of data collection and weighing various data sources require shortcuts to facilitate health care delivery. Often the shortcut is the physician's knowledge base: multiple cases allow the physician to understand the clinical evidence and make rapid and effective clinical decisions. The vulnerability of this approach is that physicians' treatment patterns are heavily influenced by where they received their medical training and where they practice and may not reflect best practice. Training and peers expedite the analysis process; instead of determining treatment plans on a case-by-case basis, providers rely on established rules. The disadvantage of medical training and peer consultation is that these sources of information can lag advances in health care practice. Research shows that health care advances can take 17 years to enter mainstream medical practice. Shortening this lag is one goal of practice policies.

If Eddy's medical decision-making model were followed for every patient, an enormous amount of time would be consumed by physicians explaining options to patients and patients attempting to explain their preferences to their doctors. The culmination of the process, attempting to integrate the view of the medically trained provider and subjective views of patients into a treatment decision, would be time consuming and difficult. Although it is not practical to carry out this process for most cases, it highlights the two fundamentals of medical decision making. First, treatment options should be based as much as possible on existing medical evidence, and second, the treatment choice should be based on what is important to the patient. Practice policies are intended to facilitate the decision making by centralizing data collection and analysis. Rather than each doctor having to collect and analyze data, a centralized body could monitor the literature and distribute practice guidelines. Contrary to the often expressed view that practice policies add to the physician workload, the intent of polices is the opposite. Practice policies are designed to facilitate health care delivery and improve health care outcomes by disseminating best practices.

Practice polices can also be used to reconcile any conflicts of interest that may arise in the principal-agent relationship when the patient delegates decision-making authority to a physician. The role of the physician, as an agent of the patient, is to make the same decision that the patient would make if he had complete knowledge of medicine. The preferences that are important in selecting treatment are those of the patient and not those of the provider.

The usefulness of practice policies is determined by the extent to which outcomes and patient preferences are known (Eddy 1990a). Practice policies provide less guidance if there is substantial disagreement among practitioners over outcomes or if patients hold widely differing preferences for treatments. When outcomes and patient preferences are clear, practice policies make explicit the reasoning behind the use of a particular treatment, recognize the consequences of its use, and conclude that use is desirable (Eddy 1990a).

Variety of Practice Policies

To fully understand the debate over practice policies, providers and analysts must define the terms used in the debate. First, Weiland (1997) examines the difference between clinical pathways and practice guidelines. **Clinical pathways** provide a timeline defining the services to be rendered and identifying who is responsible for providing care. Clinical practice guidelines are diagnostic and treatment guides developed by physicians for physicians. Clinical pathways involve all health care workers, are generally not limited to a specific event (such as a hospitalization), define what should occur before and after each activity, and routinely incorporate patients into the care plan through education. Clinical guidelines, on the other hand, are event-specific and are primarily geared for physician use.

clinical pathways
timelines defining treatment to be rendered and who is responsible for providing the care

Practice policies developed by physicians for physicians are the topic of this chapter. Although Weiland calls this type of policy a *clinical guideline*, this term is avoided in this chapter because *guideline* will be used to define one of three types of practice policies. Practice policies are preformed recommendations on treatment based on the level of information known about medical outcomes and patient preferences. The three types of practice policies are standards, guidelines, and options. Each of these policies was developed for the purpose of influencing decisions regarding medical treatments.

standards
practice policies built on strong evidence of medical effectiveness and near unanimous patient preferences that should be followed in almost every case

Standards are the most rigid of the three types of practice policies. A standard assumes that there is strong evidence on the clinical effectiveness of treatment and that an informed patient would in almost every case select the treatment. A medical intervention must be able to consistently produce an outcome to be clinically effective. Similarly, the outcome produced must be seen as desirable from the point of view of the patient. Standards should be followed in almost every case because of the predictability and desirability of outcomes. Failure to practice to a generally recognized standard may be sufficient to trigger a malpractice suit, in which case defense is likely to be difficult (Eddy 1990d).

Guidelines are less rigid than standards because the level of understanding of the outcomes and the level of preferences is lower. Guidelines are promulgated when there is dispute over the effectiveness of treatment or an informed patient would generally, but not always, select the treatment. In many cases there is justifiable clinical uncertainty over the desirability of similar drugs or surgeries, medical versus surgical intervention, or watchful waiting versus active intervention. Detre et al. (1984) documented that coronary artery bypass grafting, although beneficial for high-risk patients, was no more effective than medical treatment for low-risk patients. Just as there is professional disagreement over the relative effectiveness of alternative treatments, patients also hold divergent preferences for various treatments. Kaimal and Kupperman (2010) report women's preference for vaginal delivery after having a cesarean section ranged from 20% to 90% over six studies, with 56% ultimately attempting natural childbirth. A guideline is flexible but should be followed in most cases; failure to follow a guideline should not in and of itself suggest malpractice.

guidelines
practice policies that recognize disputes over medical effectiveness and/or less consistent patient preferences that should be followed in most cases

Options are built on the least amount of knowledge; consequently it is up to physicians and patients to determine whether they wish to follow an option. When treatment options are provided, there may be no evidence to support the effectiveness of one treatment versus others, or patient preferences for treatment vary widely or are unknown. Table 11.1 highlights the relationship among evidence on outcomes, patient preferences, and practice policies and emphasizes that when uncertainty over the fundamental elements of a decision increases, the latitude of providers and patients increases.

options
practice policies that recognize there may be little or no evidence to recommend one treatment over another and/or unknown or widely divergent patient preferences that leave treatment choice to physicians and patients

Table 11.1 Practice Standards, Guidelines, and Options

	OUTCOME		
Preferences	**Known**	**Disputed**	**Unknown**
Unanimous	Standard	Guideline	Option
Generally Similar	Guideline	Guideline	Option
Diverse or Unknown	Option	Option	Option

Table 11.1 demonstrates that there is little need for physicians to be concerned with a loss of authority or with being forced to practice "cookbook" medicine. Standards offer the least discretion in selecting a treatment plan due to the fact that there are clearly documented outcomes and an informed patient would almost every time select the treatment.

Given these factors, there is little reason for physicians to ignore evidence supporting the superiority of one treatment over others or over the preferences of patients. Many have pointed out the thin evidence base that undergirds medical practice. For example, James (1993) reports that only 10% to 20% of medical practice is based on published scientific evidence, so these conditions may be met only in a small percentage of cases.

Patient preferences are perhaps even more difficult to categorize than outcomes, given the different views that people display toward medical care and risk. Different groups (males vs. females, blacks vs. whites, young vs. old) place widely divergent values on medical treatment. In a study of guidelines, Chong et al. concluded that 36.6% of practice policy references cited treatment effectiveness research, while only 6.0% of references addressed patient preferences (2009, 979–980). They cite a number of reasons why policies do not incorporate patient preferences, including the belief that preferences are inherently individual, the lack of a generally accepted method to synthesize this information, and the lack of agreement on whether incorporation will improve medical practice (Chong et al. 2009). Again, the question of whether medicine is an art or a science arises and the answer is it is both.

Table 11.1 shows that practice policies become restrictive only when there is a high degree of agreement on outcomes and homogeneity of patients' preferences, but the determination of these preferences depends more on art than science. The patient compliance literature documents how compliance changes depending on how patient input is solicited. McNeil et al. (1982) documented how patient treatment choices change when outcomes are framed as the probability of living versus the probability of dying. Guidelines should be used when there may be strong outcome evidence but patients do not always desire the treatment or when there is a dispute over the effectiveness of treatment. Resolving disputes over effectiveness may again require more art than science; how do the particular circumstances of the patient change the probability of success of potential treatments? Finally, if patient preferences are diverse or there is little evidence to elevate one treatment over another, doctors and patients have complete discretion to select a treatment. With guidelines and options, the role of the provider is to ensure that patients understand the risks and benefits of the selected treatment. Table 11.1 demonstrates that physicians will continue to have great influence over treatment choice since in the majority of cases practice policies will provide only additional information to facilitate decision making.

Practice Policy Components

Eddy (1990c) outlines thirteen components that should be addressed when a practice policy is written. The first component is the *summary*. The summary should provide readers with a concise understanding of the policy, including why it was written, its main operational elements, and when it should be used. Whether the policy is a standard, guideline, or option should be clear. The second element is the *background*. The background allows the policy authors to elaborate on why the policy was written. Often policies are written due to the frequency of a disease or injury, the advent of new technologies that could be used to treat the disease or injury, or quality concerns including wide variation in treatment patterns or poor outcomes relative to a benchmark. The third component defines the *health problem*: What issue is the target of the policy? The policy target identifies the disease or injury to which the policy should be applied, the intervention (including preventive, diagnostic, or treatment issues), the alternatives available to practitioners, the target patient population, and any restrictions on the type of providers who should provide treatment or the setting in which it can be delivered.

The fourth component is the *health and economic outcomes*. This element describes current survival rates, disability rates, relief of pain, the cost of current treatment, and other pertinent issues to build a case for change. Kahan et al. found that physicians were more receptive to change when the scientific and professional aspects of care were emphasized. Physicians were less receptive to practice policies when the rationale was built on administrative or economic issues (Kahan et al. 2009, 1220).

The fifth, and possibly the most vital, component of the practice policy is the *evidence* assembled supporting the proposed medical intervention and the effect it will have on medical and economic outcomes. The practice policy should explain the current treatment process and the desired process. Eddy states that this section should describe what supporting evidence was considered, how it was interpreted, and what, if any, subjective judgments were incorporated into the final decision (Eddy 1990c, 2240). Evidence and the weight given to it should be determined by how it was collected. The highest form of evidence would be the results of multiple randomized clinical trials (RCT), followed by a single RCT, and finally expert opinion. Tricoci et al. (2009) evaluated practice policies and concluded that 11.4% were based on multiple RCT, 39.4% on a single RCT, and 47.5% on expert judgment. They conclude that "the current system generating research is inadequate to satisfy the needs of caregivers and patients in determining benefits and risks of drugs, devices, and procedures" (Tricoci et al. 2009, 837).

Table 11.2 Practice Policy Components

1.	Summary
2.	Background
3.	Health problem or issue
4.	Current health and economic outcomes
5.	Supporting evidence
6.	Expected effect on health and economic outcomes
7.	Evaluation (strength of) clinical effectiveness
8.	Evaluation of patient preferences
9.	Patient-specific tailoring of guideline and options
10.	Conflicts with other practice policies
11.	Comparison with interventions used for other health problems
12.	Caveats
13.	Authors

Source: DM Eddy, 1990, Clinical Decision Making: From Theory to Practice, Guidelines for Policy Statements: The Explicit Approach, *JAMA* 263 (16): 2239–2243.

The sixth component examines the expected *effect on health and economic outcomes.* While the fourth component examined the current outcomes, this section should establish what the expected benefits of the change will provide. How much is the policy expected to improve health outcomes (higher survival rates; lower complications, infections, and morbidity rates; lower readmission rates), and will any new side effects arise? Policies should address economic issues, what new costs will arise, what costs will fall, and whether total treatment costs will increase or decrease. Eddy recommends that these estimates should be quantitative and recognize the probable range of potential outcomes when possible.

The seventh and eighth components, *evaluation (strength of) clinical effectiveness* and *evaluation of patient preferences* are designed to provide essential information to readers of the policy to help them determine how much weight they should place on the policy. Should the policy be considered a standard, a guideline, or an option? The discussion of outcome estimates should describe the statistical methods used to calculate the expected outcomes. How strong is the evidence and what range of outcomes have been observed across studies? Similarly, preference judgments should be made explicit; who made the judgment and why? Readers should know who made the decision and their rationale whenever there is a need to subjectively weigh scientific evidence. If a subjective judgment is used to determine the desirability of a particular outcome, readers should know whether the preference was determined by physicians or by patients and know the method used to identify the preference.

Eddy also suggests that practice policies should include instructions for *tailoring the policy* when the policy is not a standard. This section should explore how differences in patient characteristics should compel changes in treatment and in the differences in expected outcomes. The tenth component should explore *conflicts with other policies*. In researching the policy, the authors should uncover and consider other practice policies if the recommended treatment deviates substantially from past treatment. When conflict arises, the authors of the proposed policy should explain the difference in treatment and their rationale for one approach over others. Irreconciled differences with past treatment recommendations have the potential to generate conflict and confusion and to undermine the credibility of the policy. It is vital to recognize whether the policy should be considered a standard, in which little deviation should be expected, or whether it is a guideline or option, in which legitimate disagreement will arise from clinical and patient preference judgments.

The eleventh component, *comparison with other interventions*, explores how the current policy compares with similar treatments. Eddy provides the example of comparing a policy on breast cancer screening with screenings for other types of cancers. The purpose of the comparison is to identify commonalities and differences between interventions that will improve the reader's understanding of the policy. The last two components, *caveats* and *authors*, are aimed at establishing the pedigree of the policy. Caveats attempt to recognize potential changes in the medical field—for example, research, technological, or pharmaceutical advances—that may require revisiting the policy and issuing a new policy. Eddy suggests that definitive dates be established for reviewing promulgated policies that could be substantially affected by new developments. The last section, authors, states who wrote the policy and allows readers to evaluate their qualifications and any potential conflicts of interest. As seen in the continuing debates over approval of new pharmaceuticals, justifiable questions are raised when people with ties to pharmaceutical companies sit on the approval panels or when evidence is supplied by research funded by pharmaceutical companies.

Implementation of Practice Policies

Development of a policy is only the first step in changing how care is delivered. Improving care requires effective dissemination of the policy and, ultimately, use at the patient bedside. One of the most common complaints about practice policies is the passive way they have been disseminated to providers. Simply publishing a policy will only be effective if a provider has a current interest in the condition being addressed or is treating a case and has a question on how it should be handled. If neither condition is met, the policy will likely be filed or discarded. How the information is relayed to providers has a major influence on whether the policy will improve care processes and patient outcomes.

Practice policies have had limited success in changing medical practice. Cabana et al. (1999) identified the three barriers to use: knowledge, attitudes, and behavior. *Knowledge* recognizes that a policy can be useful only if a physician is aware of its existence. Cabana et al. found that lack of awareness was the second greatest barrier to implementation (54.5%). *Attitude* refers to the fact that even if a physician has knowledge of a policy, she must agree with it before she will utilize it. Finally, if knowledge and agreement are present, a policy can still fail to have an effect if there is resistance its implementation. Cabana et al. found that the greatest barrier to use was lack of familiarity (56.5%). Other factors cited for not using practice polices were lack of self-efficacy, inability to overcome inertia of previous practice, and lack of time or resources. The authors concluded that policies will not be followed if they are difficult to use, inconvenient, cumbersome, or confusing, or if they are inconsistent with patient preferences or incompatible with organizational resources.

Active implementation processes involving multiple parties will enhance the probability of a policy being applied in practice. While the top-down approach is frequently used by payers and government, individual organizations can take steps to develop their own guidelines or adapt a policy created by another organization.

Carnett (1999) sets forth nine steps to improve patient care, of which only four steps will be discussed due to the similarity of Carnett's nine steps to other improvement processes. The first step is to identify an improvement opportunity. It matters little whether the awareness of the need for improvement emanates from a policy received from an external party or from internal dissatisfaction with a process. As discussed in the section on practice policy components, a convincing case must be made for change; the outcomes of the present process and the expected improvements to be reaped from the new process must be part of that case. It is essential for staff to recognize that performance can be improved and to be willing to pursue improvement.

Second, an interdisciplinary team should be formed. The team assembled to study and improve a process should include personnel who perform all major functions in the process. In health care, the primary decision-makers are physicians, and they should comprise the largest group in the team. Other health care workers who must be involved include nurses, pharmacists, and others involved in the process being studied. In addition to health care workers, the team must have members of upper management (to demonstrate high-level commitment to the project) and staff members familiar with quality management theory and tools. Other industries often include end users in the team to incorporate the customer view into the process; so patients and payers may be included.

Third, the organization must collect and analyze its prior performance. It does not matter whether the policy to be implemented is received from an external party or is going to be developed internally. Past performance establishes the baseline against which the new policy will be evaluated. If the organization is performing better than the current outcomes established in an externally received policy, expected improvement should be lower; the opposite is also true. The key is to demonstrate to employees that improvement can be achieved, and this begins by demonstrating a performance gap.

Organizational commitment to a practice policy will be determined by how strong a case for change can be made. To move employees from a position of contentment with current processes to one where change is not simply accepted but actively pursued requires pointing out the deficiencies and failings of the current system. Sometimes the incentive comes from publicized data (Chapter Thirteen discusses the publication of cardiac surgery outcomes in New York), but publicly available information often lacks depth, so organizations must endeavor to demonstrate why change is required, using a competent and exhaustive analysis of their own data. Health care providers are responsive to persuasive demonstrations that their mortality, morbidity, infection, or readmission rates are higher than similar providers. A primary roadblock to implementing new practice policies is the lack of information on outcomes for groups of patients and the willingness of providers to dismiss aberrant results for individual patients as isolated events.

The next step in the implementation process is the formulation of corrective actions or enhancements and the selection of an alternative. Regardless of the impetus for change (external guideline or internal desire), the way the practice policy will be implemented will be decided by the interdisciplinary team. While an externally generated practice policy may provide a starting point for how the process will change, the team will be responsible for determining how the policy fits with local practice patterns. Implementation will be more difficult as the degree of change required from current practice to desired practice increases.

One strategy worth pursuing when multiple changes are deemed desirable is to introduce changes over an extended period of time. This strategy prevents providers from being overwhelmed at a single point in time and provides the opportunity to evaluate the effect of one change or a small number of changes on patient outcomes.

Prior to starting implementation, personnel must undertake a thorough examination of issues that may impede implementation. Behavioral change is always difficult, and the health care industry must contend with long-standing traditions of physician autonomy and authority. The team should anticipate where they will encounter opposition (inertia, vested interests, time constraints, cost of implementation), understand the concerns of the opposition, and undertake whatever steps are necessary to alleviate these concerns while continuing to pursue the expected benefits of the change.

Practice policies should be actively disseminated to providers rather than mass mailed, to increase the probability that professional behavior will change (Grimshaw et al. 1995). Provider education should include targeted seminars, outreach visits, and endorsement by opinion leaders. Greater involvement of patients in the care process, including sending physicians reminders for recommended preventive care for their patients and patient-mediated interventions, has been demonstrated to be effective in altering provider behavior. Other strategies that have been demonstrated to be effective include provider feedback, financial incentives, and peer review. Kahan et al. (2009) note that physician adherence can be increased by implementing computer reminders, feedback, small-group sessions, and academic detailing.

After the guideline has been disseminated, compliance must be monitored: Has the process changed, and have outcomes improved? The team must identify process indicators that are easy to measure and have already been collected or that can be collected with minimal effort. If no monitoring is in place, it is vain to think that people will change from historical behaviors to new patterns.

Change management requires that those who are trying new things see that the new methods are improving outcomes. If the change does not improve outcomes, why bother? Change management specifies that results should be disseminated quickly to encourage workers to stay the course. Results also demonstrate that the process is being monitored and that the goals being pursued justify continual management attention.

Like the PDCA cycle, refinement of practice policies will be a continual process. Advances in health care practices continue at a rapid pace, and it is not reasonable to assume that present treatment practices will be acceptable in the future. Margo (2004) concluded that of 17 guidelines reviewed, about half were outdated in six years.

Implementation Approaches to Avoid

Implementation approaches to be avoided include: across-the-board training, big teams, too many teams, delegated implementation responsibility, and starting a project at the wrong time (Goetsch and Davis, 2010, 774–776). Across-the-board training has been used to demonstrate that all employees were trained, with bureaucrats duly documenting completion of the training. The first problem with such an approach is that the one-size-fits-all approach seldom adequately addresses the informational needs of disparate groups of employees, and the very attempt to train different employees at the same time often creates problems. Physicians do not want to be trained with nurses or other health care workers, and the divergence in status at these educational meetings may inhibit lower-level employees from voicing their concerns and opinions. The second problem is that introducing information in advance of need often results in rapid loss of information. "Use it or lose it" applies: information should be delivered when employees need it to ensure that desired procedural changes are immediately practiced. The problem with providing treatment plans for infrequent events is physicians may not read or remember the information when a case arises.

The problem with big teams is that optimal group size has been demonstrated to be five or seven people. Small groups ease communication and reduce the probability of coalition building, and groups of odd numbers cannot deadlock. Organizations must also avoid implementing a shotgun approach, in which multiple initiatives are simultaneously pursued. The problem with too many groups and too many projects is that energy dissipates and priorities become unclear when multiple quality improvement initiatives are operating at the same time. If employees do not believe that management is committed to change, the probability of successful action is greatly reduced.

Another factor that reflects the commitment of management and that decreases the likelihood of success is when top management delegates responsibility for implementation downward. If quality improvement is not important enough to upper management to be actively engaged, employees will not commit themselves.

Premature start of a quality initiative occurs when the need for change has not been created among staff, the appropriate people are not enlisted in the effort, baseline and comparative data have not been collected, potential solutions are not identified, and so on. If the organization culture is not prepared for change, if new procedures are introduced prior to their need, or if the chosen solution is inappropriate, the chance of successful implementation is minimal. Organizations may find their employees refuse to perform the new procedures or have forgotten their instruction. On the other hand, implementation cannot be delinquent; if an organization waits too long, the sense of urgency may be lost and employee enthusiasm and commitment will wane.

Uses and Barriers of Practice Policies

Because they attempt to define appropriate medical practice, practice policies can facilitate multiple goals. Eddy highlights six uses to which practice polices can be applied (Eddy 1990b). The first is supporting physician-patient interactions. Studies often report the failure of patients and physicians to communicate on the same level, with high rates of patients not receiving their doctor's instruction and physicians not communicating important information. A practice policy can support physician-patient interactions by providing concrete documentation of what should be done. A written practice policy increases patients' knowledge, narrows the information gap between provider and patient, and reduces the probability that the physician may fail to communicate import aspects of care.

A second use is defining who should deliver care. A policy could specify the type of provider (physician, physician assistant, nurse) or the level of certification required to deliver a service. Third, the policy may specify how a service should be performed. Performance criteria could include minimum standards of technical competence. Fourth, given the proliferation of ambulatory surgical centers and in-office surgery and their lower ability to respond to catastrophic events, policies may stipulate whether care should be performed inpatient or outpatient. Payers, including Medicare and managed care, also specify that services that do not require inpatient care will not be reimbursed if performed in an inpatient setting.

Fifth, the policy should note for whom the policy has been written. As discussed earlier, policies cannot be written for every potential combination of patient characteristics, but policies can be specified for a desired population. Policies should clearly specify the patient indicators for which they were designed. Finally, the policy, if written by a third party, can specify the conditions required for the services to be paid. Third-party payers, besides dictating the location of care, may specify coverage conditions and demand preservice approval of care (precertification), concurrent review, and retrospective review.

Practice policies have encountered stiff resistance and have been slow to be adopted. Besides the common problems that bedevil improvement initiatives in all organizations, a variety of implementation barriers specific to health care have thwarted widespread practice policy adoption:

- A history of autonomous decision making
- Socialization of physicians
- Uneven and conflicting evidence
- Fear of performance assessment and economic credentialing
- Mistrust of goals improving quality or lowering resource cost
- Legal issues
- Changing technology and outdated standards
- Time to familiarize oneself with a policy and questions of value
- Competing practice policies

Practice policies will continue to be underutilized, and the benefits they promise will go uncaptured until these problems can be reconciled.

Computer Decision Support

Osheroff et al. state that the goal of computer decision support (CDS) is to "provide the right information, to the right person, in the right format, through the right channel, at the right point in the workflow to improve health care decisions and outcomes" (2007, 142). The recognition that practice policies have often been ineffective led Patwardhan et al. (2009) to examine how CDS can enhance their use. The strengths of computers are their ability to collect and interpret data. It is natural that a data-intensive industry such as medicine should strive to incorporate computers into diagnosis and decision making, monitoring of treatment, and research.

We continue to encounter false starts where CDS fails to achieve its expected goals. Patwardhan et al. suggest that this failure is due to implementation problems and suggest six steps to enhance success. First, identify stakeholders and their goals. Second, catalog the current information system. Third, select CDS interventions to achieve stakeholder goals. Fourth, implement. Fifth, test. Sixth, evaluate and improve as needed. Patwardhan et al. also provide 7 general system requirements, 13 clinician-system interaction requirements, 12 clinician communication content requirements, 4 patient decision support requirements, and 4 auxiliaries. In addition to the requirements, the authors provide examples of how each requirement could be implemented in practice (Patwardhan et al. 2009, 276–278).

Evidence suggests that CDS increases the percentage of patients who receive care consistent with guidelines. To achieve this result, employees must overcome the barriers of nonconformance with current processes, slow and inflexible system performance, information overload, and nonintegrated data.

Goldstein (2008) examined CDS use for hypertension due to the substantial gaps between care delivered and proven best practices. One of the major problems undermining care was that physicians were not aware of patient nonadherence to recommended lifestyle changes and medication regimes. Patient reminders, which notify specific patients of specific medical recommendations, have shown mixed success. Reminders often achieve higher adherence to process but often have limited success in improving outcomes. Goldstein notes two of the primary limitations of reminders: rule systems cannot account for all the complexities of medical knowledge, and systems often provide easy routes to circumvent reminders. An additional concern is that CDS-driven changes to practice require new workflows and the new workflow can introduce new sources of error. Given the frequent provider nonadherence, CDS must provide an opportunity for physicians to state their reason for nonadherence; understanding these reasons is essential to advancing the use of CDS. In Goldstein's study, physicians noted that patients' disbelief of test results (for example, disbelieving that their office BP reading was indicative of their normal readings) and their nonadherence to prior recommendations stopped physicians from offering patients additional recommendations. Goldstein reminds us that building a CDS that can capture the complexities of medical care is a major undertaking, and once accomplished, the system must still overcome provider and patient resistance to its recommendations before health outcomes will improve.

Cases and Applications

Changing practice patterns is a mammoth undertaking, and evaluating success presents many challenges. Success can be judged by monitoring processes—ascertaining whether actual treatment corresponds to recommended treatment—but the true test is whether patient outcomes improve. Process and outcome measures often defy easy analysis; moreover, they are time consuming and expensive to monitor in real time, and retrospective audits are expensive and may not convey the urgency or context of real-time delivery of care. In a meta-analysis of practice policy projects, Grimshaw et al. concluded that 81 studies reported improvements out of 87 studies that examined the effects of practice policies on the process of care. A much lower number of studies reported on outcomes. Only 17 studies reported outcomes, out of which only 12 could demonstrate improvements

(Grimshaw et al. 1995, 60). Locally generated policies, as opposed to external policies, were effective in two of four studies.

Study 1: Adult Respiratory Distress Syndrome (ARDS)

Brent James explored the role of physicians in implementing a practice policy for patients with adult respiratory distress syndrome (ARDS). He noted that most policies lack sufficient detail to be implemented and that users must add "detail and definition that allow specific practice recommendations and measurement" (James 1993, 7). James highlights two key points. First, a policy will be implemented within an existing process that must be understood before implementation begins. Second, besides knowing what has been done and what we want the new process to include, providers must know what will be measured, what medical interventions are expected, how they will be measured (performed/not performed, performed with a defined time frame, performed according to a generally recognized standard, etc.), and what outcomes are sought. If outcomes will be measured, how will they be measured?

Quality improvement efforts have a checkered record for improving care, which James attributes to micromanagement and meaningless measurement and reporting. Both problems stem from misguided managerial efforts that do not understand processes and that fail to obtain commitment among the workforce, pursue changes that do not improve outcomes, and establish reporting systems designed to satisfy the demands of external parties rather than produce information that will benefit patients and providers.

ARDS affects 15,000 patients annually and kills approximately two-thirds of those affected; among high-risk patients the survival rate falls to about 10%. In the 1980s a procedure was developed for oxygenating and removing CO_2 from a patient's blood outside the body ($ECCO_2R$) since the lungs of patients with ARDS have difficulty accomplishing these tasks. James's team, while preparing to run a clinical trial to determine the effectiveness of this procedure, recognized that ventilator use varied considerably in their department. The divergence in use was so great that a single physician would treat similar patients differently between morning and evening shifts and between days.

The team's first task was to generate a detailed protocol, including ventilator management, but in researching the literature they determined that there was often nothing more than consensus to support parts of the promulgated guideline. Accordingly, a system was put in place that provided maximum flexibility to providers to practice as they saw fit, and that allowed for deviations from the prescribed guideline to be used as learning opportunities to build consensus among the treatment team. Ventilator compliance rates began below 50% and by the end of the study were commonly over 80%.

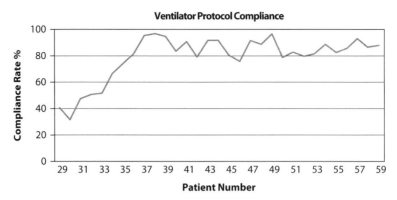

Figure 11.2 Ventilator Compliance and Practice Policies

In addition to their success in standardizing treatment, the team achieved substantial improvements in outcomes. Patient survival in high-risk groups increased to 44% for their stabilized ventilator management protocol versus 38% for $ECCO_2R$ and the 9% to 15% previously observed. The other benefits resulting from the project were that time to manage cases was reduced as decisions did not have to made on an individual basis but could be made for groups of patients. This led to more consistent and predictable treatment, which benefited the entire patient care team. Second, patients that survived left the ICU sooner, which James attributes to the ability to progress a patient through the protocol without requiring a physician order. Finally, stabilized ventilator management, besides having a superior survival rate (44% versus 38%) had a lower cost, $120,000, versus $160,000 for $ECCO_2R$.

James concludes that variation is the key problem in medical practice. When there are wide differences in the treatments that constitute the total care plan, it is impossible to identify which elements improve outcomes. Treatment must be consistently delivered to evaluate how a change affects outcomes. His second conclusion notes that everyone benefits when inappropriate variation declines; patients have higher survival rates, providers save time and achieve better outcomes, and society spends less for medical care. Finally, physicians must be intimately incorporated into the improvement effort; they must accept the rationale for pursuing a practice policy, develop the policy, and lead the initiative.

Study 2: Chronic Kidney Disease

Irving et al. (2006) used a retrospective study to determine how a clinical guideline distributed in March 2000 had affected iron management among patients with chronic kidney disease. Iron management was selected due to the high level of evidence existing on best practice, clinical relevance, the high cost of poor management, including the increased risk of hospitalization and death, and easy-to-measure performance indicators. The authors studied iron score outcomes (hemoglobin, ferritin, and TSAT) across six dialysis units in Australia in September 2004. They found consistency across the units in hemoglobin and TSAT targets although only 25% to 32% of patients achieved their hemoglobin target, while 65% to 73% reached the TSAT target. Performance on the ferritin target was low and inconsistent, with a low of 30% and a high of 68%.

The authors concluded that the process of care might affect the achievement of iron targets and that "all units had a written protocol but not all units complied with their protocol" (Irving et al. 2006, 312). Process factors that were positively correlated with adherence to the treatment policy included nursing autonomy, agreement on protocol, effective decision aids, degree of physician reliance on protocol, and a proactive versus reactive protocol. Adherence decreased with an increase in the number of treating physicians. While this study documents the problems associated with the passive distribution of guidelines, it did not attempt to track the lack of adherence to patient outcomes. The authors found that commitment to a policy will be lacking if providers do not see clear and convincing evidence that adherence to the protocol will improve patient outcomes. Their failure to track patient outcomes to protocol adherence represents a lost opportunity to determine if and how much outcome may change when protocols are followed.

Study 3: Antibiotic Practice Guidelines

Pestotnik et al. (1996) studied compliance with antibiotic practice guidelines in a Utah hospital from January 1988 through December 1994, with a total of 162,196 patients studied. The prime motive for defining a guideline was the research finding that up to 50% of antibiotic use is inappropriate and results in antibiotic resistance, adverse drug reactions, and higher cost.

The authors reported lower mortality rates and antibiotic costs after implementation of a computer-assisted decision support system. The computer system was designed to provide alerts and suggestions based on the presence of resistant pathogens, untreated infections, and incorrect dose, route, or interval of an antibiotic. Prophylactic antibiotic doses within two hours of surgery increased from 40% in 1988 to 99.1% in 1994. In 1985 the hospital recorded 19 antibiotic doses per patient; by 1994 doses per patient had fallen to 5.3. One of the prime drivers of antibiotic guidelines was overuse, and the dramatic reduction in the number of doses highlights the previous failure of providers to discontinue antibiotics when they were not needed.

After documenting lower antibiotic use, the authors examined how outcomes changed. Antibiotic-associated adverse drug events decreased from 26.9% in 1989 to 18.8% in 1994. Mortality rates for patients treated with antibiotics fell from 3.65% in 1988 to 2.65% in 1994. The daily antibiotic dose per 100 occupied beds decreased from 35.9 in 1988 to 27.7 in 1994, and cost per patient fell from $122.66 to $51.90 (adjusted for inflation).

Study 4: Diabetes Mellitus Guidelines

A study by Hetlevik et al. (2000) on the effect of clinical guidelines for diabetes mellitus found no significant change in doctors' behavior or patient outcomes. A CDS was implemented to facilitate use of the clinical guideline. The only statistically significant finding was a 2.3 mm Hg reduction in diastolic blood pressure in the intervention group that used a guideline to model care. Statistically insignificant differences in favor of the intervention group included lower HbA1c levels and systolic blood pressure; however, the control group had lower rates of smoking, decreased body mass index, and lower risk scores for myocardial infarction. Poor provider adherence to the guidelines was attributed to confusion over whether the guidelines were optional or standard and to time demands when current health problems take precedence over risk intervention.

The James and Pestotnik et al. projects emphasize several essential points. First is the need for local consensus. Both studies dealt with receptive providers who recognized the medical cost of continuing present practice and actively participated in the development of the practice policy. Each study involved an extensive literature search, developed clear practice expectations with associated process and outcome metrics, and continually fed back information to providers. Their success was built on the fact that the interventions they advocated were seen as essential to providing high-quality care and as facilitating, rather than encumbering, the health care delivery process.

Summary

Variability is inherent in a system that deals with complex problems in trying circumstances with insufficient data. The degree of variability in health care arising from conflicting research or lack of research and from differences in patient preferences requires tools to minimize variation to the extent possible. Practice policies are one tool to reduce variation by incorporating evidence and preference into treatment decisions.

For practice policies to change physician practice patterns, they must address the questions physicians have regarding the need to change and the degree of improvement to be expected. In addition to meeting these information requirements, once a persuasive case for change can be made, policies must be disseminated to providers and effectively implemented. Some of the primary barriers to the effective utilization of practice policies are providers' lack of knowledge of their existence and the difficulty of incorporating new processes into existing practices. If information technology can collect and interpret data in a way that facilitates patient care without burdening providers, it may overcome past barriers to practice policy use.

This chapter documents how practice policies have led to better health outcomes and lower costs, but it also describes initiatives that achieved meager or no improvement. The reader should take away the knowledge that health care can be improved, reduction in variation should improve care, and practice policies are one way to reduce variation and improve care. The challenge to practitioners is to successfully build the case for practice policies and adapt them to their work culture.

KEY TERMS

Clinical pathways

Guidelines

Options

Practice policies

Standards

REVIEW QUESTIONS

1. What are the six steps of the clinical decision-making process?

2. What are the differences among a practice standard, a guideline, and an option?

3. What information should be discussed in a practice policy?

4. How can an institution increase the probability that a practice policy will be embraced by providers?

5. What are the typical barriers to practice policies?

6. To support practice policies, what features should a computer system include?

7. How successful have practice policies been?

References

Cabana MD, Rand CS, Powe NR, Wu AW, Wilson MH, Abboud PA, and Rubin HR, 1999, Why Don't Physicians Follow Clinical Practice Guidelines? A Framework for Improvement, *JAMA* 282 (15): 1458–1465.

Carnett WG, 1999, Clinical Practice Guidelines; A Tool to Improve Care, *Quality Management in Health Care* 8 (1): 13–21.

Chong C, Chen I, Naglie G, and Krahn M, 2009, How Well Do Guidelines Incorporate Evidence on Patient Preferences? *Journal of General Internal Medicine* 24 (8): 977–982.

Detre KM, Peduzzi P, Takararo T, Hultgren H, Murphy M, and Kroncke G, for the Veterans Administration Coronary Artery Bypass Surgery Cooperative Study Group, 1984, Eleven-year Survival in the Veterans Administration Randomized Trial of Coronary Artery Bypass Surgery for Stable Angina, *New England Journal of Medicine* 311 (21): 1333–1339.

Eddy DM, 1990a, Clinical Decision Making: From Theory to Practice, Anatomy of a Decision, *JAMA* 263 (3): 441–443.

Eddy DM, 1990b, Clinical Decision Making: From Theory to Practice, Practice Policies—What Are They? *JAMA* 263 (6): 877–880.

Eddy DM, 1990c, Clinical Decision Making: From Theory to Practice, Guidelines for Policy Statements: The Explicit Approach, *JAMA* 263 (16): 2239–2243.

Eddy DM, 1990d, Clinical Decision Making: From Theory to Practice, Designing a Practice Policy: Standards, Guidelines and Options, *JAMA* 263 (22): 3077–3084.

Evidence-Based Working Group, 1992, Evidence-Based Medicine, *JAMA* 268 (17): 2420–2425.

Goetsch DL and Davis SB, 2010, *Quality Management for Organizational Excellence*, 6th ed., Prentice Hall, Upper Saddle River, NJ.

Goldstein M, 2008, Using Health Information Technology to Improve Hypertension Management, *Current Hypertension Reports* 10 (3): 201–207.

Grimshaw J, Freemantle N, Wallace S, Russell I, Hurwitz B, Watt I, Long A, and Sheldon T, 1995, Developing and Implementing Clinical Practice Guidelines, *Quality in Health Care* 4 (1): 55–64.

Hetlevik I, Holmen J, Krüger O, Kristensen P, Iversen H, and Furuseth K, 2000, Implementing Clinical Guidelines in the Treatment of Diabetes Mellitus in General Practice: Evaluation of Effort, Process, and Patient Outcome Related to Implementation of a Computer-based Decision Support System, *International Journal of Technology Assessment in Health Care* 16 (1): 210–227.

Ioannidis JP, 2005, Contradicted and Initially Stronger Effects in Highly Cited Clinical Research, *JAMA* 294 (2): 218–228.

Irving MJ, Craig JC, Gallagher M, McDonald S, Polkinghorne KR, Walker RG, and Roger SD, 2006, Implementing Iron Management Clinical Practice

Guidelines in Patients with Chronic Kidney Disease Having Dialysis, *Medical Journal of Australia* 185 (6): 310–314.

James BC, 1993, Implementing Practice Guidelines through Clinical Quality Improvement, *Frontiers of Health Services Management* 10 (1): 3–37.

Kahan N, Kahan E, Waitman D, Kitai E, and Chintz D, 2009, The Tools of Evidence-Based Culture: Implementing Clinical-Practice Guidelines in an Israeli HMO, *Academic Medicine* 84 (9): 1217–1225.

Kaimal A and Kupperman M, 2010, Understanding Risk, Patient and Provider Preferences, and Obstetrical Decision Making: Approach to Delivery after Cesarean, *Seminars in Perinatology* 34: 331–336.

Margo CE, 2004, Quality Care and Practice Variation: The Roles of Practice Guidelines and Public Profiles, *Survey of Ophthalmology* 49 (3): 359–371.

McNeil, B, Pauker S, Sox H, and Tversky A, 1982, On the Elicitation of Preferences for Alternative Therapies, *New England Journal of Medicine* 306 (21): 1259–1262.

Osheroff JA, Teich JM, Middleton B, Steen EB, Wright A, and Detmer DE, 2007, A Roadmap for National Action on Clinical Decision Support, *Journal of the American Medical Informatics Association* 14 (2): 141–145.

Patwardhan M, Kawamoto K, Lobach D, Patel U, and Matchar D, 2009, Recommendations for a Clinical Decision Support for the Management of Individuals with Chronic Kidney Disease, *Clinical Journal of the America Society of Nephrology* 4: 273–283.

Pestotnik SL, Classen DC, Evans RS, and Burke JP, 1996, Implementing Antibiotic Practice Guidelines through Computer-assisted Decision Support: Clinical and Financial Outcome, *Annals of Internal Medicine* 124 (10): 884–890.

Tricoci P, Allen JM, Kramer JM, Califf RM, and Smith SC, 2009, Scientific Evidence Underlying the ACC/AHA Clinical Practice Guidelines, *JAMA* 301 (8): 831–841.

Weiland D, 1997, Why Use Clinical Pathways Rather than Practice Guidelines? *American Journal of Surgery* 174 (6): 592–595.

CHAPTER 12

CASE, DISEASE, AND OUTCOMES MANAGEMENT

Introduction

Chapter Twelve, in combination with Chapters Eleven, Thirteen, and Fourteen, introduces the reader to medical practice management tools that are used to improve health care outcomes by systematizing processes, enhancing a team approach to patient care, and providing information. This chapter reviews case, disease, and outcomes management, which aim at improved patient care through coordination of care processes. Case, disease, and outcomes management focus on two important truths about health care and health expenditures.

First, a small number of patients account for the lion's share of total medical spending. One percent of patients accounts for 22% of total medical spending in the United States, while the bottom 50% of the population accounts for only 3% of spending (Druss et al. 2002). Figure 12.1 shows the percentage of total spending by various consumers of health care; note that the top 5% of the population consumes 49% of all spending. Case, disease, and outcomes management recognize that focusing managerial attention on the patients consuming the highest amount of resources could improve health outcomes and reduce medical spending. U.S. health spending is an example of the Pareto rule in action: 20% of patients account for 80% of all medical spending. Given the roughly 33,600,000 annual admissions, monitoring 20% of patients or 6,720,000 admissions may be unachievable. Paying close attention to the 5% of patients who are the most expensive to treat may be possible and could lead to cost savings. To realize cost savings, the expected reduction in use of health care resources must be less than any added review and management costs.

LEARNING OBJECTIVES

1. Examine the distribution of U.S. health care spending

2. Understand the aim, structure, and application of case management

3. Understand the aim, structure, and application of disease management

4. Understand the aim, structure, and application of outcomes management

5. Perform PubMed literature searches

A second truth is that a small number of medical conditions account for a large share of total spending. The 15 top medical conditions accounted for 44% of total medical spending in 1996 (Druss et al. 2002, 106). Studying and managing these conditions offers the hope that care can be improved and cost reduced by providing optimal care at the right time in the right setting by the appropriate provider. The shift in medical care away from acute care and toward long-term chronic care has been one of the prime drivers of the rapid run-up of health care spending. The most expensive patients and conditions overlap and provide an opportunity to improve outcomes while simultaneously managing resource use.

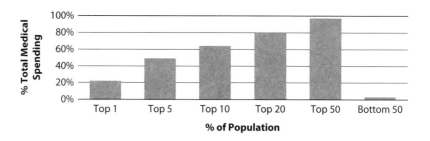

Figure 12.1 Distribution of U.S. Medical Spending across U.S. Population

Figure 12.1 shows that 1% of the U.S. population accounts for more than 20% of all medical spending and that 20% of the population accounts for four of every five dollars spent on health care. The 50% of the population that uses the least health care, column six, accounts for only 3% of total spending. Figure 12.1 shows how skewed the distribution of spending is and the potential benefit that could be reaped from focusing on a small percentage of patients.

Case, disease, and outcomes management differ in their scope and in how patients or care processes are selected. Case management is the most individualist of the three tools, focusing on particular patients, conditions, or combinations of conditions that could result in poor outcomes or high resource use and cost. Case management may begin prior to admission with a patient who is identified as high risk based on his or her condition or prior medical history, for example, a high-risk pregnancy or transplant patient. Often case management is initiated after a patient reaches a particular LOS or cost threshold or encounters a series of adverse events signaling that additional attention should be devoted to the case.

Disease management asks more systemic questions: What health conditions typically generate high costs? How can patients with or at risk for these conditions be treated to improve care or to lower cost (or both)?

Disease management relies on research and best practice to determine prospectively how a group of patients should be treated.

Outcomes management, unlike case and disease management, emphasizes outcome measures (versus process) and is more universal in its aims. At the macro level it aims at establishing a nationwide database that patients, physicians, and payers could use to determine what treatments were applied in the past and what outcomes achieved. At a micro or patient level, outcomes management focuses on a particular desired outcome, for example, length of stay, patient satisfaction, condition-specific measures, or cost per case, and it modifies the health care delivery process to achieve the desired outcome.

These tools address the essential duality of today's health care environment: how to produce the best outcome for individual patients while practicing responsible stewardship of resources at the system level. All three management processes share the common goal of improving patient outcomes and the subsidiary goals of increasing patient satisfaction and efficient use of resources. All employ similar processes involving assessment, planning, education, implementation, coordination, monitoring, and evaluation to achieve their goals. Figure 12.2 uses a Venn diagram to emphasize the similarities and differences among the three tools. The overlap of case, disease, and outcomes management highlights the core functions used to plan and coordinate health care.

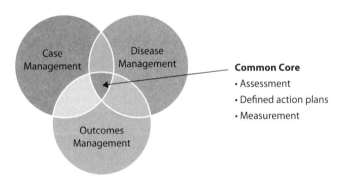

Figure 12.2 Case, Disease, and Outcomes Management

Effective use of these tools requires integrated information systems and appropriate incentives. This chapter emphasizes the traditional "management" side of quality management; that is, management defined as coordinating a production process and monitoring a system in operation. The functions of a manager are often summarized as planning, organizing, leading, and controlling. In medical care, these functions are diagnosing, establishing the treatment plan, overseeing care, evaluating the effects of care, and modifying treatment as necessary. In human activity many roads often lead to the same destination. The question for providers is: Are different courses of treatment equivalent in the health outcomes they produce and resources they consume? Case, disease, and outcomes management examine these questions and attempt to illuminate the path that should be taken.

Case Management

Case management (CM) is an outcome-driven approach to patient care, involving all appropriate health care professionals in planning and delivering treatment for specific patients (Nash, Coombs, and Leider 1999, 8). The American Nurses Association (ANA) in 1991 defined CM as "a health delivery process whose goals are to provide quality healthcare, decrease fragmentation, enhance the quality of the client's life, and contain costs" (Gallagher and Truglio-Londrigan 2004, 27). The first definition provides a process view, while the second identifies the outcomes expected to be produced from the process.

CM frequently occurs in the confines of a hospital, where the hospital recognizes that tighter control over patient consumption of health care resources could improve patient outcomes and financial performance in the DRG reimbursement environment. Under a reimbursement system that pays a flat rate per case, hospitals recognize that their financial health could be improved by ensuring that required services are delivered in a timely manner and by eliminating unnecessary tests, medications, procedures, and hospital days.

Yamamoto and Lucey provide a more expansive description of CM goals by focusing on desired outcomes: "nurse case managers can optimize client self-care, decrease fragmentation of care, provide quality care across a continuum, enhance patients' quality of life, decrease length of hospitalization, increase patient and staff satisfaction, and promote the cost-effective use of scarce resources" (Yamamoto and Lucey 2005, 162). CM is a dramatic change in how health care is delivered, shifting oversight and coordination from physicians to nurses.

Figure 12.3 shows how the case manager interacts with the three primary parties involved in patient care. Case managers are intermediaries in the traditional physician-patient relationship as they may assist providers in patient assessment and self-care instruction. Case managers also serve as a point of contact and information for patients who cannot or do not want to contact their physician. In the second and third interactions, between patients and their third-party payer and between providers and payers, case managers facilitate understanding between patients and providers regarding what are covered services and any restrictions on coverage. The medical expertise of the case manager may smooth the interaction between non-medically astute patients and third-party payers, and similarly the case manager's insurance acumen may be useful in mediating problems between providers and payers.

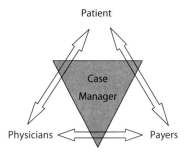

Figure 12.3 The Role of a Case Manager

The two major forms of CM are internal, or intraprovider, typically within a hospital, and external, or interprovider, typically performed by insurers and third-party payers. While this distinction may lose its significance given the growth of integrated delivery systems where a health system is as concerned about the efficient movement of a patient across providers as what occurs in a particular episode, the distinction still informs the way CM is performed and the goals pursued by a provider versus a third-party payer. Providers are typically concerned with an episode of care, while a third-party payer is concerned with the total cost of care across all episodes. Reimbursement systems will continue to determine the degree to which a health care provider's goals parallel those of a third-party payer.

The primary functions of a nurse case manager include performing case findings and screening; assessing the biological, psychological, and social needs of the patient and his or her family; assessing coping and adaptive abilities; identifying formal and informal support systems; evaluating self-care abilities; serving as a liaison and facilitating communication; coordinating care and services; information gathering and synthesizing interdisciplinary problem identification; identifying and linking the patient with the best appropriate resource, person, or institution; critical thinking and problem solving; procuring services; making eligibility decisions; authorizing hospitalization, rehabilitation, or home care needs; documentation; and monitoring and evaluating the patient's outcome (Girard 1994). Michael and Cohen (2004) make a further distinction based on the patient's abilities. Their definition of case management parallels those given above; however, they target CM on patients whose self-care capacity is limited. This distinction emphasizes defining a care plan based on the capabilities of each patient. This chapter will use the term CM for all patients, regardless of capacity for self-care.

Case managers must develop the skills of an assessor, planner, facilitator, advocate, and cost and reimbursement analyst. As an assessor, the case manager must be able to interview and gather data, anticipate problems, issues, and obstacles, and develop education based on the patient's capabilities. The key skills needed are critical thinking and analytical skills. As a planner, the case manager develops long- and short-term goals and identifies the problems to be addressed, the interventions needed, and the availability of interventions. Facilitation requires connecting patients to providers to ensure that needed services are delivered on a timely basis. Alliotta (2001) states that the role of the case manager, acting as an advocate, is to develop the patient's self-sufficiency. These roles demand knowledge of the medical condition and health care delivery system, empathy, and communication skills to deal effectively with all health care decision-makers. Rossi (2003) adds cost and reimbursement analysis to this list, recognizing that case managers often negotiate a torturous path to determine the cost of services and ability to pay, including establishing third-party insurance eligibility.

The role of a case manager in a hospital is to ensure a smooth transition for a patient from admission to discharge. The case manager must be able to identify problems, coordinate care, decrease LOS by coordinating transfer to lower-acuity facilities when appropriate, refer the patient to community support services, and provide patient education to reduce complications.

Kurtz, Cookson, and Mattie (2008) note that case managers are often integral to setting expectations for patients, their families, and providers. In addition, they should perform the role of educator by identifying best practices and educating staff. At the point of care they should coordinate care and identify and remove barriers to patient progression.

Case Management Functions

The four major functions of CM are assessment, planning, monitoring, and discharge planning. *Assessment* involves the continuous data gathering on the patient, his family, and resources. To facilitate planning, the case manager must gather patient demographics, medical history, current health status, financial and insurance resources, functional and mental abilities, cultural and religious beliefs, language skills, and education. Environmental assessments should be performed examining the patient's lifestyle, living arrangements, and employment. The goal of assessment is to determine the level of care required.

Case managers require a wide range of skills to obtain and evaluate the various sources of patient information, including interviews with patients, family, and care givers, record reviews, observation, case conferences, and consultations. Various assessment tools have been developed to facilitate data collection, including the Functional Independent Measures (FIM), covering self-care, sphincter control, locomotion, communication, and other factors, and the Medical Outcomes Study Short Form (SF36), focusing on physical functioning, physical and mental role limitations, social functioning, pain, mental health, vitality, and health perception (Rossi 2003).

Once input has been received from all involved parties, the second step is to incorporate the data into a care plan. *Planning* requires analysis and documentation of what should be done, communication with affected parties, and eliciting approval for the care plan. The care plan includes the primary physician, diagnosis and prognosis, tests and procedures, special needs, medications, mobility issues, diet and elimination, behavioral issues, and discharge plans (Rossi 2003).

Rossi provides ten questions a case manager should address in creating a treatment plan:

1. Is the patient in the correct health care setting?
2. What will be the cost of each service?
3. What is the frequency and intensity of service required?
4. Are necessary providers available?
5. What training is required for the patient and their care givers?
6. What equipment is required?
7. Will the patient encounter any physical or architectural barriers?
8. Is a second opinion needed?
9. What is the ultimate outcome expected?
10. Would the patient outcome be the same without CM? (2003, 39–40)

The first nine questions aim at clarifying a treatment plan and removing obstacles to carrying out the plan. Question 10 addresses the value added by CM: Are outcomes expected to be superior due to the use of CM? Does CM improve the health care delivery process, or would providers produce the same outcomes at the same cost without CM? If CM cannot demonstrate superior outcomes, the resources consumed by it would be better employed in other uses.

Monitoring, the third function, requires the case manager to assess the performance of the treatment plan and change the plan as necessary. The case manager must monitor a patient's condition and progress, determine whether interventions were undertaken and what their effect was, and whether targets are being reached. The promise of CM will be realized only if superior practices are identified and providers can be convinced to use these practices at the patient bedside. An institution's ability to assess whether interventions are performed as ordered and outcomes are realized will play a primary role in determining whether bedside practice can be changed. Benson et al. (2001) note that an effective variance tracking system requires measures, multidisciplinary input on tracked elements, and simple-to-use data collection methods. Monitoring is essential to determine the causes of variance: Is a failure to provide a service or realize a desired outcome due to clinical factors, action or inaction by the provider or the patient, or procedural or system weaknesses?

The tracking of deviations is necessary to understand when and how the treatment plan should be changed due to the failure to reach targets or the emergence of new needs. From the quality improvement standpoint, this data should also be employed to recognize natural variation, common weaknesses in the system, and the emergence of new phenomena in the system known as special cause variation. Understanding desired outcomes and monitoring performance is the only way to ensure that current and future patients receive maximum benefit from health services.

The final function is discharge planning. *Discharge planning* is contingent upon monitoring and assessing a patient's readiness for discharge. Once targeted outcomes are achieved, the case manager must coordinate transfer to other environments. Regardless of a destination, the case manager must anticipate the patient's needs, provide self-care education as needed, and identify other health care providers to ensure continuity of care.

Measurement and Accountability

While the CM functions provide a logical overview of the process, successful implementation requires clear and measurable goals. Table 12.1 provides a roadmap case managers should use to direct care (intermediate outcomes) and measure success (final outcomes).

Table 12.1 CM Functions and Intermediate and Final Outcomes

Functions of Case Management→	Intermediate Outcomes of Case Management→	Final Outcomes of Case Management
Assessment	Patient Knowledge	Health Outcomes
Planning	Patient Involvement	Quality of Care
Facilitation	Patient Empowerment	Cost of Care
Advocacy	Patient Adherence	Coordination of Care

Source: Case Management Society of America Council for Case Management Accountability, 1997, Figure 37.1, in EL Cohen and TG Cesta, 2001, *Nursing Case Management*, Elsevier/Mosby, St. Louis, MO, 418.

It is easy to speak in generalities about what should be done, but specifying exactly what should be measured and how an individual case manager should be evaluated is more difficult. Foster (2003) provides clarity by attaching specific measures to CM competencies.

Competency	Measure
Management of care	Effective care plans
Position-specific functions	Provides accurate information to third-party payers
Safety	Identifies high-risk patients
Age-specific care	Assesses skin breakdown
Pain management	Monitors pain
Performance improvement	Demonstrates performance improvement
Fiscal management	Reduces costs
Compliance	Follows code of conduct
Patient satisfaction	Generates positive guest relations

These nine competencies and the related measures define precisely what is desired in terms of performance. The safety competency can be conceptualized as recognizing a patient as high risk before an undesirable outcome occurs, for example, identifying expectant mothers before a premature birth occurs.

Case Management Cases

While it is easy to lay out the parameters of a CM system and describe the skills needed by a case manager, true understanding of the complexities and nuances of the process can be obtained only by examining patient cases. The following cases describe key elements and insights gained by applying the tool.

Study 1: Rheumatoid Arthritis

Boyer (1999) examined CM for a patient with rheumatoid arthritis (RA), who after months of pain, was diagnosed and prescribed a nonsteroidal anti-inflammatory. Over time the symptoms progressed and when the patient could barely walk, she contacted a rheumatologist. The rheumatologist prescribed prednisone and methotrexate, which provided temporary improvement but led to worsening side effects. The patient's situation is common for RA patients: temporary relief is achieved but drugs lose their efficacy over time and lead to worsening side effects. RA treatment thus requires multiple and continuous interventions. RA is a condition ripe for CM as patients require education through the changing circumstances of their disease.

The impact of RA is devastating, with bone erosion occurring in 90% of patients within two years of diagnosis. As RA progresses, functional impairment increases; 50% of patients report severe functional impairment within six years of their first visit. Similarly, 50% to 60% of patients become unable to work over time. Emotional and psychological problems also accompany the pain and fatigue of RA. Medical care costs are estimated to be $5,000 per patient per year, while losses from decreased productivity are estimated at $200 million per year in the United States.

A case manager must be familiar with the variety of medications used to treat RA, their side effects, and their effectiveness over time. The first issue that must be addressed is how effectiveness is measured. Boyer measured effectiveness using the Larsen score, which assesses joint erosion and narrowing on a 100-point scale. A second measure is treatment costs. Medications are integral to care and comprise approximately 23% of treatment costs. Initially, prednisone and corticosteroids are prescribed for pain and to slow the rate of joint damage. Disease-modifying antirheumatic drugs (DMARDs) have been shown to produce better outcomes and reduce the need for joint replacement, so the treatment rule is that these medications should be prescribed as soon as possible. However, DMARDs lose their efficacy over time and are associated with toxicity. Tests for toxicity have been estimated to account for 80% of the cost of drug therapy. One of the recent innovations in treating RA is tumor necrosis factor (TNF). TNF-inhibiting drugs work in conjunction with the patient's body to reduce joint inflammation. At the time of Boyer's study, TNF-inhibiting drugs had not demonstrated the declining efficacy of DMARDs.

Besides familiarity with medications, the case manager must consider the type of provider the patient should see. Should the patient see a generalist or a rheumatologist? Rheumatologists have been shown to elicit better functional outcomes from patients but they increase the cost of treatment by 3%. This relationship, better outcome and higher cost, highlights a prime consideration that medicine is only beginning to grapple with: Are better outcomes worth the price?

Boyer also points out another contribution of case managers that is often lost in academic discussions: case managers often achieve a higher level of trust and familiarity with patients and serve as a communication conduit with physicians. Boyer suggests that case managers may be better able to obtain accurate information on patient compliance, response to treatment, and general functioning. Boyer emphasizes the human element, never veering from the impact of the disease on the physical and psychological well-being of the patient. The author also emphasizes the role of medicine. Her use of graphs to show the results of early- versus late-starting DMARDs therapy and the effectiveness of TNF therapy over time demonstrates the need for case managers to stay abreast of medical advances to ensure that patients receive the optimal care.

Study 2: High-Risk Pregnancy

Handley and Stanton (2006) emphasized assessing accomplishment and benchmarking in treating high-risk pregnancy. Measurement is essential to assess progress, and the authors provide precise measures to evaluate disease indicators, functionality, comfort (pain), complications, and self-care ability (skills and knowledge).

The authors provide a clean overview of the CM process and measures in a 4 × 4 table (Table 12.2), following the CM functions of assessment, intervention, monitoring, and evaluation across four outcomes categories: clinical, psychological, functional, and spiritual. This table presents a large amount of information and highlights a key CM issue: volumes of information exist for clinical assessment and intervention (the top left quadrants), but measures become sparser as one moves toward evaluation (downward) and nonclinical outcomes (rightward).

Table 12.2 Case Management Process for High-Risk Pregnancy

	Clinical	Psychological	Functional	Spiritual
Assessment	7 measures including indicators of constipation, indigestion, muscle wasting, hygiene, skin irritation, contractions, and infection	8 measures including privacy, depression, anxiety, boredom, intimacy, loss of communication with family and others, separation from work, and curtailment of social activities	4 measures including muscle weakness, diminished stamina, compromised healing, and ADL problems	3 measures including access to clergy, reduced prayer, and grief over pregnancy
Intervention	5 measures including diet and fluid intake, skin protection, hygiene assistance and infection, contraction protection	5 measures including diversions, marking time to delivery, visitations, phone calls, and private time	3 measures including passive activity, physical therapy, and continuation of ADL	2 measures including access to faith and clergy
Monitoring	4 measures including vital signs, dietary, fluid and bowel cycles, and assessment of fetus	3 measures including mood, visits and communication, and activity	3 measures including stamina, muscle tone, and ADL difficulties	1 measure concerning patient wishes for spiritual support
Evaluation	1 measure assessing outcomes with evidence-based practice guidelines	1 measure assessing patient's ability to cope with changes	1 measure assessing patient's ability for self-care and ADL	1 measure assessing patient's satisfaction with spiritual support

Source: M Handley and M Stanton, 2006, Evidence-based Case Management in a High-Risk Pregnancy: A Case Study, *Lippincott's Case Management* 11 (5): 245.

From the authors' perspective the absence of information on patients' psychological needs was notable. The evaluation of psychological and spiritual needs rests on a limited and subjective set of measures; provider experience may be the best guide in assessing whether these needs are fulfilled. That is, the physician may be the best judge of how a particular patient is faring relative to their other patients in a similar situation.

Optimal treatment for high-risk pregnancies depends on accurate assessment of gestational age, but a case manager must make a variety of decisions for which clinical guidelines provide minimal assistance. The article highlights the role of bed rest. Providers walk a fine line between minimizing the risk of premature delivery and excessive bed rest leading to complications. As stated earlier, guidelines often give little attention to nonclinical factors, leaving case managers to sort out patients' psychological and spiritual needs and the appropriate interventions.

Study 3: Hypercalcemia

Bernet, Shumway, and Bunin (2006) provide a purely clinical approach to CM to illustrate the diagnostic process and discuss treatment options. The case followed the treatment of a patient with symptomatic hypercalcemia. Five treatment possibilities were available, and they were evaluated in terms of how quickly the intervention worked and whether the desired outcome could be sustained. After treating the patient's acute disorder, pain, the focus shifted to diagnosis. Diagnosis depends on the probability of common causes; hyperthyroidism and malignancy account for 90% of all cases, and the appropriate screening test is one that best differentiates the two causes. The screening test could of course conclude that neither is the cause and additional tests would be warranted.

The selected screening test supported the working diagnosis of hypercalcemia, and the patient was transferred from the theater hospital to Walter Reed Army Medical Center, where a history and a physical were completed and an imaging test study was ordered. The attending physician was again confronted by the choice of possible imaging tests; the choice was based on their sensitivity, ability to identify actual positives, the rate of false positives, cost, and time. The imaging test identified a parathyroid adenoma. This led to the final clinical decision: How should it be treated? Five treatment options were available, and their costs and benefits were weighted. Parathyroidectomy was selected due to its superior long-term outcomes and the lack of clinical indicators militating against surgery. This study highlights clinical choice and reinforces the need for case managers to evaluate choices in complex cases. Figure 12.4 summarizes the duties of a case manager as described by Rossi (2003).

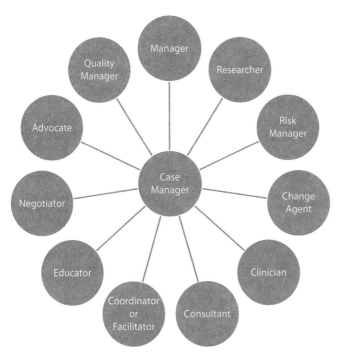

Figure 12.4 Duties of a Case Manager

Figure 12.4 illustrates the tasks a case manager may be called on to fulfill. CM that improves outcomes requires a vast set of skills and the ability to work with a broad array of personnel. The CM function may more fully embrace the idea of a holistic healing system than any other component of health care.

Disease Management

The Care Continuum Alliance (CCA) defines disease management (DM) as a system of coordinated health care interventions and communications for people with conditions in which patient self-care efforts are significant. The two primary factors in this definition are that DM is designed to serve patients with specific medical conditions and is aimed at improving the patient's ability to manage his or her condition.

The CCA (2011) cites six primary components including:

1. Population identification processes

2. Evidence-based practice guidelines

3. Collaborative practice models to include physician and support-service providers

4. Patient self-management, including primary prevention, behavior modification, and compliance or surveillance training

5. Process and outcomes measurement, evaluation, and management

6. Routine communication among patients, providers, and payers

Olin and Rhoades (2005) report that five medical conditions—heart conditions, trauma, cancer, mental disorders, and pulmonary conditions—accounted for the bulk of health care spending. Figure 12.5 shows the contribution of each condition to total medical spending and that all five conditions accounted for 32.7% of all spending in 2002.

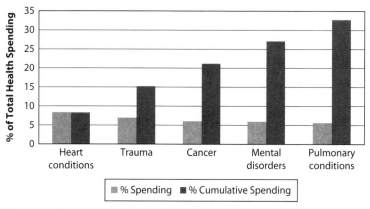

Figure 12.5 Five Most Costly Medical Conditions

Source: GL Olin and JA Rhoades, 2005, The Five Most Costly Medical Conditions, 1997 and 2002: Estimates for the U.S. Civilian Noninstitutionalized Population, *Statistical Brief* #80. Rockville, MD, Agency for Healthcare Research and Quality, http://www.meps.ahrq.gov/mepsweb/data_files/publications/st80/stat80.pdf, accessed June 8, 2013.

Figure 12.5 shows that five conditions account for roughly one-third of total medical spending and emphasizes the potential benefit to be reaped from focusing on a small set of medical conditions. While we risk the **fallacy of composition**—inferring that something is true of the whole because it is true in some of the parts of the whole—the idea behind disease management is that we can define best practice and apply it consistently to a group of patients. Although medical practice will always require customization based on a particular patient's desires and the set of conditions he or she presents with, the idea is enticing that for large groups of patients we can consistently provide optimal care, neither too little care nor too much. Of the five most costly conditions, trauma stands out, because it is an acute condition rather than a chronic condition. A primary distinction between CM and DM operates on this difference; DM deals with chronic conditions and is more likely to emphasize care across settings. DM asks what care should be delivered across time and location and how the patient can be

fallacy of composition inferring that something is true of the whole because it is true in some of the parts of the whole

trained to be an active participant in her care. Given the chronic nature of these conditions, a prime goal of DM is to build a strong patient-practitioner relationship.

Opportunities for Improvement

The need for greater standardization of care has been documented by many studies. Wennberg and his coauthors over many years have documented wide differences in the amount of care delivered across seemingly homogeneous populations. Of greater concern than the differences in care delivered was the lack of differences in outcomes achieved; that is, although care varies widely, the difference in how patients are treated has little impact on health outcomes. The problem is that without agreement on what is appropriate treatment, patients may be placed at risk of receiving too little or too much care. Besides the risk to the patient there is the corresponding question of whether scarce resources are being used effectively. Failing to provide necessary care may increase long-term cost, while the provision of unnecessary care is at best a waste of resources and in the worst case can produce adverse results that will require the expenditure of more resources.

McGlynn et al. (2003) reported that only 54.3% of patients received recommended levels of care, and their study documented how recommended care varied by medical condition. The article was a clarion call to standardize medical practice by informing physicians of what tests should be run and what treatments should be provided and documenting patient care deficiencies. Condition-specific studies routinely document treatment gaps. Diabetes care provides one example. Data collected between 1988 and 1995 (derived from the Centers for Disease Control's population-based Behavioral Risk Factor Surveillance System, as well as the National Health and Nutrition Examination surveys) reveal significant gaps in the treatment of diabetes and screening for diabetes-related complications. Nearly one in five patients with diabetes had poor glycemic control (HbA1c level > 9.5%), more than one-third had elevated blood pressure (>140/90 mmHg), and more than half had elevated LDL cholesterol levels. Use of screening measures showed similar variation, with only 28%, 55%, and 63% of diabetic patients receiving more than one HbA1c test per year or annual foot and eye exams, respectively. Systematic variation in care has been documented across racial and ethnic groups, with African Americans, Hispanics, and Native Americans more likely to die of diabetes-related complications than Caucasians.

A potential solution to this deficiency is DM. Studies frequently show that recommended care increases when clear protocols are instituted and non-physician providers are incorporated into the treatment process. Gattis et al. (1999) reported that six of ten trials that assessed the use of proven efficacious medications demonstrated significantly higher prescribing rates (or dosing) in those patients randomized to a multidisciplinary care group.

Developing a Disease Management Program

Step 1 in developing a DM program is to establish a clear definition of the disease, its scope, and impact (Ellrodt et al. 1997). The target population should first be defined by disease and then subdivided into high-risk groups based on comorbidity conditions or age. Treatment will vary based on a patient's risk classification; low-risk patients may be treated conservatively while high-risk patients should be provided more active and continuous care and monitoring. Targeted populations might include high-volume clinical services, high-cost health care expenditures, services that have great variation in clinical practice, services that pose significant risks to patients, clinical opportunities for improvement, or patient care situations in which long-term complications are linked to provider risk (Doxtator and Rodriquez 1998).

Table 12.3 Steps for Developing a Disease Management Program

1.	Define the disease, its scope, and impact
2.	Develop baseline information on treatment and resource utilization
3.	Generate specific clinical and economic questions and research the literature
4.	Critically appraise and synthesize the evidence
5.	Evaluate benefits, harms, and costs
6.	Develop guidelines for professional collaboration and patient self-management
7.	Create a system for process and outcome measurement and reporting
8.	Implement the program
9.	Complete the quality improvement cycle by continuous measurement and assessment of the program

Source: G Ellrodt et al., 1997, Evidence-based Disease Management, *JAMA* 278 (20): 1688.

The intent of implementing a DM program is to improve outcomes. To determine success, it is vital that providers understand how the health care delivery system has operated in the past. *Step 2* requires providers to define their goals. Outcomes may cover broad areas encompassing processes and resource utilization, health outcomes, and cost. Once these measures are defined, providers must review historical performance to establish the baseline against which outcomes achieved under the DM program will be compared. Did the process change, were services used more or less frequently, were patients more compliant, did patients recuperate faster or achieve better functionality after treatment, did the cost of treatment decrease?

In *step 3*, providers must question the process of care; for example, what are the most effective means of prevention or treatment, or what drugs are most effective? Has a clinical guideline been created for the condition, and what impact has it had on health care processes and outcomes? Identifying relevant literature requires providers to develop proficiency in using **PubMed** and other search engines. The difficulty in literature searches is not locating information but rather reducing a huge number of references to a relevant and manageable number.

PubMed
a free database that provides access to more than 22 million citations on medical science topics

A three-part PubMed search strategy is effective. The primary search is based on the condition or disease, followed by a second search on disease management or guideline. The third search identifies the intersection of the first two searches, entered as #1 and #2. In the event a search returns too many citations, users can use an advanced search feature to limit either of the first two searches to articles where the desired term appears in the title (or title/abstract). Limiting a search to a term found in the title (or abstract) ensures the user that the term was a primary factor in the retrieved citations rather than an incidental word used in the article.

A PubMed search (http://www.ncbi.nlm.nih.gov/pubmed) for type 2 diabetes produced 94,199 citations (searched March 14, 2013), which is too many to be helpful. To limit a search to the exact phrase, the search topic should be enclosed in quotations marks. For example, "type 2 diabetes" returned 55,458 citations. Next, a search for "disease management" returned 14,877 citations. The ADVANCED SEARCH feature of PubMed can be used to identify the union of the two search terms. For example, entering #6 and #7 (for "type 2 diabetes" and "disease management") in the search shown in Figure 12.6 generated 488 references.

Evaluating 488 references may be undesirable, so users could further limit their search again using ADVANCED SEARCH. The user could limit the search for the condition to articles where the exact phrase occurs in the title (or title/abstract). The user goes to the SEARCH BUILDER field, enters the name of the condition or disease in quotation marks, and switches the field from ALL FIELDS to TITLE. A search of "type 2 diabetes" restricted to TITLE produced 25,214 (less than half those found when ALL FIELDS was the default criterion). Searching for the title restricted to "type 2 diabetes" and "disease management" returned 212 citations. Other advanced functions allow users to limit the search by language, by type of publication (research, review, clinical trial, guideline, etc.), by date (within last five years), by full text availability, and other delimiters.

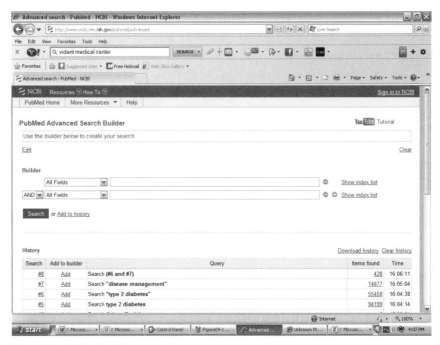

Figure 12.6 PubMed Searching

Step 4 in developing a disease management program is to evaluate and synthesize the evidence obtained in step 3. Is the information valid? Should it and can it be used in delivering patient care? Ellrodt et al. (1997) suggest that studies should be evaluated based on their design, population, intervention, and outcomes. The design of the study determines the extent to which the results can be depended on. The gold standard of research is the randomized controlled trial, in which subjects are divided into experimental and control groups with a single variable altered to assess its effect on outcomes. The study population speaks to whether the intervention will work for the intended patients. Did the study examine patients who volunteered (potential **self-selection bias**)? Were only high-risk or elderly patients studied? The study population may determine the extent to which the outcomes achieved are likely to be realized with the intended patients. For example, a study examining high-risk patients may find improved outcomes or cost savings due to their high use of resources. A similar program applied to a low-risk population may find no change in outcome or cost.

What intervention(s) did the study use? Earlier the CCA's six DM components were introduced. Did the program being evaluated incorporate one or more interventions into the patient care process? Does your organization currently utilize these interventions? If they are currently

self-selection bias
recognizes that subjects who volunteer for research studies may be more motivated to participate and their motivation, more than the intervention, may explain any results produced; differs from selection bias in that in selection bias the researcher errs in how subjects or samples are chosen

in place, then no further improvements can be expected (unless the interventions can be more effectively implemented or operated). Finally, did the study improve outcomes, and were the improvements statistically significant?

Step 5 involves evaluating benefits, harm, and costs. Given the baseline data collected in step 2, providers should be able to specify the changes in outcomes they expect from the intervention. These changes could include improved outcomes, reductions in resources used, higher patient satisfaction, or reduced costs. Any change in process may also produce harm, so where a harm could emanate from an intervention, its impact needs to be recognized and neutralized when possible or minimized when elimination is not possible.

Introduction of new costs related to the program also need to be recognized. Total cost may increase due to the addition of services, and even if total costs are expected to decrease, the distribution of costs and cost savings should be recognized. Assume that DM using outpatient follow-up is expected to reduce LOS and overall costs. However, the program will increase an outpatient department's costs. The transfer of responsibility must be recognized to avoid adding tasks to a department without increasing its resources. Similarly, if functions are being taken away from a department, their resource allocation should also be reassessed to ensure that resources are used effectively and efficiently.

Step 6 is to develop practice policies and pathways. As discussed in Chapter Eleven, practice policies describe treatment and may be rigid (standards) or flexible (options). Pathways provide a detailed accounting of what should be done by whom at what time. Treatment plans should be collaborative, incorporating all involved health care personnel and outlining self-management expectations for patients. Practice policies and pathways cannot address every complexity of medical practice, so issues will arise in which providers will not receive guidance from medical evidence. Thus they will have to rely on pathophysiological rationale, clinical judgment, and local utilization data to guide their decisions (Ellrodt et al. 1997).

Step 7 emphasizes that measurement must be incorporated into the workflow and not be a task added after the fact. Providers need to identify critical process and outcome variables and develop a data capture mechanism. Providers should know what will be measured, how it will be measured, when data collection will occur, and how the information will be used, including who will receive reports, how often, and in what format.

Chapter Fourteen provides a discussion of implementation strategies and approaches, the focus of *step 8*. Implementation requires developing a convincing rationale for change, educating providers on how the treatment process will change and on how success will be determined, providing resources to carry out the desired changes, and demonstrating commitment and resolve to carry through with recommendations. Demonstrating credibility is critical; providers must recognize that changing the delivery process is a serious effort that will be followed to its objective. Without credibility, change will be impossible to achieve.

Just as changing the delivery process must be seen as a serious process, providers should see the change as the starting point for continuous improvement, which is *step 9* of the development process. Providers must continually monitor practice and identify opportunities for improvement. The first set of questions that should be asked address program implementation: Has the program been implemented as intended? Were interventions undertaken, initiated at the correct time, and effectively carried out? If treatment plans are not being followed, providers must determine why actions are not being carried out as intended. The second set of questions should address results: If actions are completed as planned, are the expected results achieved? If expected results are not achieved, why didn't the intervention work as intended? Expectations may have been set too high or may not have been grounded on evidence, or changes in the patient populations may have neutralized or reversed the expected outcomes. If the expected results are achieved, what further improvements can be implemented? Regardless of whether the expected results are achieved, the PDCA cycle always returns to planning to initiate a continuous quality improvement cycle aimed at improving patient outcomes.

Todd and Nash (1997) move beyond the theoretical model of Ellrodt et al. and offer a model congruent with the needs of day-to-day medical practice. They suggest that seven factors are required to enhance the probability of successful implementation of a DM program, as shown in Table 12.4.

Table 12.4 Practice Requirements for Successful Disease Management

1.	Understanding the course of disease
2.	Targeting patients likely to benefit from the intervention
3.	Focusing on prevention and resolution
4.	Increasing patient compliance
5.	Increasing continuity across health care settings
6.	Integrating data management systems
7.	Aligning incentives

Source: WE Todd and D Nash, 1997, *Disease Management—A Systems Approach to Improving Patient Outcomes,* American Hospital Publishing Co., Chicago IL.

These requirements are largely absent from current medical practice. While understanding of disease processes is widespread, the remaining six requirements are often absent and present major challenges to providers. Patient targeting and increasing compliance is often absent. One-size-fits-all treatment approaches are often used without considering whether a patient is receptive. Providers are limited in their ability to demand that patients alter their behaviors and are therefore often hesitant to do so. Focusing on prevention and aligning incentives runs contrary to our predominant reimbursement systems, which pay providers based on tests and procedures and minimize payment for evaluation and management services. Similarly, the fragmentation of health care continues with the proliferation of specialists, HIPAA concerns with patient privacy, and difficulties integrating diverse information systems. Todd and Nash correctly identify the keys to successful DM practice, but achieving these requirements is hindered by the structure and history of medical practice.

Role of Self-Care

A prime component of most DM programs is patient self-management. Levich (2007) notes that all patients self-manage, some successfully, others poorly. Practitioners must recognize the supremacy of patient choice. In discussing type 2 diabetes, Nuovo (2007, 139–201) tackles management of patients and their diabetes. Promoting self-management includes six functions: assessing the patient's readiness for change, providing education and support, coaching, facilitating the development of patient-determined action plans, prescribing of medication, and ongoing monitoring. Education and support include instruction in blood testing and the proper use of medication, explaining required behavioral changes including diet and exercise, describing the social, emotional, and economic consequences of the condition, instruction on the recognition of symptoms in order to avoid complications, and providing sources of information.

A large obstacle to achieving better health outcomes is patient behavior and willingness to change. Levich (2007) recommends **motivational interviewing** to overcome patient resistance. Motivational interviewing begins with empathy; the care giver must be able to place himself or herself in the patient's condition to establish rapport, understand the patient's resistance to change, and move him to an active and positive role in self-care. If a patient continues to resist change, the provider should cultivate **discrepancy**. Discrepancy requires a patient to recognize two mutually exclusive desires. The care giver should elicit from the patient what he wants from his life (good health) and demonstrate how his goal is incompatible with his current behavior (noncompliance with diet and exercise, medication

motivational interviewing
the care giver attempts to place himself or herself in the patient position to establish rapport, understand resistance to change, and move the patient to an active and positive role in self-care

discrepancy
the care giver attempts to make the patient recognize two mutually exclusive desires, typically the incompatibility of short-term behavior and long-term health with the goal of moving the patient to a healthier lifestyle

regime). The hope is that a patient's recognition of the incompatibility of his goals and behavior will lead him to pursue the long-term goal of better health over current behavior.

Care givers should not actively oppose resistance; provider opposition often increases patient resistance and may make individuals less likely to consider changing their behavior. Confronted with resistance, care givers should explore alternatives; a helpful response to patient resistance is: Given that you are unwilling to make a proposed change, have you considered other changes? Levich calls this technique **rolling with resistance**, redirecting a patient's energy away from opposition to searching for alternatives. Finally, the care giver should promote self-efficacy. When patients believe they are in control of their condition, rather than being controlled by the condition or providers, they will be more likely to change.

rolling with resistance the care giver attempts to redirect a patient's energy away from opposition to change to searching for more desirable alternatives

Disease Management Goals

Raney (2003) identifies the five goals of DM as prevention, improving the course of disease, case management for high-risk and high-cost patients, conformance to guidelines, and statistical analysis and adjustment. Avoiding disease is the best case outcome, so high-risk individuals should be identified and their behaviors altered or medication prescribed prior to the onset of disease. DM often is initiated after the onset of disease; the goal at this point is to improve the course of disease. Improving the course of disease means reducing morbidity, complications, mortality, and the need for medical services. High-risk and high-cost patients require an active and participatory treatment model in which they and their care givers are in regular contact and their health status is closely monitored to avoid costly interventions. The fourth goal, ensuring compliance with guidelines, involves assessing whether care is being delivered consistent with known standards that produce optimal outcomes. Closing the loop is measurement and statistical analysis. Results must be monitored to determine whether expected outcomes are being realized and to determine when adjustment is necessary and what adjustments are needed.

General Structure of a Disease Management Program

The structure of a DM program is designed for a specific condition. By necessity, the following discussion provides the essential components of a program but is not representative of any particular program. The structure is based on cardiovascular disorders discussed in *Disease Management for Nurse Practitioners*, (Lippincott Williams and Wilkins 2001).

The DM program is composed of three distinct phases. The first phase defines the condition, the second establishes the treatment plan, and the final phase provides the foundation for patient self-management. This structure targets condition-specific factors and thus differs from the general model of Todd and Nash. This book provides clinical guidance for patients with specific diseases, but issues of continuity across providers, data management, and incentives are not addressed.

The first phase begins with *assessment*: identifying the patient's condition and the available baseline information. The next step is to understand *causes and pathophysiology*. The cause of the condition may emanate from disease, infection, congenital disorder, trauma, or behavior. Pathophysiology is the study of the changes in mechanical, physical, or biochemical functions as a result of the disease. The third step is documenting the *clinical presentation*, including level of pain, respiratory issues, and fatigue. The final step is determining the *differential diagnoses*, that is, the list of potential diagnoses and the final *diagnosis* based on the patient history, clinical presentation, and screening tests.

The second phase encompasses the *management* aspect of DM, including *general* control of contributing factors, *medication* choices, planning *surgery* (including its type and timing when appropriate), establishing the conditions for and making the arrangements for *referral* to specialist and other support services, and establishing *follow-up*, including specifying exams and tests and their timing.

The final phase is *patient self-management.* Self-management includes teaching patients new diet and exercise regimens, instructing them on medication use, and teaching them to identify worsening symptoms or complications, when to take action, and what action to take.

Disease Management Cases

Study 1: Type 2 Diabetes

Lairson et al. (2008) studied the impact of DM on patients with type 2 diabetes. The study was motivated by the findings of two studies that found less than 5% (study 1) or 40% (study 2) of diabetes patients received the care recommended by the American Diabetes Association. The DM program included access to a diabetes educator, patient education classes, reminder letters and phone calls to patients, and monthly reports to physicians. Patients were divided into two groups. The recommended care for the first group, the DM group, was managed with a software package, and the control group received usual care.

Patient compliance was measured based on the percentage of patients completing their recommended HbA1c, urine microalbumin, and lipid panel tests. A composite compliance percentage was compiled based on patients' completing two or more of these tests. Patient use of the certified diabetes educator was also assessed. The only measure to demonstrate a difference between the experimental and control groups was completion of HbA1c tests and this occurred only in two of the four quarters studied.

Outcome changes were assessed based on HbA1c levels achieved, percentage of patients with HbA1c levels greater than 9.5%, mean number of hospital admissions, and number of complications. There was no statistical difference in outcomes between the two groups in any quarter.

Changes in cost were determined by examining office visit costs, inpatient costs, outpatient costs, and the sum of these three measures. Costs for office visits were significantly higher in two of the four quarters examined for the DM group, and total cost was higher in one quarter for DM patients.

The authors concluded that their modest results highlight the difficulty of implementing theoretically attractive programs in actual practice. They suspected that the modest results were due to the lack of dedicated DM personnel, care givers having to juggle demands and not devoting all their efforts to the program, the loss of key personnel early in the program, and difficulty maximizing the use of the DM software.

Study 2: Telemedicine

Smith et al. (2008) studied the impact of using telemedicine to send specialty advice and evidence-based messages to physicians treating patients with diabetes. Their study randomized physicians into an experimental group, who received the tailored advice and messages, and a control group, who received generic information on cardiovascular risk. During the study 70% of patients reviewed were determined to have performance or outcome gaps in their care.

The researchers examined the effects of their telemedicine intervention on care processes, risk-factor control, and cost. In addition they surveyed physicians in the experimental group to determine if the telemedicine messages were useful and if the messages were used to manage their patients. The researchers received a 78% response rate to their usefulness and use questions; 59% of the physicians indicated the messages were useful and 49% reported they were incorporated into patient management.

Process changes were measured using the ADA-NCQA provider score. The results indicated no significant difference in care process between the two groups of physicians. Risk-factor control was assessed using 18 measures. The telemedicine messages were associated with improved risk control for 2 of the 18 factors. Patients treated by physicians receiving the telemedicine messages were 80% more likely to be not smoking or advised to quit and 99% more likely to be taking aspirin regularly. The researchers concluded, "There was no significant difference between the trial arm on the process of care, metabolic and cardiovascular risk-factor control (except for smoking cessation and aspirin use), or the estimated 10-year risk of coronary artery disease" (Smith et al. 2008).

The third outcome measure, cost, showed significant differences between groups. The total cost of care for patients treated by physicians receiving the telemedicine messages was $6,252 per patient. The cost in the control group was $8,564, a savings of $2,311 per DM patient. Outpatient cost was $288 lower in the experimental group versus the control group ($1,842 versus $2,129). The cost savings did not equal the difference between experimental and cost groups due to rounding. The cost difference was attributed to higher utilization of hospitalization for musculoskeletal pain and orthopedic surgery in the control group. Despite the lack of improvement for process and risk-factor control, the lower cost per DM patient may indicate quality improvement, that is, equivalent outcomes at lower cost.

Study 3: Review of Cost Reduction in Chronic Conditions

In a review of the DM literature, de Bruin et al. (2011) focused on the ability of these programs to reduce health care costs for patients with diabetes, depression, heart failure, and COPD. In 21 studies they found 13 concluding cost savings and 4 reporting higher costs. The largest and most consistent savings were found in heart failure and COPD, which the authors concluded was due to the likelihood of these patients with these conditions using expensive, short-term interventions. Problems associated with substandard diabetes and depression care are more likely to manifest over a longer period of time, but DM studies typically do not track costs for more than one year.

The authors conclude based on their review of multiple studies that "although it is widely believed that disease management programs reduce healthcare expenditures, the present study shows that evidence for this claim is still inconclusive" (120). As discussed in this chapter, DM programs have a variety of components, and de Bruin et al. conclude based on their review that it is difficult to determine which services reduce cost, whether there are specific conditions under which cost savings are achieved, the extent to which a program is implemented, and whether the program was fully embraced by patients and providers.

Study 4: CBO Review of Costs and Health Outcomes

A 2004 review of the literature by the Congressional Budget Office (CBO) concluded there was "insufficient evidence to conclude that disease management programs can generally reduce the overall cost of health care services" (1). This review cited work from the *British Medical Journal* to conclude DM's "impact on survival and recurrent infarction, their cost effectiveness, and the optimal mix of components remain uncertain" for congestive heart failure and coronary artery disease. (McAlister et al. 2001, 957). For diabetes care the CBO concluded that DM led to a reduction in HbA1c levels and greater patient compliance, but there was no evidence to conclude better outcomes.

The CBO noted that these studies presented many problems for assessing the potential for cost savings, including self-selected patients. Self-selected patients may be more motivated and compliant, reducing the likelihood that results will be generalizable to less motivated and compliant patients. A second problem is the selection of high-risk and high-cost patients for inclusion; given the high utilization of resources by this class of patients, it is unlikely that similar outcomes or cost savings will be achieved in lower-risk populations. A third problem is that DM studies often failed to include program costs. Studies often report cost savings from lower patient utilization of resources without adding in the costs to put the program into operation. Inclusion of program costs would lower expected program savings. A fourth problem is the potential for higher total expenditures due to longer life; in this case annual costs could be lower, but lifetime costs could increase.

Study 5: Review of Clinical and Economic Outcomes in Chronic Disease

Ofman et al. (2004) provided the most far-ranging literature review by examining not only outcomes, processes, and cost but also quantified the use of various interventions and improvement in patient satisfaction. Of note was their categorization of the different terms used for disease management. They found 14 different terms including patient care team, patient care planning, primary nursing care, case management, critical pathways, primary health care, continuity of patient care, guidelines, practice guidelines, disease management, comprehensive health care, ambulatory care, disease state management, and disease management.

Ofman et al. concluded that for coronary artery disease patients DM programs were effective in reducing nonfatal refractions. At the end of ten years, 29% of DM patients had experienced one or more nonfatal refractions compared to 40% of those who were not part of a DM program—a 27.5% lower rate. Similarly, they found that DM programs were effective in reducing cholesterol levels. More than twice as many of the DM patients, 43% versus 21%, achieved LDL cholesterol goals.

The authors reviewed nine common interventions: patient education, multidisciplinary teams, provider education, provider feedback, patient reminders, provider reminders, patient financial incentives, organization financial incentives, and provider financial incentives. The most frequently used interventions were patient education (used in 79% of the reviewed studies), multidisciplinary teams (57%), and provider education (37%). The least frequently used interventions were patient financial incentives (6%), organization financial incentives (1%), and provider financial incentives (0%).

They found that depression had the highest rate of improvement between treatment and control groups, with 48% (41 of 86 studies) showing improvement, followed by hyperlipidemia (45%), and coronary artery disease (39%). On the other hand, conditions showing the least improvement were back pain (16%), COPD (9%), and chronic pain (8%). The three outcomes showing the greatest improvements were patient satisfaction (71%), followed by patient adherence (47%) and disease control (45%). The least improvement was seen in cost reduction (14%), emergency room visits (11%), and hospitalization (11%). The authors conclude that DM programs were effective but that in many cases the clinical results were modest. The greatest improvements were seen in intermediate outcomes such as satisfaction and adherence. This review, like the previous two, concluded there was little demonstrated cost savings or reduction in the use of health care services.

Outcomes Management

Outcomes management (OM) has been defined as "an ongoing process to measure, monitor, and improve the results from significant investment of resources to provide health care" (Jones et al. 1999, 4). Nash, Coombs, and Leider defined OM as "the establishment of systems and standards for monitoring and measuring the quality of patient care on the basis of specific outcomes for patients' well-being" (1999, 9).

OM comes closest to the idea of evidence-based medicine (EBM) and in its broadest conception encompasses case and disease management. Ellwood (1988) pointed out that one of the problems in health care is that physicians, payers, and administrators have different insights into patients and these insights are not shared. The failure to share information reduces everyone's ability to understand what effect the choices of patients, physicians, and payers have on health care outcomes.

According to Ellwood, OM must use a patient-understood language of outcomes and include a national database containing clinical, financial, and health outcomes that can be accessed by patients, physicians, and payers. Ellwood's vision emphasizes that medicine must rely more heavily on standards and guidelines; variation cannot be controlled if all decision-makers plot their own course. Over the past 100 years voluminous amounts of medical data have been recorded, yet this data has failed to produce systematic change. The data collected was designed to support a single patient encounter or a series of encounters for one patient and was not recorded to make assessments across patients.

Third, a national database is needed, where the experience of millions of admissions and billions of physician visits can be used to determine the best treatments and the relationship between cost and health outcomes. The database should be able to efficiently analyze data and provide relevant information to decision-makers at their point of need. Ellwood (1988) calls this capacity for retrieval and analysis capacity a "clinical trial machine," recognizing that such a system would be able to identify appropriate patient groupings and that the constant update of clinical, financial, and health outcomes data would allow rapid assessment of treatments that deliver superior results.

While Ellwood envisions a national database serving patients, physicians, and payers, attempts at establishing OM have generally been limited to single organizations. Nelson et al. (1998) provide an intuitive overview of the process and link it to the PDCA cycle. The first step in the OM process is to identify an outcome of interest. As we have seen with case and disease management, the outcome of interest may be based on a high volume of cases, high cost, poor outcomes, data availability, a belief that outcomes could be improved, or simple curiosity. The second step is to research the existing literature to identify practical and measurable solutions. The third step is to collect baseline data to establish how the process has been operating. Anecdotal evidence (a single high-profile failure) is often biased and when used as the basis for study should be supplemented with data from similar cases. Is case volume high, or are outcomes regularly failing to meet expectations? Often numeric data will disprove common but unfounded conclusions. Steps 1 through 3 constitute the Plan aspect of the PDCA cycle.

Assuming baseline data indicates a need for change, the fourth step is to improve the process. The challenge is to bring a large group of diversely trained individuals to consensus on what should be done and implement change. The change should be clear, understandable, measurable, and have a causal or probabilistic connection to the desired outcome. Step 4 is the Do in the PDCA cycle.

Steps 5 and 6 constitute the Check function in PDCA. Step 5 requires plotting data, before and after the change is made. Has a significant change occurred in outcomes? Statistics and SPC tell us that change is constant; the question is: Has a variable of interest sufficiently increased or decreased to suggest that something other than day-to-day variation has occurred? If outcomes are significantly better, the care givers need to determine whether the difference is due to the implemented change or another cause. Are the patients in the postimplementation group equivalent to the preimplementation group? If the patients are approximately the same, we may conclude that the change was successful. If the patients are different, Nelson recommends risk-adjusting the data. The goal of risk adjustment, step 6, is to determine whether improved outcomes were due to lower-intensity patients. On the other hand, risk adjustment may indicate improvement if equivalent outcomes are achieved with a sicker population.

Step 7 is ongoing monitoring and continuous improvement, the Act in PDCA and reinitiation of the cycle. Continuous monitoring is required to institutionalize improvements and provide a basis for continuous quality improvement. As SPC and Brent James point out, CQI can occur only in a stable system where one variable is changed at a time to determine if it is effective. Step 7 assumes a health delivery team is operating over a long time horizon during which changes are given sufficient time to demonstrate their effect.

Table 12.5 Developing an Outcomes Management Program

1.	Identify outcome of interest
2.	Develop measure, practical solutions
3.	Collect baseline data (and analyze), small sample
4.	Change the process
5.	Plot data
6.	Account for differences in patients, risk adjustment, stratify, and refine
7.	Make changes while measuring key outcomes

Source: E Nelson et al., 1998, Building Measurement and Data Collection into Medical Practice, *Annals of Internal Medicine* 128 (6): 460.

Berwick and Nolan (1998) recommend a simple model of improvement based on aim, measurement, change, and testing. *Aim* defines the goal and what we want to accomplish. *Measurement* specifies how performance will be assessed or when we will know that improvement has occurred. *Change* specifies how the process will be altered to improve its performance. *Testing*, similar to the PDCA cycle, is a small-scale test to determine whether the change improved performance and achieved the desired goal. From these bare-bones models, Maljanian, Effken, and Kaerhle (2000) added depth, describing how OM should operate and the factors to be measured.

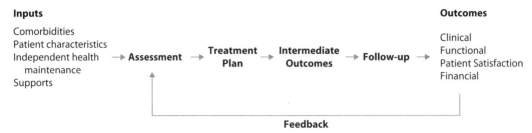

Figure 12.7 Outcomes Management Model

Their model includes clear specification of factors that affect outcomes: patient characteristics (age, gender, weight), comorbidities (depression, CVD, CHF, diabetes), risk factors (symptom control, skin/wound integrity, cognitive ability), and supports (family, community). Similarly, outcomes are clearly stated: clinical (mortality, morbidity, readmission), financial (charges, LOS), patient satisfaction, and functional outcomes (ADL). Between the inputs and outcome there is the initial assessment leading to the development of an appropriate treatment plan and an assessment of intermediate outcomes, to check whether the plan is accomplishing what was expected. Subsequent medical follow-up would be scheduled based on progress. In the study, outcomes were assessed at 3, 6, and 12 months.

Maljanian, Effken, and Kaerhle studied the implementation of their OM model for hip fracture patients and found significant process changes. Nurses were more likely to report they used aggregate patient data to revise the care they provided and to identify subgroups of patients requiring special care. The authors could not attribute any outcome changes to the OM program due to lack of baseline data, and although LOS and billing changes were observed, these changes may have been driven by managed care policy changes.

Patel and Perez (2001) defined their OM program in three steps: establishing a baseline, developing a multifactor intervention program, and monitoring. Their emphasis on intervention warrants attention. Their interventions included treatment algorithms designed for varying degrees of hyperlipidemia, physician education on treatment, newsletters for physicians, and academic detailing for the top statin prescribers. Academic detailing includes a personalized history of their prescribing practices, patient hospitalizations, and costs. The third phase, measurement of results, was scheduled for six months after the beginning of the program. While no assessment was provided, the authors conclude based on their program that outcomes management could improve patient care and be more effective than traditional care.

Outcomes Management Cases

Study 1: Cesarean Section Rates

Peters, Cowley, and Standiford (1999) studied the effect of implementing an OM program on cesarean section rates. They were motivated by the knowledge that their rate of cesarean section, 22%, was higher than the county rate of 19% and by the increased medical risk associated with the procedure. Process changes implemented to reduce the use of C-sections included internal and external cesarean section benchmarks and developing tools to ensure consistency, such as peer review criteria and Bishop scoring. Improving practice consistency was a large component of their work, as preprinted physician orders were already in place, but additional guidance was needed for their application.

The top reasons for C-section were identified as breech, repeat, and disproportion. Six strategies were created to reduce cesarean use. The first was to encourage vaginal birth after C-section through patient education and chart audits. The second strategy addressed breech presentation and the encouragement of external cephalic version. Additional strategies addressed failed induction, failure to progress, physician and staff education, and the establishment of peer review for cases that did not meet criteria. The team produced substantial clinical, financial, and patient satisfaction improvements. Within three years of establishing the program, overall cesarean section rates had fallen from 22.0% to 16.1%, and C-sections for repeats and breeches had fallen from 9.0% to 6.9%. In addition the hospital documented a savings in charges of $334,776 in the first year of the program and $631,072 in the last year.

Study 2: Clinical Pathways in Perinatal Care

Jones et al. (1999) provide a brief history of clinical pathway work in perinatal services beginning with the establishment of standing orders, initial assessment, pain management, patient and staff education, and discharge planning. The next step in practice pattern reform is targeting clinical, operational, service quality, and financial outcomes that move beyond the hospital walls in the fourth trimester.

The authors recognized the main resources required for OM were collaboration, outcome assessment, information systems, clinical practice guidelines, research, and education. They discovered that implementing change was difficult despite their textbook approach. The article is notable as it reports on the second attempt to implement an OM program for newborn care. The first attempt foundered due to physician resistance, an increase in paperwork, and lack of clarity over when actions should be taken. As a result of the initial failure and other organizational changes, a second attempt was made to institute a clinical pathway. The second attempt included reducing paperwork, consolidation of patient information into the pathway, and other changes.

The second attempt identified two areas for improvement: prolonged discharge and poor organization of follow-up home care visits. The causes of prolonged discharge were late receipt of lab results and stabilization after circumcision; both processes were changed to smooth the discharge process. The cause of the poor home care arrangement was attributed to poor information flows, which were corrected by incorporating orders into the pathway. While the program failed to reduce LOS or produce cost savings, it was deemed successful due to its ability to improve collaboration and communication, streamline the discharge process, establish protocols, implement a structure to measure process and outcomes, and reduce the number of forms and documentation time (Jones et al. 1999).

Case Studies Summary

The case studies highlight the difficulty inherent in instituting change. While case, disease, and outcomes management have intuitive appeal, their ability to improve clinical outcomes and lower health care costs has not been proven. I not wish to discourage anyone from attempting to institute one or more of these programs but rather emphasize the difficulty in successfully implementing a program and demonstrating improvement.

When one of these programs is considered, an organization must precisely define what it seeks to achieve and determine the level of improvement that is achievable. Organizations producing superior outcomes (better than average mortality rates or infection rates, shorter than average LOS, etc.) may find improvement to be small, while providers with below average outcomes may be able to achieve substantial improvement. Both types of organizations may be able to improve processes, but only the latter may be able to demonstrate significant outcome improvements. In my view, the process of assessing operations and incorporation of other members of the care delivery team and the patient into treatment planning will produce benefits even if it does not include demonstrably better health outcomes or lower costs.

Summary

The common goal of case, disease, and outcomes management is improved patient outcomes. Subsidiary goals include increasing patient satisfaction, improving communication and teamwork among members of the health care delivery team, educating and empowering patients, and reducing costs. Common processes employed to achieve these goals include assessment, planning, education, implementation, coordination, monitoring, and evaluation.

Case management focuses on particular patients and their conditions that could lead to poor outcomes or high resource utilization. Disease management focuses less on patients and more on health conditions that typically consume large amounts of health care resources. The goal of DM is not tailoring individual care but putting into place guidelines that can be used across patients. Outcomes management emphasizes results rather than process and functions at micro and macro levels. At the micro level OM seeks to modify treatment processes to achieve a particular outcome, and at the macro level it aims to establish a database where patients, physicians, and payers can determine what treatments were applied in the past and the outcomes they produced.

While these three medical practice management tools expand the roles of non-physician providers in the planning and management of care, they should be not viewed as diminishing the role of physicians but rather as assisting physicians in delivering care. Case managers should be viewed as extenders and supplements to physicians; their job is to ensure that procedures are done as expected and to lessen physicians' administrative duties. Reduced administrative burdens will allow physicians to maximize the time they can devote to patients and guiding the delivery system.

KEY TERMS

Discrepancy	PubMed
Fallacy of composition	Rolling with resistance
Motivational interviewing	Self-selection bias

REVIEW QUESTIONS

1. What are the critical activities involved in assessment?

2. What are the chief similarities among case, disease, and outcomes management?

3. What are the chief differences among case, disease, and outcomes management?

4. How successful have case, disease, and outcomes management been?

5. Perform a PubMed search on a medical condition and case, disease, or outcomes management. Describe how the advanced search features enable you to obtain a manageable number of references.

References

Alliotta SL, 2001, Key Functions and Direct Outcomes of Case Management, in *Nursing Case Management: From Essentials to Advanced Practice*, 3rd ed., edited by EL Cohen and TG Cesta, 415–422, Elsevier/Mosby, St. Louis, MO.

Benson, LM, Bowes J, Cheesebro K, Stasa C, Horst T, Blyskal S, Hoenig NM, Wolf M, Hanson C, Bangel L, Bergman K, Cyphers NK, and Duncan P, 2001, Using Variance Tracking to Improve Outcomes and Reduce Costs, *Dimensions of Critical Care Nursing* 20 (2): 34–42.

Bernet V, Shumway NM, and Bunin JL, 2006, Case Management Study: Walter Reed Army Medical Center, A 37-year-old Soldier with Right Flank Pain, *Military Medicine* 171 (7): 684–686.

Berwick DM, and Nolan TW, 1998, Physicians as Leaders in Improving Health Care: A New Series in Annals of Internal Medicine, *Annals of Internal Medicine* 128 (4): 289–292.

Boyer CG, 1999, Case Management for Patients with Rheumatoid Arthritis, *The Case Manager* 10 (4): 65–73.

CCA (Care Continuum Alliance), 2011, http://www.carecontinuum.org/dm_definition.asp, accessed June 21, 2011.

Cohen EL and Cesta TG, 2001, *Nursing Case Management: From Essentials to Advanced Practice*, 3rd ed., Elsevier/Mosby, St. Louis, MO.

CBO (Congressional Budget Office), 2004, An Analysis of the Literature on Disease Management Programs, October 13, 2004.

De Bruin SR, Heijink R, Lemmens LC, Struijs JN, Baan CA, 2011, Impact of Disease Management Programs on Healthcare Expenditures for Patients with Diabetes, Depression, Heart Failure or Chronic Obstructive Pulmonary Disease: A Systematic Review of the Literature, *Health Policy* 101 (2): 105–21, doi: 10.1016/j.healthpol.2011.03.006.

Doxtator R and Rodriquez DE, 1998, Evaluating Costs, Benefits, and Return on Investment for Disease Management Programs, *Disease Management* 1 (4): 185–192.

Druss BG, Marcus SC, Olfson M, and Pincus HA, 2002, The Most Expensive Medical Conditions in America, *Health Affairs* 21 (4): 105–111.

Ellrodt G, Cook DJ, Lee J, Cho M, Hunt D, and Weingarten S, 1997, Evidence-based Disease Management, *JAMA* 278 (20): 1687–1692.

Ellwood P, 1988, Shattuck Lecture: Outcomes Management, *New England Journal of Medicine* 318 (23): 1549–1556.

Foster, AP, 2003, Quality Management for Case Managers, in *Case Management in Healthcare: A Practical Guide*, edited by P Rossi, 734–749, W. B. Saunders, Philadelphia, PA.

Gallagher LP and Truglio-Londrigan M, 2004, Using the "Seven A's" Assessment Tool for Developing Competency in Case Management, *Journal of the New York State Nurses Association* (Spring/Summer 2004): 27–31.

Gattis WA, Hasselblad V, and Whellan DJ, 1999, Reduction in Heart Failure Events by the Addition of a Clinical Pharmacist to the Heart Failure Management Team, *Archives of Internal Medicine,* 159 (16), 1939–1945.

Girard N, 1994, The Case Management Model of Patient Care Delivery. *AORN Journal* 60 (3): 403–415.

Handley M and Stanton M, 2006, Evidence-Based Case Management in a High-Risk Pregnancy, *Lippincott's Case Management* 11 (5): 240–246.

Jones ML, Day S, Creely J, Woodland M, and Gerdes J, 1999, Implementation of a Clinical Pathway System in Maternal Newborn Care: A Comprehensive Documentation System for Outcomes Management, *Journal of Perinatal and Neonatal Nursing* 13 (3): 1–20.

Kurtz, E, Cookson, J, and Mattie, L, 2008, LOS Management: The Path to Efficiency, *Healthcare Financial Management* 62 (11): 98–102.

Lairson DR, Yoon SJ, Carter PM, Greisinger AJ, Talluri KC, Aggarwal M, and Wehmanen O, 2008, Economic Evaluation of an Intensified Disease Management System for Patients with Type 2 Diabetes, *Disease Management* 11 (2): 79–94.

Levich BR, 2007, Self-Management in Chronic Illness, in *Chronic Disease Management,* edited by J Nuovo, 9–31, Springer, New York, NY.

Lippincott Williams and Wilkins, 2002, *Disease Management for Nurse Practitioners,* Lippincott Williams and Wilkins—Springhouse Division, Springhouse, PA.

Maljanian R, Effken J, and Kaerhle P, 2000, Design and Implementation of an Outcomes Management Model, *Outcomes Management for Nursing Practice* 4 (1): 19–26.

McAlister FA, Lawson FM, Teo KK, and Armstrong PW, 2001, Randomised Trials of Secondary Prevention Programmes in Coronary Heart Disease: Systematic Review, *BMJ* 323 (7319): 957–962.

McGlynn EA, Asch SM, Adams J, Keesey J, Hicks J, DeCristofano A, and Kerr EA, 2003, The Quality of Health Care Delivered to Adults in the United States, *New England Journal of Medicine,* 348 (26): 2635–2645.

Michael C and Cohen, EL, 2005, Two Strategies for Managing Care: Care Management and Case Management, in *Nursing Case Management: From Essentials to Advanced Practice,* 4th ed., edited by EL Cohen and TG Cesta, 33–37, Elsevier/Mosby, St. Louis, MO.

Nash DB, Coombs JB, and Leider H, 1999, Pre-Course Reading for: The Three Faces of Quality, American College of Physician Executives, Amelia Island, FL.

Nelson E, Splaine M, Batalden P, and Plume S, 1998, Building Measurement and Data Collection into Medical Practice, *Annals of Internal Medicine* 128 (6): 460–466.

Nuovo J, 2007, *Chronic Disease Management,* Springer, New York, NY.

Ofman J, Badamgarav E, Henning J, Knight K, Gano A, Levan R, Gur-Aire S, Richards M, Hasselblad V, and Weingarten S, 2004, Does Disease

Management Improve Clinical and Economic Outcomes in Patients with Chronic Diseases? *American Journal of Medicine* 117 (3): 182–192.

Olin GL and Rhoades JA, 2005, The Five Most Costly Medical Conditions, 1997 and 2002: Estimates for the U.S. Civilian Noninstitutionalized Population. *Statistical Brief* #80. Agency for Healthcare Research and Quality, Rockville, MD. http://www.meps.ahrq.gov/mepsweb/data_files/publications/st80/stat80.pdf, accessed June 8, 2013.

Patel B and Perez, HE, 2001, A Means to an End: An Overview of a Hyperlipidemia Outcomes Management Program, *American Journal of Medicine* 110 (6A): 12s-16s.

Peters C, Cowley M, and Standiford L, 1999, The Process of Outcomes Management in an Acute Care Facility, *Nursing Administration Quarterly* 24 (1): 75–89.

Raney G, 2003, Disease Management, in *Case Management in Healthcare: A Practical Guide*, edited by P Rossi, 511–523, W. B. Saunders, Philadelphia, PA.

Rossi P, 2003, *Case Management in Health Care*, 2nd ed., Saunders, Philadelphia, PA.

Smith SA, Shah ND, Bryant SC, Christianson TJ, Bjornsen SS, Giesler PD, Krause K, Erwin PJ, and Montori VM, 2008, Chronic Care Model and Shared Care in Diabetes: Randomized Trial of an Electronic Decision Support System, *Mayo Clinic Proceedings* 83 (7): 747–57.

Todd WE and Nash D, 1997, *Disease Management—A Systems Approach to Improving Patient Outcomes*, American Hospital Publishing Co., Chicago, IL.

Yamamoto L and Lucey C, 2005, Case Management "Within the Walls": A Glimpse into the Future, *Critical Care Nursing Quarterly* 28 (2): 162–178.

CHAPTER 13

PROFILING, ECONOMIC CREDENTIALING, AND RISK ADJUSTMENT

Introduction

Medicine has historically operated as an activity built on strong interpersonal relationships founded on trust. The physician-patient relationship and the assumption of trust have been diminished by rapid changes in society, including increasing mobility of patients, the emergence of health care as an industry, increasing patient expectations, and expanding information outlets. These changes have fractured long-term care relationships and stimulated the discussion of whether patients and society are receiving value for their health care dollars. Expanding information sources amplify the effect of isolated health care failures and often lead to unwarranted and uninformed conclusions about the effectiveness of the overall system.

No doubt health care providers are responsible for the often skewed perceptions the public and lawmakers have of the performance of their industry. Health care has achieved dazzling successes yet has never been required to systematically justify its performance. Health care information continues to be unorganized, unstandardized, and inaccessible, rendering it impossible for providers, patients, and lawmakers to compare providers and treatments, identify outliers, and make sound policy. In 1999 Marshall titled an editorial "Time to Go Public on Performance?" The answer to that question is emphatically yes. Patients, payers, and the public have the right to know before treatment is started what the probability of success is. But the devil is in the details. This chapter explores the details: What has been learned

LEARNING OBJECTIVES

1. Understand the goal, structure, and effects of physician profiling

2. Understand the goal, structure, and effects of academic detailing

3. Understand the goals and challenges of economic credentialing

4. Incorporate risk adjustment into comparisons of treatments and providers

5. Explain the structure of the Medicare MS-DRG system

6. Explain the factors other than treatment that affect health outcomes

from preliminary attempts to report medical performance, and what are the challenges moving forward?

In the early twentieth century Ernest Codman annually published patient outcomes one year after their discharge from his End Result Hospital. The idea did not capture the imagination of the medical community, and public reporting of patient outcomes languished. The idea came to prominence again in 1989, when the state of New York began collecting, analyzing, and reporting mortality rates for coronary artery bypass graft surgery (CABG).

The state of New York believed that public reporting of results would allow patients to make better choices when selecting a provider and encourage providers to improve their outcomes. Assessing outcomes on the basis of raw mortality rates always draws the criticism that rates are not comparable due to differences in the underlying patient populations. Physicians or institutions with high mortality rates insist that their patients are sicker than average, and therefore poorer outcomes do not reflect differences in performance but rather the lower probability of survival for their patients. Aristotle noted that "the worst form of inequality is to try to make unequal things equal"; his observation stands as a warning against simple and unwarranted comparisons.

The New York study anticipated that providers with higher mortality rates would argue their patients were sicker than other providers and attempted to identify preoperative risk factors and calculate a predicted mortality rate based on these underlying medical factors. Forty-two factors were incorporated into their risk adjustment model. The publicly released report did not simply rank institutions from lowest (best) to highest (worst) mortality rate but rather based rankings on hospitals' actual outcomes compared against their expected, risk-adjusted performance. The department of health issued annual reports on hospital performance, including number of cases, crude mortality rates, and risk-adjusted rates, and identified hospitals whose risk-adjusted mortality rates were significantly higher or lower than expected. The department initially refused to issue reports identifying individual physicians but finally released this information after losing a freedom of information lawsuit filed by the newspaper *Newsday*.

It appears that New York reaped large benefits from the public release of data. From 1989 through 1992 the volume of CABGs in New York increased by 30.6%, and the expected mortality rate increased from 2.62% to 3.57%, an increase of 36.3%. While the expected number of deaths was increasing, actual mortality rates fell, suggesting improved performance. The risk-adjusted mortality rate fell from 4.17% in 1989 to 2.45% in 1992, a reduction of 41.2%, shown in Table 13.1.

Table 13.1 CABG Mortality Rates in New York

	1989	1990	1991	1992
Volume	12,269	13,946	14,944	16,028
Actual Mortality Rate	3.52%	3.14%	3.08%	2.78%
Expected Mortality Rate	2.62%	2.97%	3.16%	3.54%
Risk-adjusted Mortality Rate	4.17%	3.28%	3.03%	2.45%

Source: EL Hannan et al., 1994, Improving the Outcomes of Coronary Artery Bypass Surgery in New York State, *JAMA* 271 (10): 761–766.

In the first two years of the program, actual mortality rates exceeded the expected rate; however, to improve comparability risk, adjusted rates should be used. Risk-adjusted rates are used for comparison with expected rates because they recognize high-risk patients should have higher mortality rates and thus providers treating high-risk patients may have higher actual mortality rates than those serving low-risk patients and yet providing superior care. In 1989 the risk-adjusted mortality rate was 4.17% versus a 2.62% expected rate, demonstrating that patient outcomes were less than expected. In the third and fourth years the results were reversed: risk-adjusted mortality rates were lower than expected. In the fourth year, the risk-adjusted mortality rate was 2.45% versus an expected rate of 3.54%.

Widespread improvements were seen across hospitals, with 27 of 30 hospitals achieving lower risk-adjusted mortality rates and the number of hospitals with mortality rates significantly greater than the expected rate declining from five in 1989 to one in 1992. While the improvement in performance cannot be definitively attributed to the release of performance data, it is undeniable that public reporting of outcomes precipitated changes in CABG programs.

One hospital began to identify patients at risk for poor outcomes. Discovering that these patients were often admitted through the ER, the hospital altered its processes to improve patient stability prior to surgery. Other programs began to refer high-risk patients to physicians with superior outcomes, reduce the number of physicians with small caseloads, withhold surgical privileges from physicians with persistently poor outcomes, and replace chiefs of service and reorganize programs (Hannan et al. 1994).

The release of physician information drew fierce resistance from some physicians, who suggested hospitals should refuse to provide information that would allow individual physicians to be identified. Some of the resistance was an understandable concern with the accuracy of data and the validity of risk adjustment, but other resistance was simply aversion to attempts to increase accountability and reduce professional authority.

Public release of performance data threatens the power delegated to physicians to regulate medical practice. Echoing the resistance encountered by Florence Nightingale, many commentators implied that patients could be placed at risk if physicians attempt to game the system by refusing to accept high-risk patients or by sending them out of state for treatment. While no evidence exists to document patient shifting, it remains a commonly voiced response to attempts to establish public reporting systems.

Physician Profiling and Report Cards

report cards

a set of measures and benchmarks to evaluate physician performance; another term for a physician profile

Attempts to measure the performance of medical providers have expanded greatly since 1992. The growth in managed care programs during the 1990s gave rise to physician profiling, or **report cards**, where a third-party payer (with access to thousands of patient claims) could compare the use of medical services for their subscribers and provide reports to doctors documenting their performance against comparable physicians. One of the potential benefits of physician profiles was the ability to discard intrusive utilization reviews performed on a case-by-case basis with an aggregated measure of performance. Physicians would not have to concern themselves with justifying a single outlier case and would be subject to review only for a series of cases that failed to meet quality standards or that indicated excessive resource use.

The goal of physician profiles is to identify a set of measures and benchmarks that provide a valid and reliable indicator of performance. The uses to which the profiles could be applied include assisting patients with provider selection by increasing patient access to information on resource use and outcomes, reducing practice variation by identifying practice patterns inconsistent with quality guidelines or substantially different from care delivered by similar providers and disseminating this information to physicians, and reducing unnecessary resource usage and cost.

The issue of variation has been widely researched by Wennberg (see Chapter Two) and others who documented wide differences in utilization of medical services between relatively homogenous geographic areas. Selecting an appropriate referent is essential when assessing the performance of physicians; for example, should the processes and outcomes of specialists be evaluated against those of generalists? When pursuing quality improvement, the answer should be yes; all patients should receive the best care regardless of which physician they seek treatment from. On the other hand, specialists and generalists are significantly different in terms of their medical training and in the patients they treat and may not be capable of producing equivalent outcomes.

Krein et al. (2002) examined the question of the drivers of variation: Is variation due to the physician, or does it arise from the provider group in which physicians work or from the facility at which they practice? They studied diabetes patients treated in VA facilities to determine the effect of the facility, the physician practice group, and the individual doctor on **process measures**, intermediate outcomes, and resource use. The authors found moderate physician-level effects that explained 8% to 10% of the variance in ordering HbA1c, LDL, and lipid profile tests, but the prime differences in resource use and intermediate outcomes occurred at the facility level. There were not large differences in the way treatment was delivered within a facility, but there were large differences between facilities. Physicians within a facility tend to treat patients similarly and thus quality improvement efforts should be aimed at minimizing facility-level (versus physician-level) variation. Their findings echo the earlier conclusions of Wennberg and his colleagues, who identified practice style (physicians tending to practice medicine similar to the peers they interact with) and medical training as the primary determinants of procedure use.

process measures assessment of the degree to which providers deliver care that has been demonstrated to produce desired outcomes

Developing a Practice Profile

The first step in developing a physician profile is to determine the measures that affect the health condition one wishes to improve. The measures selected will depend heavily on the medical condition or group of providers one seeks to profile. As stated earlier, the primary foci are: what should take place (that is, the care process), what outcomes are desired, and what resources should be consumed. When studying diabetes care, Krein et al. (2002) identified process, intermediate outcomes, and **resource use measures**. The process measures included the ordering rate for three lab tests. Intermediate outcomes examined five test results, including HbA1c and LDL levels and whether they were within recommended values, and resource use measured the cost of care in four areas. Their use of twelve measures is notable; those who create profiles must be sensitive to potential users and not overwhelm them with information.

resource use measures assessment of the amount of inputs consumed to treat a patient

Table 13.2 Implementing a Practice Profile

Step 1	Select measures and establish performance thresholds
Step 2	Collect data: who, where, when, and how
Step 3	Analyze data and identify outliers
Step 4	Communicate

Miller and Saigal (2009) evaluated care given to VA patients with prostate cancer using Donabedian's structure-process-outcome model. Four structural factors were measured, including number of patients and board certification. Seven process factors were monitored, including **severity** and functional assessments, blood loss, and follow-up. The outcomes measures were presence of PSA after surgery, patient assessment of urinary, sexual, and bowel function, and patient satisfaction—16 measures in total.

Once the essential variables are identified, how they will be measured must be defined. For process measures, the measure is typically the rate at which a physician's patients complete recommended tests. **Outcome measures** are more complex as they often record not only the results of tests but evaluate the results against a standard to judge the effectiveness of medical management. For example, what level of blood pressure, LDL, or HbA1c constitutes ineffective management of hypertension, cholesterol, or diabetes? Does an HbA1c level greater than 9.0 indicate ineffective management, or should a higher or lower value be used? The threshold is important as the desired outcome is a measure of the percentage (rate) of patients with ineffective management. Providers who measure the number of patients with a HbA1c greater than 9.0 will have a significantly higher rate of nonconformance than providers using a threshold of 9.5. Developers of thresholds must consider medical evidence and what benchmarks are available when selecting clinical outcome thresholds. Resource and cost measures are generally easy to measure as they usually record monetary amounts.

Step 2 requires the collection of data: Where will the information for the measures identified in step 1 be located, and who will collect it? There are three primary data sources: administration or billing systems, medical record systems, or provider or patient reporting. The administrative or billing systems typically provide data on the use of resources and process type information. The standardization of charge codes and well-defined and long-established information systems make the data collection easy and inexpensive. Data on treatment cost is generally limited; most administrative systems provide reliable information on charges, but the relationship between cost and charge is tenuous due to a history of setting charges to maximize income rather than to reflect the underlying cost of treatment.

Data on medical outcomes such as test results typically must be drawn from the medical record system. Final outcome determination, such as response to treatment, is typically a time-intensive and expensive process requiring individual record review. The question of when data will be collected must be addressed; should the earliest, latest, best, or worst measure be used when multiple measurements are available? As with outcome thresholds, developers of profiles must be sensitive to existing practices and

---

severity

assesses the contribution to risk due to the patient's overall state including individual characteristics and the sum of her medical conditions

outcome measures

assessment of the degree to which desired outcomes are achieved

structure the profile to maximize its generalizability. Questions of legibility, multiple terms used to describe the same phenomena, different record recording processes, and oversight make data collection highly subject to error.

Finally, issues of posttreatment functionality (30-day, 60-day, one-year follow-up) and patient satisfaction require the creation of additional data collection systems since these measures are not typically captured in administrative or medical record systems. Posttreatment data is highly susceptible to failure of the respondents to reply or complete all the required fields. The patient satisfaction literature also indicates that patient assessments of their satisfaction may be more influenced by nonclinical factors (bedside manner of care givers, food service, etc.) than medical treatment. A large challenge facing those attempting to create physician profiles is to combine information from various data sources.

After collecting data, the analyst must put it into a usable from. The goal is to create a report that compares similar things, apples to apples. A report comparing apples to oranges will be neither useful nor a good use of data or time. One of the first issues the analyst must consider is whether raw or risk-adjusted numbers should be reported. The argument for raw numbers is that they have not been altered and let the audience make their own judgments. The counterargument is that reports should consider differences in patient risk factors and adjust accordingly. The second issue is establishing comparison groups: Should all physicians be compared, or should physicians be divided by specialty and location? The analyst must recognize the need for transparency in risk adjustment so everyone can evaluate the soundness of the methodology. I suggest that reports should include both raw and risk-adjusted numbers and compare physicians against all other physicians as well as against subgroups.

The last step is to communicate the findings to users. The reports should clearly identify outliers and emphasize goals. As mentioned before, outliers are outcomes that substantially differ from average performance, and the presence of a single outlier in a small group can significantly alter a comparison between providers. On the other hand, there is little to be gained by focusing on small differences, because small differences in performance between providers is expected and should not be the basis for recommending practice changes. Reports should be a single page to avoid information overload. O'Connell, Henry, and Tomlins (1999) state that **effective feedback** must be an active and repeated process that offers clear alternatives to current practice, is part of a larger strategy to change behavior, provides information close to the time at which decisions are made, and is delivered by a credible and respected authority.

effective feedback
a communication tool to alter behavior by providing information on alternative actions at the point decisions are made delivered by credible authorities

Jamtvedt et al. (2006) in examining the effect of audit and feedback on behavior note that the effect is likely to be greater when the feedback intensity is high. The intensity of feedback is determined by the recipient, format, source, frequency, duration, and content. The authors conclude that feedback is more effective when the recipient receives it close to the time decisions are made and when the recipient's performance is substantially different from the desired performance. Overall, they conclude that audit and feedback have modest effects.

Glabman (2005) reported on a hospital-generated profiling system that was developed to understand the performance of its physicians to proactively respond to any data that might be forthcoming from external agencies. The hospital system also sought to standardize practice and shorten the time needed to incorporate medical advances into medical treatment. The profile created incorporated quality (adherence to treatment guidelines and recommendations), clinical effectiveness (mortality, LOS), and finance (cost per admission, denials).

The profile, shown in Figure 13.1, compares individual physicians against other members of their specialty and the overall hospital and provides threshold and target performance levels. The report is easy to interpret, displaying the number of conforming events (Num) and total events (Denom) and tracks year-to-year progress. The profiled physician is exceeding targets on five quality measures, meeting target on two others, and was not evaluated on three others. In terms of clinical effectiveness, she is exceeding target performance for ALOS for DRG 194, the highest volume DRG, and meeting targets for mortality, overall ALOS, and Medicare ALOS. Her financial performance exceeds the target for denied days and Lab/CT ratio and meets target on direct cost per admission.

The hospital system uses the profile to identify outliers defined as the lowest performing 10%. The lowest 10% are called in to discuss their results and to elicit from the physician their concerns. The reports are not used to put doctors on the spot, and the report is distributed only to the physician, his or her department chair, and the medical staff office; a fourth copy is filed. The system intends to add measures of patient satisfaction and readmissions to future reports.

A drawback of profiles is that they must be limited to a small number of measures to avoid data overload, generally a single page to encourage providers to study the information. Due to this self-imposed limitation, profiles may be more applicable to practices that provide a limited number of services and are procedure oriented.

The use of profiles elicits charged debate. Kassirer (1994) suggests that the appropriate uses of profiles are for the physician's own information and

Dr. Jane Doe: Cardiologist

Quality Measures

Quality Measures	Physician Jan-Dec 2004	Physician Num/Denom	Jan-Dec 2003	Num/Denom	Group Jan-Dec 2004	Specialty Jan-Dec 2004	Hospital Jan-Dec 2004	Benchmarks Threshold	Target	Maximum
Indicator Description										
AMI - Aspirin at Arrival	100%	12/12	88%	7/8	97%	93%	88%	95%	98%	99%
AMI - Aspirin at Discharge	100%	2/2	50%	1/2	100%	94%	88%	96%	98%	99%
AMI - ACE Inhibitors for LVSD	n/a	n/a	100%	1/1	n/a	100%	91%	81%	95%	98%
AMI - Beta Blockers at Discharge	100%	2/2	100%	2/2	86%	94%	89%	91%	97%	99%
AMI - Beta Blockers at Arrival	91%	10/11	86%	6/7	93%	85%	93%	91%	95%	98%
HF - LVF Assessment	100%	13/13	100%	17/17	98%	95%	84%	94%	98%	99%
HF - ACE Inhibitors for LVSD	100%	4/4	67%	2/3	100%	88%	96%	85%	93%	97%
SIP - Prophylactic antibiotic received within 1 hours prior to surgical incision	n/a	n/a	n/a	n/a	n/a	n/a	88%	69%	85%	92%
SIP - Prophylactic antibiotic discontinued within 24 hours prior after surgery end time	n/a	n/a	n/a	n/a	n/a	n/a	83%	46%	75%	88%
CPOE	26-50%	1541/4231	26-50%	2702/7866	0-25%	0-25%	0-25%	26-50%	51-75%	79-100%

Clinical Effectiveness

Clinical Effectiveness	Physician Jan-Dec 2004	Physician Num/Denom	Jan-Dec 2003	Num/Denom	Group Jan-Dec 2004	Specialty Jan-Dec 2004	Hospital Jan-Dec 2004	Benchmarks Sev Adj NJ Avg	Sev Adj NJ Top 25th	Sev Adj NJ Top 10th
Indicator Description										
Overall Mortality	3.3%	4/121	5.5%	7/128	3.2%	3.1%	3.6%	4.2%	2.0%	0.8%
All Payer Overall Average Length of Stay	4.53	548/121	4.65	595/128	4.97	4.83	4.67	5.01	4.09	3.44
ALOS for Highest Volume APR-DRG 194 - Heart Failure	5.44	87/16	5.00	100/20	6.00	5.88	6.16	4.22	6.04	5.43
Medicare Overall Average Length of Stay	5.06	349/69	5.01	411/82	5.52	5.38	5.97	5.27	4.26	3.61

Finance

Finance	Physician Jan-Dec 2004	Physician Num/Denom	Jan-Dec 2003	Num/Denom	Group Jan-Dec 2004	Specialty Jan-Dec 2004	Hospital Jan-Dec 2004	Benchmarks Threshold	Target	Maximum
Indicator Description										
Clinical Denials - % of Managed Care Denied Days	3.4%	6/174	19.5%	25/129	5.8%	10.6%	7.3%	6.3%	6.1%	5.9%
LAB-CT Ratio	1.09	12/11	1.70	17/10	1.15	1.41	2.00	1.60	1.50	1.40
Overall Direct Cost per Admission	$2,720	125 cases	$2,519	128 cases	$3,228	$3,225	$3,526			

Legend:
- Below Threshold
- Between Threshold and Target
- Between Target and Maximum
- Meets or Exceeds Maximum

Ocean Medical Center

Figure 13.1 Physician Profile

for the identification of outliers. Limiting use to self-improvement reduces the need for data precision. Inappropriate uses of profiling include basing clinical privileges and recertification on profiles. If profiles will be used for these purposes or publicly distributed, they must meet higher data accuracy standards. The debate revolves around the idea of formative and evaluative use (Weiss and Wagner, 2000). Formative use is for the personal use of a physician to compare his or her practice against others and decide for himself or herself when change is required. Evaluative use refers to the use of the information by others to control the practice of the physician. While formative use should be the overwhelming objective of profiling, there will be times when physicians demonstrating inappropriate variation from practice norms or standards will need the guidance of evaluative use.

Profiling Cases

Balas et al. (1996) in a meta-analysis of twelve studies on physician profiling concluded that peer comparison and feedback had a small effect on patient-physician contacts and that the benefit of the profiling was unlikely to exceed its cost. They raise an interesting point, noting that research often focuses on averages and "anecdotal evidence suggests that high utilizers decrease utilization and low utilizers increase utilization. . . and this [focus] may fail to have a significant impact on the average" (588). Based on their observation, profiling may be achieving two objectives: reducing inappropriately high utilization and increasing care to patients being underserved without changing "average" practice.

The research on the effect of physician profiling and feedback has been mixed. Multiple researchers—Evans, Hwang, and Nagarian (1995), Ross, Johnson, and Castronova (2000), and Noetscher and Morreale (2001)—have attributed length of stay reductions to physician profiling. A study by Zemencuk et al. (2006), documented a statistically significant reduction in length of stay of 0.32 days and one-third of physicians reported that profiles influenced their practice. A second focus of their research was physician perception. Almost half, 45%, of physicians prior to being profiled held a negative view of the practice. After being profiled, those holding a negative view fell to 28%. Before profiling, 34% and 46% believed profiling would cause physicians to discharge patients earlier than normal and to order fewer tests and procedures. After profiling, these percentages fell to 8% and 14%.

Schectman et al. (1995), O'Connell, Henry and Tomlins (1999), and Mainous et al. (2000) found conflicting evidence on the effect of profiling on pharmaceuticals use. Schectman et al. (1995) examined prescribing patterns between physicians who received education only, education and feedback on prescribing patterns, and a control group. They found the experimental groups changed their prescribing habits but there was no difference between the education-only group and the education and feedback group. Their model initially examined academic and nonacademic physicians separately; when these groups were combined, the change in prescribing patterns was significantly different between group model and network physicians.

A study of prescribing patterns in Australia undertaken by O'Connell, Henry, and Tomlins (1999) found that feedback of prescribing rates had no effect on prescribing rates. Mainous et al. (2000) examined antibiotic overuse and concluded that practice profiling had no effect on prescribing patterns based on the increase in antibiotic use between the pre- and postintervention periods. However, they noted that "prescribing in the patient education group and the patient education and feedback group increased at a significantly lower rate than in the control group" (22).

Hofer et al. (1999) studied the effect of physician practice on care for diabetic patients and concluded that physicians accounted for 8% of the variance in inpatient care and 13% in outpatient care after risk-adjusting for age and gender. After adding additional factors to account for socioeconomic status, duration of diabetes, and **health status**, the percentage of variation explained by physician practice fell to 1% for inpatient and 4% for outpatient. The Hofer et al. study suggests that practice profiles may have little effect on practice style given that much of the variance in medical care lies outside the control of doctors.

Greenfield et al. (2002) in studying diabetic care recognized that failure to consider physician-level **clustering** could distort quality evaluations. Clustering is the idea that groups of similar patients will select certain physicians so there will be distinct differences in outcomes unrelated to patient intensity. Drawing on statistical theory, clustering violates the assumption that patients within a practice are statistically independent observations.

The impact of clustering was seen in their findings that processes (compliance with recommended care) and outcomes were significantly better for endocrinologists than generalists. Subsequent analysis demonstrated that there were significant differences in patients between endocrinologists and generalists. Patients of endocrinologists were younger, more educated, had had diabetes longer, and were more likely to be using insulin. When adjustments for case mix and clustering were made, process and outcome differences were insignificant. They concluded that "comparing the quality of care provided by different physicians may be inaccurate if careful attention

health status
assesses the contribution to risk due to the patient's overall state including severity of illness, physical capability, social support, emotional status, and other measures

clustering
a statistical problem where similar patients select certain physicians and thus differences in outcomes may be related to provider choice more than treatment; related to self-selection

is not paid to patient case-mix and physician-level clustering" (115). Given their finding that quality is different, the larger questions remain: Who is responsible, and what can be done to improve care?

Concerns over the Use of Practice Profiles

Kassirer (1994) highlighted many of the problems and concerns physicians have with profiles, including the source of data, potential for incorrect data, general absence of baseline data, no ability to correct for lack of patient compliance, and risk adjustment. An unintended but expected consequence of assessing physicians using profiles is that physicians may change their behavior in undesirable ways to improve their report. One of the most common fears is that physicians may refuse to treat high-risk patients who are more likely to have poor outcomes or who will consume large amounts of resources. A second fear is that physicians could attempt to game the system by overstating disease severity or downplaying physical or psychosocial functioning or health status, to make it appear that patients are more ill than they are (Hofer et al. 1999).

Beside the concerns of physicians, what is the real-world effect of profiles? Do patients access and use information on physicians when choosing a provider? Cristianson et al. (2010) note that the usefulness of physician report cards will be determined by their availability, credibility, and applicability. Availability addresses whether consumers have access to reports. Reports on hospital performance are more numerous than physician reports, as many state hospital associations produce reports while no state physician association produce reports. Health plans produce many reports, but access is often restricted to subscribers. Credibility is determined based on who produces the report and how trustworthy the information is. Cristianson et al. note that health plan information is seen as less credible than information produced by health care associations, yet the majority of reports were produced by health plans—91 out of 161 hospital reports and for 71 out of 103 physician reports. Applicability examines what services are reported and which providers are profiled. Hospital reports include mortality and complications for a small number of conditions, typically heart attack, heart failure, pneumonia, and infection, while physician reports include clinical process measures but do not monitor patient satisfaction, cost, or efficiency measures. Physician reports were generally limited to diabetes and heart disease and were not useful to a majority of patients.

Schneider and Epstein's 1998 study encapsulates the problems facing those who want to see public reporting influence patients' choice of providers. Their study examined the level of information that Pennsylvania CABG patients had prior to surgery. Pennsylvania began releasing reports on CABGs in 1992, and patients who underwent CABG surgery from July 1995 through March 1996 were surveyed; n = 474. The results were disappointing; only 19.6% reported they were aware of the performance data, and only 11.8% were aware of the information prior to surgery. Only 3.8% and 1.5% reported they knew the hospital and physician ratings. Unfortunately, a large number of patients who thought they knew the ratings of their hospital or physician were incorrect, and only four patients, 0.8%, knew the correct rating of their hospital and surgeon and reported that it had a moderate or major effect on their selection of providers.

The preceding discussion presents an interesting picture of physician profiles. Profiling is a tool that could provide systematic reporting of performance and increase information to patients and doctors to enhance provider selection and identify areas for investigation and improvement. On the other hand, profiles have a host of methodological problems which require caution in their use, and it is clear that neither providers nor the general public have embraced their use. Cristianson et al. note that availability is a key issue and the proliferation of information on the Internet may encourage greater use of physician performance data. Profiles will produce the maximum benefit within the health care industry only if providers embrace them and actively utilize the information profiles convey. A potentially promising variation on physician profiling is **academic detailing**, which does not seek a comprehensive measure of performance but focuses on a single medical intervention.

academic detailing
a communication tool aimed at increasing physicians' use of a specific medical intervention that has been demonstrated to produce superior patient outcomes

Academic Detailing

Academic detailing is a more focused type of profiling, while profiling attempts to assess the overall effectiveness and efficiency of a practice; academic detailing generally is concerned with a specific medical intervention. The common focus of academic detailing is processes rather than outcomes, which minimize the impact of factors outside the control of physicians. Academic detailing often is performed as one-on-one educational outreach on a specific medical intervention, such as use of diuretics and beta blockers for hypertension or the use of broad spectrum antibiotics, with the expressed purpose of changing a provider's behavior. In some cases the goal is to increase usage of the target intervention (screening), other times it targets reducing the use of a service (broad spectrum antibiotics), or it may aim to switch a physician from the use of one drug or procedure to another that is more effective, lower cost, or both.

The Academic Detailing Process

The first step in the process is to identify an area of improvement. Is there credible and reliable evidence to support a particular treatment? Curry et al. (2011) identified colorectal cancer screening for academic detailing due to colorectal cancer being the second leading cause of cancer death and estimates that 50% to 60% of deaths could be prevented if individuals over the age of 50 received regular screenings. Despite the evidence on effectiveness, only 61% of targeted individuals receive timely screenings. Compliance was measured as completing one screening in the past year.

Data was collected from four primary care practices in Pennsylvania from February 2008 through January 2009. A sample of 323 patients established baseline performance and demonstrated that 17% had been screened in the last year in the preintervention period and this increased to 35% postintervention.

The third step was to determine how providers compared to the recommended standard. Unlike physician profiling, which often focuses on providers significantly lower and higher than average, academic detailing targets all providers at variance with the recommended standard. Since multiple studies document the underprovision of preventive services, this often results in across-the-board detailing visits.

The fourth step is communication, including crafting the message and selecting the messenger. The messenger must be credible (peer-to-peer is optimal), able to explain the evidence underlying the standard, and able to encourage change. The study provided visits to each practice and covered four areas: screening guidelines, reimbursement and referral issues, counseling patients, and screening alerts and reminders. A sample of 301 patients was reviewed postintervention, showing that overall screening had increased insignificantly, from 56% to 60%. The practice with the lowest screening rates in the preintervention period showed significant improvement, jumping from 21% to 53%, $p < 0.01$. The number of patients screened in the last year increased significantly in all four practices in the postintervention period. A third outcome was that the educational visits highlighted a screening innovation with which the majority of physicians had been unfamiliar prior to the study.

Academic Detailing Cases

Simon et al. (2005) studied hypertension and found rates of diuretic or beta blocker use increased 12.5% to 13.2% in academic detailed practices that received face-to-face visits versus an increase of 6.2% in the control group, who received the information by mail. In the second year of the study, practices in which academic detailing was performed in a group setting had increases similar to the control group, 11.3% versus 10.1%. Providers that received one-on-one academic detailing continued to increase their use of diuretic or beta blockers at substantially higher rates than the control group, 14.7% versus 10.1%. The authors note that their results are similar to other studies that saw the effect of academic detailing diminish after six months and suggest that sustained improvement may require continuous reminders.

Witt et al. (2004) sought to increase the use of inhaled steroids and reduce the use of β2-agonist in children with asthma. A guideline was developed, prescription profiles were created, and visits were arranged between the study authors, who were physicians, and doctors to discuss their practice and the recommended guideline. Control groups were not visited but received mailed information. In the twelve postintervention months, visited groups achieved higher rates of inhaled steroid use in eleven months than the control group, but the difference was insignificant. The authors concluded that academic detailing had no effect on steroid or β2-agonist use and suggest that the result may be due to lack of reinforcement, as only one detailing visit was undertaken between the authors and physicians.

Shaw et al. (2003) wanted to determine if academic detailing could reduce the number of errors occurring while prescribing drugs of addiction. Their intervention included a one-on-one visit, a summary of prescribing requirements, and a follow-up interview; the control group had no intervention. At the end of the study the experimental group saw prescription errors fall from 41% to 24%, while the control group saw their error rate increase from 25% to 28%. This study focused its intervention on an institution with a high error rate; as mentioned before, studies often show greater improvement accrues to organizations that have the largest performance gaps. It is interesting to note that the error rates at the end of study were similar for the experimental and control groups given the higher preintervention rate of error in the experimental group.

Siegel et al. (2003) studied the effect of academic detailing on antihypertensive prescribing patterns. The intervention included one-on-one meetings with a pharmacist who reviewed the physician's prescribing pattern, provided verbal and written information on national treatment recommendations, and discussed barriers to change. The effect of the intervention was measured by the change in prescription rates pre- and postintervention across four types of hypertension. The authors found that recommended beta blocker use increased by 6% to 12% and the sought-after reduction in calcium antagonist use fell from 6% to 11%. All changes were statistically significant.

Solomon et al. (2001) were concerned with the overuse of broad spectrum antibiotics and whether academic detailing could curtail prescriptions. The study divided 17 medical groups into experimental and control groups and created and distributed prescription recommendations. The experimental groups' prescriptions for levofloxacin and ceftazidime were reviewed, and if deemed inappropriate the prescriber would be contacted by the academic detailer, who discussed case-relevant data and the clinical literature. During the baseline period, the experimental groups recorded 8.5 days of unnecessary antibiotic use and the control group averaged 7.6 days. Postintervention, the experimental groups' average fell to 5.5 days while the control group increased to 8.8. The risk of unnecessary antibiotic use fell by a statistically significant 41% in the experimental groups.

These five cases raise a number of issues in how academic detailing is performed: across-the-board intervention versus focus on inappropriate practice, who delivers the guideline and discusses the evidence (pharmacists versus physician), how many visits are undertaken (one, two, or three), and whether education is delivered in a group or individual setting. The studies also demonstrate a wide range of results from no effect to short-term effects. Long-term impacts could not be determined due to the limited amount of time covered in these studies. The takeaway message is that academic detailing can be undertaken in a variety of formats and that program choice may have profound impacts on effectiveness. At this time the literature does not provide definitive evidence on the effectiveness of academic detailing.

Economic Credentialing

Economic credentialing
incorporation of economic criteria including cost of treatment and revenue generated into physician assessment

physician cost profiling
assessment and comparison of physicians based on their use of resources in treating their patients

Economic credentialing and **physician cost profiling** are the terms used to represent the dark side of physician profiling. The terms suggest that the goal is not quality improvement but rather cost reduction. Economic credentialing epitomizes the fears of many health care practitioners that organized medicine is losing control of the field and that physicians and patients will be subjected to treatment decisions made by managers or bureaucrats with minimal knowledge of medicine or the patient. As discussed in physician profiling, some of the opposition arises from simple aversion to oversight. Oversight is necessary and overdue, and it is essential that patients have the right to access more information. But physicians are entitled to accurate assessment, and they should understand the goals of assessment, understand how analysis is performed, and be given access to data when issues arise. Hershey defines economic credentialing as "the practice of applying economic data and

efficiency criteria to hospital medical staff appointment and reappointment decisions" (Hershey 1994, 3). Appointment and reappointment
decisions hit at the heart of the ability of physicians to earn a living and
justifiably raise physicians' concern.

The AMA defines economic credentialing as "the use of economic criteria unrelated to quality of care or professional competency in determining an individual's qualifications for initial or continuing staff membership
or privileges" (AMA 2013, http://www.ama-assn.org/ama/pub/physician-
resources/legal-topics/medical-staff-topics/economic-credentialing.page).
This definition draws the battle line: the AMA will oppose any attempt to
inject non-quality or non-competency factors into any decision affecting
if and how a physician functions with a hospital or health plan. (The AMA
does not oppose competency-based factors for assessing a physician's right
to practice medicine.) On the other hand, AMA Policy E-4.07 recognizes
"the mutual objective of both the governing board and the medical staff is
to improve the quality of care and efficiency of patient care in the hospital"
(AMA 2013, http://www.ama-assn.org/ama/pub/physician-resources/
medical-ethics/code-medical-ethics/opinion407.page). While these two
pronouncements appear to be clear and distinct, in reality, quality and efficiency are integrally related to cost and resource use.

The motivation for economic credentialing is reimbursement. Under
cost and charge reimbursement, hospitals did not have to concern themselves with the economic impact of staff physicians. If excessive resources
were consumed or patients were hospitalized for extended periods of time,
the cost of the resources used would be recouped from the government
or private payers. With the advent of DRG reimbursement for Medicare
patients and the adoption of non-charge-based reimbursement by private
insurers and utilization review to determine whether care was appropriate,
hospitals had an incentive to monitor and evaluate the performance of their
medical staff.

Hospitals not only have the right to consider economic impacts but in
order to ensure continued operation also have a responsibility to monitor
use of resource. Hofer et al. (1999) note that 80% of physician practices that
use capitation reimbursement profile their doctors. The authors also note
that it is highly likely that physician practices engaged in profiling prior to
its adoption by hospitals or health plans.

The growth in proprietary ambulatory surgery centers has created
an additional issue for hospitals. The emergence of physician-owned
ambulatory surgery centers creates a situation in which physicians can
direct high-reimbursement patients to their own practices and send
no-pay or low-reimbursement patients to hospitals. The physicians'

conflict of interest
a situation in which opportunity for personal gain gives rise to behavior that is contrary to professional duty

conflict of interest could deprive hospitals of profitable patients and saddle them with unrecoverable costs.

Economic credentialing raises the issue of what are legitimate and illegitimate economic issues that physicians should and should not be held accountable for. Legitimate issues include treatment decisions, including not following guidelines (unnecessary treatment; inappropriate, excessive, and redundant testing; failure to use indicator lists for diagnostic studies) and the use of resources (use of more expensive devices, refusal to use formularies) (Hershey 1994, 5, 7). Denial of payment is a questionable area; some argue the denial has no effect on the need for care or quality of care delivered. However, failure to follow the procedures required to secure payment is avoidable, and repeated failure to comply may unnecessarily place an institution in jeopardy. Repeated denials is an appropriate objective of profiling: Is the provider advancing or jeopardizing the interest of the organization?

medical staff independence
the ability of physicians to provide the best treatment for their patients without interference from nonmedical personnel

Generally recognized illegitimate issues include payer mix (a high percentage of low- or no-reimbursement patients), low patient volume or revenue, patient dumping, and/or conflict of interest. Prior to the emergence of physician-owned facilities, courts tended to side with physicians on dumping and conflict of interest issues, but with the emergence of physician-owned facilities, which place physicians in direct competition with hospitals, courts are starting to recognize hospital interests in restricting privileges.

exclusive contracts
limitation on the number of parties and individual can trade with

The legal issues involve **medical staff independence**, **exclusive contracts**, conflict of interest, and patient volume. Physicians seeking redress have two legal remedies: **antitrust** and **procedural due process**. Antitrust, typically restraint of trade challenges, have historically met with little success. Procedural due process challenges have met with modest success based on claims that physicians were denied hearings and procedural rights guarantee to them under medical staff bylaws. Procedural challenges have to prove not only that the physician was denied due process but that he or she would prevail on the merits of the case (Hershey 1994, 5).

antitrust
a term to describe a broad range of behavior and practices intended to reduce competitiveness in a market

procedural due process
a defined set of actions designed to regulate conflict between two or more parties and ensure aggrieved parties are given the right to define their case and be judged on its merits

Risk Adjustment

The goal of risk adjustment is to recognize differences in patient populations existing *prior* to treatment that could affect health outcomes. If all other things were equal except treatment, then differences in outcomes could be attributed to the care delivered. When assessing outcomes, we do not want to give praise for superior outcomes or blame for substandard outcomes to treatments or providers if the cause of the outcome is not driven by the care delivered or the skill with which the treatment is rendered. Health care comparisons are complicated by the fact that no two patients are identical; the assumption of "all other things being equal" cannot be made, so comparison must consider the differences that patients introduce into the treatment process.

While the majority of the profiling discussion in this chapter focused on clinical processes and outcomes, appropriate resource use is routinely profiled, and risk adjustment has been used to determine reimbursement to providers based on what they should expend, that is, based on what they produce, rather than on the resources they used. When Medicare moved from cost-based reimbursement to MS-DRG payment for inpatient services, it was faced with the problem of what hospitals are producing and how they should be paid. When the DRG system was created it had 467 categories; the release of the 25th version provides for two levels of comorbidities and complications and has over 900 categories, and has been designated as MS-DRGs. Medicare set payment by estimating how much care should cost, and the first step was to divide medical services into major diagnostic categories (MDC). MDCs divide care by body system, reasoning that treatment for the respiratory system (MDC 4) would be significantly different from treatment for the circulatory system (MDC 5).

After dividing medical care by body system, the second step was to divide treatment within each MDC into medical or surgical care, recognizing that surgery generates higher resource use and cost. The third distinction made was based on the type of surgical or medical service delivered. The fourth adjustment recognized the presence of complications or comorbidities, because patients presenting for care with preexisting conditions or comorbidities will have a higher probability of adverse outcomes and of consuming more resources.

Figure 13.2 diagrams the DRG system for MDC 21—Injuries, Poisoning and Toxic Effects of Drugs. Of particular interest is the DRG number and weight, which indicate how much higher or lower than average a hospital is paid for treating a patient in that category. A DRG weight of 1.00 would indicate average payment. A DRG weight of 5.20 (DRG 901, Wound w/ MCC) indicates the hospital would receive 420% more than the average payment, whereas a weight of 1.22 (DRG 903 Wound w/o CC) would pay a provider 22% more than the average payment. Assume the average reimbursement for a case with a DRG weight of 1.00 is $5,000, a patient classified as DRG 901 would produce a payment of $26,000 to the hospital. Hospitals receive equal amounts for treating similar cases although total reimbursement is adjusted for medical education expenses, disproportionate share, cost of living, and other factors that effect a hospital's operating expenses. The relationship between DRG 901 and 903 is significant; the identification of a major complication or comorbidity (MCC) increased reimbursement over the wound without complications or comorbidities (w/o CC) by 426% (5.20/1.22).

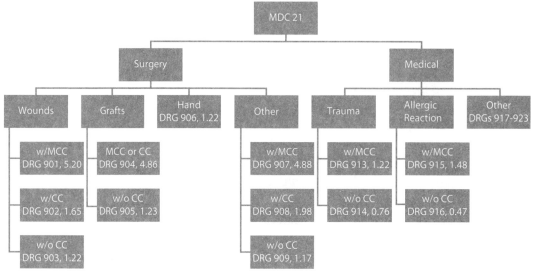

Figure 13.2 Structure of Medicare MS-DRG Reimbursement System

First, the DRG system explicitly recognizes that some types of surgical or medical services are more expensive to treat than others (Wound w/ MCC, 5.20 > Grafts w/MCC or CC, 4.86). Second, surgical care is more expensive to provide than medical care (Wound w/MCC, 5.20 > Trauma w/ MCC, 1.22). Third, the system recognizes that costs change systematically with the level of complications and comorbidities a patient brings into a care episode (Wound w/MCC, 5.20 > Wound w/CC, 1.65 > Wound w/o CC, 1.22). Providers seeking to maximize revenue have an incentive to provide surgical care and to identify complications and comorbidities to increase reimbursement. Inappropriate identification of complications and comorbidities is described as **up-coding** and could result in a Medicare fraud and abuse investigation.

The purpose of risk adjustment within the Medicare MS-DRG system is to establish payment, and consequently it does not incorporate many factors that could affect other outcomes. Medicare primarily covers patients over the age of 65, so there is little need to incorporate age into their reimbursement system, but as the purpose of risk adjustment expands beyond reimbursement and the patient population becomes more heterogeneous, the number of factors must increase.

up-coding

the inappropriate identification of complications and comorbidities that do not affect the cost of providing care but produce higher revenue for a provider

Risk Factors

Iezzoni (2003) notes that risk adjustment starts by obtaining the answers to four questions: the risk of what, over how long, for what population, and for what purpose? *The risk of what* recognizes that there are a multitude of outcomes, both clinical and nonclinical, that should be tracked. The most visible clinical outcome is mortality, but mortality is only one clinical outcome. Risk adjustment must examine the factors that affect other clinical outcomes as well as predicting resource use and patient satisfaction. Iezzoni identifies five clinical outcomes (mortality, **acute clinical stability**, severity/extent of **principal diagnosis** and comorbidities, complications and iatrogenic illness, and **physical functional status**) and three nonclinical outcomes (resource use, satisfaction, and health-related **quality of life**).

Over how long addresses the issue of outcomes changing over time. The mortality rate for bariatric surgery has been reported as 0.5% at discharge but may be as high a 51.0% one year after surgery for men over the age of 75 (Flum et al. 2005, 1906). Flum et al. reinforce the point Codman made in 1916: the effectiveness of care should not be assessed at the point of discharge but rather at a more distant point in time. The goal of medical care is to return patients to their predisease or injury status, so performance should be assessed at 3, 6, or 12 months after treatment.

For what population speaks to the variety of patients treated in a health care system. Health outcomes vary substantially by age, gender, and race and ethnicity. Life expectancy varies dramatically by gender; in 2007 females in the United States had a life expectancy of 80.4 years versus 75.4 for males (*Statistical Abstract of the United States*, 2012). If differences in gender affect outcomes, then the precision with which we can define a population will allow us to make better predictions about "the risk of what over what time period."

For what purpose refers to a primary goal of risk adjustment, which is to make comparisons. Non-risk-adjusted comparisons of the effectiveness of treatments or providers are valid only when the patients being treated are similar. One use of risk adjustment is to encourage providers to treat patients with high probabilities of poor outcomes by explicitly recognizing factors other than treatment that affect outcomes. Providers with older and sicker patients need to know that their performance and the outcomes of their patients will not be compared against a younger and healthier population without adjustment. Similarly, assessments of efficiency and cost should be adjusted to reflect expected resource use for specific populations. When reports are publicly released, they should account for factors outside the providers' control. It is likely a provider with a 2.0% mortality rate may

acute clinical stability
the immediate physiological functioning of the patient measured by vital signs, serum electrolytes, hematology findings, arterial oxygenation, and neurological functioning

principal diagnosis
the reason the patient entered the health care system

physical functional status
assessment of a patient's sensory and motor functions

quality of life
a measure of the value patients place on their health status and quality of life

be producing superior outcomes to another provider whose mortality rate is 1.5% when other factors are considered.

Outcomes are the results of three major types of input factors. The first are the factors a patient brings into treatment. Overlapping in some particulars with Iezzoni's five clinical outcomes, these patient inputs can be divided into five clinical factors (acute clinical stability, severity and extent of comorbidities, the principal diagnosis and its severity and extent, physical functional status, and demographic factors) and four nonclinical factors (health-related quality of life; socioeconomic status; cognitive, psychological, and social functioning; and attitudes and preferences).

The other two major inputs are the choice of treatment and the effectiveness with which it is implemented, and random events. The medical decision-making model and small area variations were introduced in Chapter Two to highlight the fact that many medical conditions have a wide variety of treatment options. A primary goal of risk adjustment is to evaluate the choice of treatment and how it is delivered: What treatment produces the best medical outcomes and uses resources efficiently? How effectively is it delivered? The optimal treatment may not produce the desired outcome if problems arise in communication and coordination or if human or equipment failures arise.

The final input is random events. Random events attempt to recognize the positive or negative outcomes that cannot be attributed to patient factors or treatment. Random chance may explain why one patient has an adverse reaction to a drug when the overwhelming majority of patients receive its therapeutic benefit; for example, severe allergic reaction to the measles, mumps, and rubella vaccine occurs in four patients per million vaccinations (http://www.cdc.gov/vaccines/pubs/vis/downloads/vis-mmrv.pdf). Chance may also explain why some patients recover from illnesses or injuries that are typically fatal.

Figure 13.3 graphically represents the three inputs that affect health outcomes and documents the range of patient factors and health outcomes that should be considered when assessing the effectiveness of treatment. It also hints at the complexity involved in comparing treatments and providers, as treatment is only one of the major factors affecting health care outcomes. Figure 13.3 forces those making comparisons to recognize that if they cannot quantify the effect of patient factors and random events, their conclusion on medical effectiveness may be based on a flimsy foundation. As mentioned earlier, is important to note that multiple factors appear both as patient inputs and as outcomes, which highlights the need to identify these conditions prior to treatment to avoid mischaracterizing a factor as an outcome when it was an input, or as an input when it was the result of treatment.

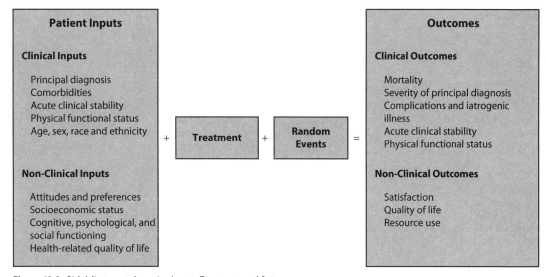

Figure 13.3   Risk Adjustment: Assessing Inputs, Treatment, and Outcomes

Source: L Iezzoni, 1997, *Risk Adjustment for Measuring Healthcare Outcomes*, 2nd ed., Health Administration Press, Chicago, IL, 46.

Clinical Patient Inputs

Two of the earliest measures used to risk-adjust patients were *age* and *gender* as both were easy to observe, readily available, and had intuitive relationships with outcomes. Older patients generally have more health issues and lower recuperative ability than younger people, leading to higher resource use and poorer clinical outcomes. *The Statistical Abstract of the United States* (2012) demonstrates that a 40-year-old in 2007 was expected to live an additional 39.9 years, while a 60-year-old was expected to live only another 22.5 years. The apparent inconsistency is due to the fact that a person born today will be expected to have an average life expectancy, a 60-year-old alive today having already survived childhood diseases and other injuries that could have killed him or her now has a high probability of living longer than average. The lower life expectancy of older people negatively affects the probability of successful medical treatment and should be considered when evaluating treatment.

Similarly, life expectancy varies dramatically between men and women. A 60-year-old woman is expected to live an additional 23.9 years, while a man of the same age is expected to survive and additional 20.9 years.

A third factor is *race and ethnicity. The Statistical Abstract* documents large differences between black and white life expectancy. At birth a white child is expected to live 78.4 years, while a black child is expected to survive 73.6 years. Many studies have documented the differences in prevalence for medical conditions across races and ethnic groups.

Table 13.3 Leading Causes of Death by Race: 2007

White	Deaths	%	Black	Deaths	%	Hispanic	Deaths	%
Diseases of heart	516,883	26.6	Diseases of heart	71,461	24.9	Diseases of heart	28,921	21.7
Malignant neoplasms	455,978	23.4	Malignant neoplasms	62,475	21.8	Malignant neoplasms	26,633	20
Lower respiratory diseases	111,559	5.7	Cerebrovascular diseases	16,882	5.9	Accidents	12,052	9.1
Accidents	108,886	5.6	Accidents	13,684	4.8	Cerebrovascular diseases	7,005	5.3
Cerebrovascular diseases	91,830	4.7	Diabetes mellitus	12,671	4.4	Diabetes mellitus	6,287	4.7
Intentional self-harm (suicide)	64,660	3.3	Assault (homicide)	8,902	3.1	Liver disease and cirrhosis	3,592	2.7
Diabetes mellitus	50,950	2.6	Nephritis or nephrosis	8,334	2.9	Assault (homicide)	3,524	2.6
Nephritis or nephrosis	46,419	2.4	Lower respiratory diseases	7,657	2.7	Lower respiratory diseases	3,310	2.5
Assault (homicide)	33,208	1.7	HIV	6,767	2.4	Influenza and pneumonia	2,966	2.2
HIV	27,952	1.4	Septicemia	6,045	2.1	Perinatal conditions	2,804	2.1
All causes	1,944,617		All causes	286,581		All causes	133,004	

Source: Statistical Abstract of the United States, 2012, http://www.census.gov/compendia/statab/2012/tables/12s0118.pdf.

Table 13.3 highlights the three major races or ethnic groups in the United States have very different causes of death. The top two causes, heart disease and cancer, are the same across all three groups, but the remaining top eight are substantially different. Whites are the only group in which suicide (#6) falls in the top ten causes, while septicemia (#10) falls in the top 10 for blacks and no other group. Hispanics have three causes of death in their top ten that are not shared with blacks or whites: liver disease (#6), influenza and pneumonia (#9), and conditions originating in the perinatal period (#10).

Adjustments for age, gender, and race or ethnicity create a conundrum for risk adjustment: Are these factors the cause of different outcomes, that is, are they risk factors? Or do they indicate different treatment? The question regarding different treatment allows two conclusions: discrimination may be present, or the different treatment may be the result of different patient preferences. The higher life expectancies of the young and of females and whites could indicate that providers deliver more care to these patients, or that older, male, and black patients do not want intense medical interventions, among other possibilities.

These demographic variables present two issues: patient inputs should be recognized in order to avoid attributing poorer clinical outcomes to treatment, and clinical outcomes that are the result of inappropriate treatment, for example, discrimination, should be recognized. If outcomes are different because health care providers are actively limiting care to certain classes of patients, risk adjustment would explain the difference and fail to identify an opportunity to improve care.

On the other hand, if patient preferences are systematically different between classes of patients and no risk adjustment is undertaken, providers treating patients who prefer less intense care and have worse outcomes may be labeled as low-quality providers when they are actually honoring patient preferences. The difficulty in untangling these factors is that they probably reflect all three possibilities: age, gender, and race and ethnicity are a cause of different health outcomes and also reflect differences in patient preferences, and providers might treat each group differently. Preferences and processes may be mutually reinforcing; for example, providers may observe that males typically want to limit their interaction with the health care system and may suggest less frequent follow-up visits for all males. As seen in root cause analysis and statistical process control, identification of variance is only the start of the process. The quality analyst or provider must then determine where, why, and how the variance arose and whether it was appropriate or inappropriate.

Health outcomes vary dramatically based on the **principal diagnosis** and its **severity**. The principal diagnosis is the reason the patient entered the health care system and its impact on mortality rates, resource use, and cost is well established. Not only does the Medicare MS-DRG system not only base reimbursement on diagnosis but the Center for Medicare and Medicaid also provides the geometric mean for LOS for each DRG. For example, patients with heart failure may be treated medically or surgically, including transplantation. Medical treatment for heart failure and shock w/cc is DRG 292 with a weight of 1.03 and a geometric LOS of 3.5 days, while surgical treatment involving the permanent implant of a cardiac pacemaker (DRG 243) carries a weight of 3.06 and LOS of 3.1 days. Obviously, the type of treatment employed will affect health outcomes. Surgery entails more risk than medical care, and treatment should be determined by the severity of disease.

Severity of disease addresses the questions of at what point the disease was identified and treatment was started and whether this will affect outcomes. Among the best known severity systems is the five-stage model used to classify cancer. The National Cancer Institute notes that staging is important to select the appropriate treatment, develop a patient's prognosis, identify appropriate clinical trials for a patient, and facilitate the exchange of information among providers. Five stages are recognized; stage 0 identifies carcinoma that has not spread beyond its original site while stage 4 recognizes a cancer has spread to other organs. Staging considers the site of the primary tumor, the size and number of tumors, lymph node involvement, cell type and tumor grade, and the presence of metastasis (National Cancer Institute). Table 13.4 shows the stage distribution and relative five-year survival rate for kidney cancer (2003–2009).

Table 13.4 Cancer Staging

Stage at Diagnosis	% of Patients	5-Year Relative Survival
Localized (confined to primary site)	63%	91.7%
Regional (spread to regional lymph nodes)	17%	64.2%
Distant (cancer has metastasized)	17%	12.3%
Unknown (unstaged)	3%	33.5%

Source: Stage Distribution and 5-Year Relative Survival by Stage at Diagnosis for 2003–2009, All Races, Both Sexes, SEER.

Table 13.4 shows that the five-year survival rate increases dramatically with early detection and treatment. The outcomes of physicians treating patients with metastasized cancers will not be as good as those of physicians treating patients with localized cancers. The question for risk adjustment is whether the delay in detection was a result of a physician failing to order appropriate screening tests or whether it was due to the failure of a patient to regularly visit a physician or complete screening recommendations?

Comorbidities are diseases other than the principal diagnosis that affect outcomes. In 2000, it was estimated that 64 million Americans had one chronic condition and another 61 million Americans had more than one chronic condition. In total, almost 45% of the population had one or more chronic conditions. Comorbidities produce unstable outcomes and may limit the effectiveness of care and must be considered when comparing treatments and providers.

In the MS-DRG system there are three levels of severity based on secondary diagnosis codes: MCC (Major Complication or Comorbidity) reflecting the highest level of severity; CC (Complication or Comorbidity), the next level of severity; and Non-CC (Non-Complication or Comorbidity) cases which have no secondary diagnoses that will significantly affect severity of illness or resource use. Complications are the direct result of the primary diagnosis, and the challenge to providers is to determine if the complication was the result of the disease or of the treatment.

The MS-DRG system clearly lays out the expected effect of complications and comorbidities on cost of treatment and reimbursement. For example, DRG 299 Peripheral Vascular Disorder w/MCC has a DRG weight of 1.0973 with an expected LOS of 3.7 days. At the next level of severity w/ CC (DRG 300) the weight falls to 0.8596 with an expected LOS of 3.3 days while w/o CC (DRG 301) has a weight of 0.6427 and LOS of 2.5 days. For peripheral vascular disorder, the MS-DRG system expects major complication or comorbidity will increase resource use by 71% over care without complications or comorbidity. This pattern, with similar changes in reimbursement, is seen across the 999 DRG categories.

Acute clinical stability reflects the immediate physiological functioning of the patient measured as vital signs, serum electrolytes, hematology findings, arterial oxygenation, and neurological functioning. Acute clinical stability factors include a relatively small set of measures that are routinely collected and that routinely predict short-term death in gravely ill patients. Iezzoni concludes that "the value of acute physiological parameters in assessing patient risk for imminent clinical outcomes is undisputed"; however their ability to predict a broader set of outcomes, such as resource use, is more uncertain. (Iezzoni 1997, 61–62).

Physical functional status and limitations may arise from congenital or acquired factors; may be permanent or transient, systemic or localized; may involve sensory and motor functions; and may be physical or psychosocial (Iezzoni 1997, 78). The degree of limitation, like severity of the principal diagnosis, can be a prime predictor of medical outcomes. Researchers have documented that patients' ability to walk is a significant predictor of 30-day mortality rates for Medicare beneficiaries treated for pneumonia and congestive heart failure.

Iezzoni also notes that measuring functional status raises several methodological issues, including lack of readily available data, inability to detect changes in functionality, change in results based on the data collection method, the need for disease-specific measures given the inapplicability of generic measures for all medical conditions, the inappropriateness of a single number to represent functionality, and change in results based on whether the physician or the patient performs the assessment (Iezzoni 1997, 84).

Nonclinical Patient Inputs

Health-related quality of life is the measure that attempts to determine the value patients place on their health status and quality of life. This measure is an amalgam of severity of illness, physical functioning, and other factors. The assessment of health status can be used to determine the need for care, guide treatment decisions, and predict outcomes. The value patients place on their health status will affect what they seek from medical care and determine whether the desired outcome is to improve their perception of the quality of their life. Iezzoni notes that "the best predictor of future health status is prior health status" (1997, 92).

Socioeconomic status includes income, occupation, high-risk behavior (smoking, drinking, drug use, sexual behavior) and other factors. Low income may indicate restricted access to health care and poorer health outcomes, or low income may be the result of other factors, such as low educational achievement, that predict lower income and worse health outcomes. The point is we must be careful to recognize whether income is a cause of poor health outcomes or if poor health and low income are the result of other factors.

Occupations have been shown to be correlated with certain illnesses. Workers exposed to airborne contaminants are more likely to have respiratory illness while those employed in high-stress positions may experience higher rates of heart disease and hypertension. Engaging in risky behavior increases the probability of disease or injury and may indicate unwillingness to comply with recommended treatments. Iezzoni notes that compliance rates are especially poor among patients of low socioeconomic status, which in turn limits outcomes (1997, 97). Again, the question arises: Should providers take additional measures to increase compliance, or should they respect the choices made by these patients?

Cognitive, psychological, and social functioning refers to patients' ability to interact with their environment and understand medical information, and assesses their access to social support. After a patient is released from care, adequate cognitive, psychological, and social skills are imperative for those who must undertake self-care or be cared for by others. Multiple studies show that patients living alone have higher mortality rates (Iezzoni 1997, 87).

Attitudes and preferences is a category that includes a distillation of experience, beliefs, goals, health status, quality of life, and understanding of treatment options. Attitudes and preferences affect what the patient seeks from medical care and may predict outcomes. Attitudes and preferences are by definition personal and may distinguish a patient from other patients of similar age, gender, race and ethnicity, and socioeconomic status. As mentioned earlier, compliance rates are lower among members of low socioeconomic status, but we must guard against making the fallacy of composition, assuming that what is true of part of the whole is true for every part of the whole. Determining patient preferences is one of the greatest challenges in medicine. Although most members of a particular group may prefer a certain treatment, not every member will have the same preference. The duty of providers is to determine as accurately as they can what the patient would do if he or she had complete knowledge of his or her medical situation.

Treatment

The patient-physician relation is a principal-agent relationship in which patients recognize their lack of knowledge in medicine and delegate decision-making power to physicians in order to maximize their well-being. A physician acting as a perfect agent should select the treatment the patient would choose if he or she were fully informed in medicine. The physician should understand the patient's preferences but, as stated in Chapter Two, this is a very high and perhaps unachievable standard; patients may not know or be unable to articulate their preferences, and physicians may not have sufficient time to elicit the patient's preferences before treatment must begin.

The other major input to treatment selection is medical science: evidence that supports the efficacy of treatment. One of the goals of practice policies and evidenced-based medicine is to more rapidly incorporate medical advances into medical care, a lag estimated to be 17 years. The hope is that more effective use of currently available knowledge will promote more effective treatment and improve outcomes over those resulting from potentially outdated practices learned in medical school training or from ineffective local practice styles.

Complicating treatment selection is the fact that outcomes are nondeterministic; that is, treatment does not always result in identical outcomes across patients. Drugs that are efficacious for most patients can create life-threatening conditions for a small number of patients. When physicians and patients compare outcomes, it is essential that they recognize the inherent risk of treatment and the possible interactions with comorbidities, age, functional status, and other patient factors. One of the advantages of profiling versus utilization review is its emphasis on average outcomes rather than on single, exceptional events.

Random Events

In Chapter Six natural variation was defined as differences in performance that can be probabilistically predicted. That is, based on past history we know the range of outcomes produced and can determine if an outcome was the result of special cause variation. The definition of special cause variation is central to the idea of random events. SPC reminds us that even after we identify "abnormal" variation, we cannot consider this conclusive evidence of superior or inferior performance; the underlying cause of the variance must be identified before judgment is made.

Regression analysis incorporates an error term to account for unexplained changes in the dependent variable due to omitted variables. Random events in risk adjustment can be seen as unrecognized and unmeasured variables. Developing a complete model of medical care is impossible, but even if it were possible, it would be uneconomical. Identifying all factors that could affect outcomes would be an extremely time-consuming process and would probably defeat the purpose for which it was designed, namely, to identify factors that can be used to improve care. Before hard conclusions are drawn, limitations should be recognized; because unmeasured factors will always be present, quality improvement should focus its efforts on common factors across cases.

Outcomes

Just as patient inputs are multidimensional, the desired and undesired outcomes of these inputs, treatment, and random effects encompass many factors. As detailed earlier, Iezzoni identifies five clinical and three nonclinical outcomes. These outcomes can be seen through the lens of the five Ds introduced in chapter one: death, disability, disease, discomfort, and dissatisfaction. The purpose of risk adjustment is to inform the evaluation of treatment and of providers by identifying outcomes that could be improved. The highest-profile *clinical outcome* is mortality, the first D. Death is an infrequent but not unexpected result of care, and unlike utilization review or root cause analysis, the goal of risk adjustment is to identify providers whose performance over groups of patients and over time is significantly different from that of their peer group. The second D, degree of disability, relates to *physical functional status,* which is aimed at improving the patient's ability to complete everyday activities such as dressing, eating, toileting, walking, and maintaining a home. When improvement in functionality is unachievable, the desired result may be to arrest or slow the decline in a patient's capabilities.

The third D, disease, aims at reducing the *severity of principal diagnosis* or improving *acute clinical stability.* Severity of disease can be reduced through changes in lifestyle, and through treatment, medication, or rehabilitation. Disease assessment can be gauged by identifying significant vital signs and physiological markers and determining whether they have improved.

The unintended effects of treatment are the occurrence of *complications and iatrogenic illness.* The adverse effects may be due to medical error or oversight, or they could be an inevitable result of disease or treatment in which the benefit of care is valued more highly than the known side effects. For example, the failure to identify a medication allergy may not be possible in the first instance, but prescribing the same medicine more than once would be a medical error. On the other hand, a drug with known side effects may be prescribed if the main therapeutic effect is considered more beneficial than the harm that may arise as a side effect.

The fourth and fifth Ds address nonclinical outcomes, discomfort and dissatisfaction. These parallel Iezzoni's categories of *health-related quality of life* and *satisfaction*. While pain management has obvious clinical implications, satisfaction in this case is concerned with how pain affects a patient's perception of his or her quality of life. Given the inherent subjectivity of peoples' attitudes toward quality-of-life issues, there is inconsistency in how it is defined and how it should be measured.

Iezzoni's final outcome is *resource use,* which has clinical and quality implications as well as implications for efficiency, a possible sixth D for dollars. In my opinion, quality and efficiency are inseparable. The primary clinical implications for resource use deal with whether guidelines were followed and whether too many, too few, or inappropriate resources were employed to treat a patient. Given the demands on health care providers to lower costs, it is essential that providers recognize the effects of their decisions on patients and institutions. Patients and institutions have limited resources, and any use of resources that does not create a benefit equal to or greater than the cost of the service undermines the ability of the health care system to maximize health. Waste in one part of the system reduces spending in other parts of the health system or economy. The provider thus must make a judgment call between a potential loss, for example, a lack of preventive care driven by limited funds, and a potential waste, for example, running a test that does not alter a treatment plan or performing a procedure that does not improve outcomes.

A strong point of risk adjustment is the incorporation of multiple factors. Again, however, the fact that several factors are both inputs and outcomes—namely, severity and extent of principal diagnosis, acute clinical stability, physical functional status, and health-related quality of life—highlights the need to assess patients prior to treatment to avoid concluding that the outcomes of treatments are inputs, such as a treatment that has adversely affected functional status being retrospectively labeled a preexisting condition. Likewise, we must avoid concluding that inputs are outcomes; we must recognize, for example, a poor outcome that is a probable result of the severity of the patient's principal diagnosis. Iezzoni's *Risk Adjustment for Measuring Healthcare Outcomes* (2003) provides a comprehensive discussion of risk adjustment and is recommended reading.

Risk Adjustment Systems

This section provides the reader with a brief view into how a risk adjustment system operates. The two systems selected for review are **APACHE II** and the **Charlson Index** score. APACHE II collects twelve routine physiological values, such as hematocrit, WBC, and arterial pH, previous health status, and age to calculate an acute physiology score (APS). The APS can range from 0, lowest risk, to 71, highest risk. The APACHE system estimates the risk of death for ICU patients based on the idea that the severity of disease can be measured by the degree to which a patient's physiological variables vary from normal. Weights are assigned to each variable and increase as the patient's measurements vary in either direction from normal values. The APS is calculated using the worst physiological values recorded in the first 24 hours of admission.

APACHE II
a risk-assessment tool that assesses severity based on how far a patient's physiological values vary from normal

Charlson Index
a risk-assessment tool that assesses severity based on the presence of comorbid conditions

Physiological Variable	+4	+3	+2	+1	0	+1	+2	+3	+4
Temperature	>41°	39–40.9°		38.5–38.9°	36–38.4°	34–35.9°	32–33.9°	30–31.9°	<29.9°
Blood Pressure	>160	130–159	110–129		70–109		50–69		<49
Heart Rate	>180	140–179	110–139		70–109		55–69	40–54	<39
Respiratory Rate	>50	35–49		25–34	12–24	10–11	6–9		<5
8 Other Variables									

Figure 13.4 Scoring the APS in the APACHE II System

Figure 13.4 shows how the APS is scored. A patient with a normal temperature would receive a score of 0 versus scores of 4 for patients with temperature less than 29.9°C or greater than 41°C. The value of the APS is determined by its ability to distinguish different probabilities of death. Knaus et al. (1985) reported a mortality of rate of 1.9% for patients with APS scores of 0–4, compared to 3.9%, more than twice as high, for patients with scores between 5 and 9. At the upper range of the scale, the mortality rate was 73% for patients with scores from 30 to 34 and 84% for those with scores greater than 35.

The goal of APACHE II was to improve treatment of care for critically ill patients and further research by ensuring that control and experimental groups were similar. Physician profiling faces the same difficulty as research: When we compare the outcomes of two physicians, are their patients similar? The structure of APACHE II provides insight to physician comparisons and stands as a warning against superficial evaluation.

The Charlson Index (Charlson et al. 1987) examines 19 comorbid conditions and assigns weights of 1, 2, 3, or 6, based on their observed relationship with one-year mortality in a group of patients. For example, myocardial infarction is assigned a weight of 1.0, severe liver disease a 3.0, and AIDS a 6.0. The resulting comorbidity index is the sum of the weights, and it ranges from 0, lowest risk, to 33, highest risk. When the developed weights were used to predict mortality in a second group of patients, the researchers found that patients with scores of 0 had an 8% chance of death, those with 1.0, 25%, 2.0, 48%, and those with scores of 3.0 or more, 59%. This index is easy to use, can be completed using administrative data, and emphasizes that all comorbid conditions are not equal in their effect on outcomes.

Quach et al. (2009) compared APACHE II and the Charlson Index to determine how well they predicted death in ICU patients. Their conclusion was that APACHE II performed better and that adding the Charlson comorbidities did little to improve the predictive power of the reduced model that used only age, sex, and APS or the full APACHE II model. The different performance between APACHE and Charlson was not surprising since APACHE was developed for ICU patients and Charlson was developed for medical patients. Differences in the target group could require different weights on the comorbidity conditions, and advances in treatment could also indicate Charlson's 1987 weights are no longer appropriate. The authors conclude that the use of the Charlson Index may be beneficial in the absence of other risk adjustment systems.

Risk adjustment highlights the factors that should be recognized when comparing outcomes across treatments or providers. While this discussion of risk adjustment covered only two systems, readers should understand there are multiple systems. Iezzoni identified 17 systems that were created to serve different purposes. Potential users need to identify the appropriate system based on the target population, their goals, and the availability of data.

Summary

The establishment of greater oversight and accountability of health care providers is necessary and inevitable. This chapter highlights the details: any attempt to make comparisons across providers must consider the potential causes of poor outcomes other than the treatment provided. As

Aristotle stated, "The worst form of inequality is to try to make unequal things equal." Demands that all physicians produce identical outcomes ignore the host of issues that render this impossible.

Risk adjustment provides insight into the multitude of clinical and non-clinical inputs that should be considered when comparing providers and forces us to recognize that these factors can be inputs as well as outcomes. In addition to risk adjustment difficulties, comparisons across physicians are often dogged by problems of patient clustering, comanagement of patients, small sample sizes, and limited areas of applicability. These problems present grave challenges even to those seeking comparisons across physicians who treat similar patients for similar conditions. Despite the methodological challenges, the goal of improved health outcomes must drive continued efforts to produce better reports.

This chapter discussed the process and goals of physician profiling, academic detailing, and economic credentialing and demonstrated how these tools were implemented in practice. While providers remain resistant and public use is limited, it is clear that, properly utilized, these tools could be a potent force in reducing variation and improving health care. To overcome resistance and obtain the benefits these tools promise, we must make appropriate comparisons and use the results with care.

KEY TERMS

Academic detailing	Outcome measures
Acute clinical stability	Physical functional status
Antitrust	Physician cost profiling
APACHE II	Principal diagnosis
Charlson index	Procedural due process
Clustering	Process measures
Conflict of interest	Quality of life
Economic credentialing	Report cards
Effective feedback	Resource use measures
Exclusive contracts	Severity
Health status	Up-coding
Medical staff independence	

REVIEW QUESTIONS

1. What types of information should be compiled for a physician profile?

2. What is the difference between a physician profile and academic detailing?

3. What can the developers of physician profiles do to enhance the receptiveness of providers to these tools?

4. What is economic credentialing?

5. What are the goals of risk adjustment?

6. Briefly describe each of the six patient clinical factors that can affect outcomes.

7. Briefly describe the four nonclinical patient factors that can affect outcomes.

References

American Medical Association (AMA), 2013, http://www.ama-assn.org/.

Balas EA, Boren SA, Brown GD, Ewigman BG, Mitchell JA, and Perkoff GT, 1996, Effect of Physician Profiling on Utilization: Meta-analysis of Randomized Clinical Trials, *Journal of General Internal Medicine* 11 (10): 584–590.

Charlson ME, Pompei P, Ales KL, and MacKenzie CR, 1987, A New Method of Classifying Prognostic Comorbidity in Longitudinal Studies: Development and Validation, *Journal of Chronic Diseases* 40 (5): 373–383.

Cristianson J, Volmar KM, Alexander J, Scanlon DP, 2010, A Report Card on Provider Report Cards: Current Status of the Health Care Transparency Movement, *Journal of General Internal Medicine* 25 (11): 1235–1241.

Curry WJ, Lengerich EJ, Kluhsman BC, Graybill MA, Liao JZ, Schaefer EW, Spleen AM, and Dignan MB, 2011, Academic Detailing to Increase Colorectal Cancer Screening by Primary Care Practices in Appalachian Pennsylvania, *BMC Health Services Research* 11: 112 (9 pages).

Evans JH, Hwang Y, and Nagarian N, 1995, Physicians' Response to Length-of-Stay Profiling, *Medical Care* 33 (11): 1106–1119.

Flum DR, Salem L, Elrod JA, Dellinger EP, Cheadle A, and Chan L, 2005, Early Mortality Among Medicare Beneficiaries Undergoing Bariatric Surgical Procedures, *JAMA* 294 (15): 1903–1908.

Glabman M, 2005, Keeping Score: Scorecards, Profiles, and Report Cards Rapidly Expanding to Track Physician Performance, *The Physician Executive* 31 (6): 26–31.

Greenfield S, Kaplan S, Kahn R, Ninomiya J, and Griffith J, 2002, Profiling Care Based on Different Groups of Physicians: Effects of Patient Case-Mix (Bias) and Physician-Level Clustering on Quality Assessment Results, *Annals of Internal Medicine* 136 (2): 111–121.

Hannan EL, Kilburn H Jr, Racz M, Shields E, and Chassin MR, 1994, Improving the Outcomes of Coronary Artery Bypass Surgery in New York State, *JAMA* 271 (10): 761–766.

Hershey N, 1994, Economic Credentialing: A Poor Title for a Legitimate Assessment Concept, *American Journal of Medical Quality* 9 (1): 3–9.

Hofer TP, Hayward RA, Greenfield S, Wagner EH, Kaplan SH, and Manning WG, 1999, The Unreliability of Individual Physician "Report Cards" for Assessing the Costs and Quality of Care of a Chronic Disease, *JAMA* 281 (22): 2098–2105.

Iezzoni, L, 1997, *Risk Adjustment for Measuring Healthcare Outcomes*, 2nd ed., Health Administration Press, Chicago, IL.

Iezzoni, L, 2003, *Risk Adjustment for Measuring Healthcare Outcomes*, 3rd ed., Health Administration Press, Chicago, IL.

Jamtvedt G, Young JM, Kristoffersen DT, O'Brien MA, and Oxman AD, 2006, Does Telling People What They Have Been Doing Change What They Do? A Systematic Review of the Effects of Audit and Feedback, *Quality and Safety in Health Care* 15 (6): 433–436.

Kassirer J, 1994, The Use and Abuse of Practice Profiles, *New England Journal of Medicine* 330 (9): 634–635.

Knaus WA, Draper EA, Wagner DP, and Zimmerman JE, 1985, APACHE II: A Severity of Disease Classification System, *Critical Care Medicine* 13 (10): 818–829.

Krein SL, Hofer TP, Kerr EA, and Hayward RA, 2002, Whom Should We Profile? Examining Diabetes Care Practice Variation among Primary Care Providers, Provider Groups, and Health Care Facilities, *Health Services Research* 37 (5): 1159–1180.

Mainous AG, Hueston WJ, Love MM, Evans ME, and Finger R, 2000, An Evaluation of Statewide Strategies to Reduce Antibiotic Overuse, *Family Medicine* 32 (1): 22–29.

Marshall MN, 1999, Time to Go Public on Performance? *British Journal of General Practice* 49 (446): 691–692.

Miller DC and Saigal CS, 2009, Quality of Care Indicators for Prostate Cancer: Progress toward Consensus, *Urologic Oncology* 27 (4): 427–434.

National Cancer Institute, Cancer Stages, http://www.cancer.gov/cancertopics/factsheet/Detection/staging, accessed June 9, 2013.

Noetscher CM and Morreale GF, 2001, Length of Stay Reduction: Two Innovative Hospital Approaches, *Journal of Nursing Care Quality* 16 (1): 1–14.

O'Connell DL, Henry D, and Tomlins R, 1999, Randomised Controlled Trial of Effect of Feedback on General Practitioners' Prescribing in Australia, *BMJ* 318 (7182): 507–511.

Quach S, Hennessy DA, Faris P, Fong A, Quan H, and Doig C, 2009, A Comparison between the APACHE II and Charlson Index Score for Predicting Hospital Mortality in Critically Ill Patients, *BMC Health Services Research* 9:129, 8 pages.

Ross G, Johnson D, and Castronova F, 2000, Physician Profiling Decreases Inpatient Length of Stay Even with Aggressive Quality Management, *American Journal of Medical Quality* 15 (6): 233–240.

Schectman JM, Kanwal NK, Schroth WS, and Elinsky EG, 1995, The Effect of an Education and Feedback Intervention on Group-Model and Network-Model Health Maintenance Organization Physician Prescribing Behavior, *Medical Care* 33 (2): 139–144.

Schneider EC and Epstein AM, 1998, Use of Public Performance Reports: A Survey of Patients Undergoing Cardiac Surgery, *JAMA* 279 (20): 1638–1642.

SEER (Surveillance Epidemiology and End Results), Stage Distribution and 5-Year Relative Survival by Stage at Diagnosis for 2003–2009, All Races, Both Sexes, http://seer.cancer.gov/statfacts/html/kidrp.html#survival, accessed June 9, 2013.

Shaw J, Harris P, Keogh G, Graudins L, Perks E, and Thomas PS, 2003, Error Reduction: Academic Detailing as a Method to Reduce Incorrect Prescriptions, *European Journal of Clinical Pharmacology* 59 (8–9): 697–969.

Siegel D, Lopez J, Meier J, Goldstein MK, Lee S, Brazill BJ, and Matalka MS, 2003, Academic Detailing to Improve Antihypertensive Prescribing Patterns, *American Journal of Hypertension* 16 (6): 508–511.

Simon SR, Majumdar SR, Prosser LA, Salem-Schatz S, Warner C, Kleinman K, Miroshnik I, and Soumerai SB, 2005, Group versus Individual Academic Detailing to Improve the Use of Antihypertensive Medications in Primary Care: A Cluster-Randomized Controlled Trial, *American Journal of Medicine* 118 (5): 521–528.

Solomon DH, Van Houten L, Glynn RJ, Baden L, Curtis K, Schrager H, and Avorn J, 2001, Academic Detailing to Improve Use of Broad-Spectrum Antibiotics at an Academic Medical Center, *Archives of Internal Medicine* 161 (15): 1897–1902.

Statistical Abstract of the United States, 2012, http://www.census.gov/compendia/statab/.

Weiss KB and Wagner R, 2000, Performance Measurement through Audit, Feedback, and Profiling as Tools for Improving Clinical Care, *Chest* 118 (2 Suppl): 53s–58s.

Witt K, Knudsen E, Ditlevsen S, and Hollnagel H, 2004, Academic Detailing Has No Effect on Prescribing of Asthma Medication in Danish General Practice: A 3-Year Randomized Controlled Trial with 12-Monthly Follow-ups, *Family Practice* 21 (3): 248–253.

Zemencuk JK, Hofer TP, Hayward RA, Moseley RH, and Saint S, 2006, What Effect Does Physician "Profiling" Have on Inpatient Physician Satisfaction and Hospital Length of Stay? *BMC Health Services Research* 6: 45, 8 pages.

CHAPTER 14

BENCHMARKING AND IMPLEMENTATION

Introduction

It is difficult to improve when you have nothing but your-self to emulate. Imagine a college student who decides to take up swimming to improve his physique and health status. After going to the student athletic facility, he finds himself alone in an Olympic-size pool. Although he took swimming lessons in his preteen years, he has forgotten most of the information, so he jumps in and swims 36 laps. Concluding that he must be at least an adequate swimmer, since he is capable of swimming more than a mile, he sees no need to evaluate or improve his technique. Swimming becomes a part of his daily routine.

After college, he moves to a new city and a new pool. Not only does this pool have other swimmers but the lanes are shared by two or more people. Two days after starting to swim at the new facility, one of the other swimmers, who is more than 30 years his senior, says, "You are a strong swimmer, but your technique is lousy. You need to buy goggles and put your head in the water." The suggestions makes perfect sense, as having one's head out of the water results in dragging the legs and increasing water resis-tance. He buys goggles and promptly increases his speed and reduces effort. The pool is divided into fast, medium, and slow lanes. Since his speed is average among the "fast" swimmers, he concludes he must be a good swimmer. Self-satisfied complacency sets in again, and he sees no further reason to evaluate his technique.

Employment takes him to another city and pool, where again he is surprised when another swimmer, only 20 years older, comments on his strength but dismisses his form. Having already heard remarks to the same effect and made adjustments, he is skeptical. What does this

LEARNING OBJECTIVES

1. Explain the goals and process of benchmarking

2. Understand the structure of balanced scorecards and how to use them

3. Understand the structure of dash-boards and how to use them

4. Apply implementation strategies and post-execution controls and incen-tives to increase the probability that desired changes will be incorporated into everyday routines

person know? The woman proceeds to tell him he is taking 18 strokes to complete one 75-foot length (a measurement) and he should take only 11 strokes (a benchmark). His first task was to determine the credibility of the source. How many strokes was he taking, since it had never occurred to him to count strokes? To this point he had been content to count distance (an outcome, not a process). Impressed by the fact that the woman knew the number of strokes he was taking, he accepted her conclusion that a good swimmer would complete the distance in eleven strokes.

Given the variance between where he was and where he should be, he recognized the need for improvement and although doubtful he could reduce his number of strokes by 38.9% (−7/18), he opened himself to suggestions for improvement. A few modest changes brought the number of stokes down to 13, but, as the law of diminishing returns dictates, the elimination of the two remaining strokes took considerable attention and effort.

This example demonstrates three truths about quality improvement. The first is that you cannot manage what you cannot measure. In this example, the lack of understanding of the process prevented the swimmer from recognizing the deficiency in his technique. The second truth is that without a standard it is impossible to determine how much improvement is needed. The third truth deals with capturing low-hanging fruit and the law of diminishing returns. The further you are away from a target, the easier the improvement. As you approach your goal, more effort is required and the return will be lower. The purpose of this chapter is to explore the benchmarking process, **balanced scorecards** and **dashboards**, and to provide guidelines for implementing quality improvement initiatives.

balanced scorecard
a tool to communicate an organization's goals and define the plan for achieving these goals

dashboard
a tool to track and monitor a single process or set of activities

Benchmarking and Best Practice

Benchmarking is commonly seen as a process of comparing an organization's processes and outcomes against those of other organizations. Benchmarking is a shorthand and ongoing method of improvement that does not require an organization to discover better ways of doing things or reinvent practices already in use by others. Camp and DeToro state that benchmarking "ensures the best practices are uncovered, adopted and implemented" (Camp and DeToro 1999, 12.2). BusinessDictionary.com defines best practice as "a method or technique that has consistently shown results superior to those achieved with other means."

Benchmarking can also be performed internally. Goals can be based on the performance of other departments or the historical performance of a single department. The goal in either case is to determine how an organization is performing and to identify areas in which improvements can be made. If an external benchmark is used, the initial target could be to achieve the average performance of the industry. Once an organization achieves average industry performance, it should set its sights on reaching the performance of organizations deemed best-in-class. One of the advantages of benchmarking is the establishment of credible improvement goals. Employee awareness that superior performance has been achieved in other places (or by rivals) should encourage them to improve.

Table 14.1 describes the four types of benchmarking an organization may undertake. The type of benchmarking performed will be determined by the organization's goals and the availability of information. **Internal benchmarking** is the fastest and easiest to undertake because the organization controls the information. For example, the infection rates of one surgical nursing unit could be compared to its historical rates or to the performance of similar units in the same organization during the same time period.

internal benchmarking comparing performance across units of a single organization

Organizations using industry benchmarking compare their performance against the average for their industry or the top performers in their field. The complication in implementing **industry benchmarking** is locating data; is industry data available through trade associations or in published reports? If data is available, the organization should begin by striving to equal or surpass average industry performance. If the organization is already above average or performance improvement has produced better than average results, the organization should strive to meet the performance of industry leaders.

industry benchmarking comparing organizational performance to the industry average or top performers in the field

Table 14.1 Types of Benchmarking

1.	Internal: easiest, comparison of one department or division with another
2.	Industry: comparison against industry performance
3.	Competitive: comparison against rival
4.	Functional: identification and comparison against a recognized leader in performance of a process; may not be in the same industry

Competitive benchmarking seeks to meet or exceed the performance of competing organizations. The obvious problem in implementing competitive benchmarking is that, in order to guard their competitive advantage, competitors do not share information. The goal of every organization should be to provide its customers with value superior to that of its competition; moreover, knowledge of an organization's superior performance can provide the basis for an effective marketing campaign. Similarly,

competitive benchmarking comparing organizational performance against other organizations vying for the same customers

recognizing a competitor's superior performance can provide the impetus to motivate employees to improve performance.

The final type of benchmarking is functional, which requires the organization to identify a recognized leader in the performance of a process. An advantage of **functional benchmarking** is that the recognized leader may not be in the same industry and may be willing to share their methods. For example, hospitals have multiple different functions, such as room scheduling, guest relations, and food service. The best performers in these functions may be found in the hospitality industry, and hotels and restaurants may be willing to share their expertise with health care organizations.

functional benchmarking

comparing organizational performance for a process against that of the recognized leader in the process from inside or outside the industry

The Benchmarking Process

The first step in the benchmarking process is to determine what to benchmark. Providers must understand why patients patronize one organization over others. Is it due to the outcomes they achieved, the price of their goods or services, the selection of products offered (breadth of care), patient service (how care is provided), timeliness of care, the environment in which care is delivered, or a combination of these factors?

The second step is to identify a benchmark that the organization will strive for. What should be the goals or targets the organization will attempt to achieve? As Table 14.1 suggests, external benchmarks may be derived from rivals, in which case the goal is to achieve a competitive advantage over other organizations operating in the same market, or it may be derived from the industry, in which case the goal may be to achieve better than average performance or best-in-class performance.

The third step is to determine how the targets will be achieved. Assume an organization seeks to be a leading performer and a gap exists between its current performance and that of the best-in-class performer. The recognition of a performance gap simultaneously encourages change and raises questions as to how the gap can be narrowed. Rivals, of course, will not be willing to share trade secrets that could decrease their competitiveness, but a health care organization may be able to find a provider in another geographic region that is willing to share information. The probability of information exchange will be increased if the information-seeking organization offers the opportunity for collaborative benchmarking. Collaborative benchmarking involves a two-way flow of information in which each organization is recognized as having superior performance in a given area and each organization can learn from the other. Collaborative benchmarking provides the potential for partnership and mutual gain.

Table 14.2 Benchmarking Steps

Step 1	Determine from the customer perspective what makes a difference between one supplier of a good or service and another
Step 2	Set performance targets
Step 3	Determine how to achieve targets
Step 4	Organize resources and motivate staff to achieve or exceed targets

Source: J. Beckford, 1998, *Quality: A Critical Introduction*, Routledge, New York, NY, 257.

On the other hand, functional benchmarking is used to identify a best-in-class performer from inside or outside the industry. Identifying a best-in-class performer from outside one's industry does not raise competitive concerns and may increase the willingness of the best-in-class performer to share information. A prime example of process benchmarking was the recognition that LL Bean had a world-class order processing system. This reputation led other companies, Xerox and Chrysler to name but two, to study and adopt LL Bean's order-filling process (Heizer and Render 1996). The focus of process benchmarking is not what is produced but rather how operations are run; thus organizations producing copiers and automobiles can learn how to improve their order-filling process from a retail firm specializing in clothing and outdoor equipment.

Finally, the organization must reorganize its resources to achieve its targets. The organization must maintain leadership to ensure that staff is motivated toward achieving the targets and must institute monitoring systems to continually judge and communicate performance to employees. After determining what needs to be done, it is management's job to ensure it is carried through.

There are four primary prerequisites essential to benchmarking (Goetsch and Davis 2010). The first is that an organization must be committed to the process and have the will to follow benchmarking to its conclusion. Upper management must understand the benefits of benchmarking, be committed to the process, and be actively involved to demonstrate to other employees why benchmarking should be embraced by everyone in the organization. If upper management announces a benchmarking program and delegates its operation to lower-level employees, the message that the program is not important to senior staff will be heard by subordinate employees who will similarly assign it a low priority.

Second, benchmarking programs must be consistent with the organizational vision and its strategic objectives. As mentioned earlier, Step 1 in the benchmarking process requires organizations to understand their customers; in health care this requires providers to recognize what attracts patients. If benchmarking compares product or service attributes that patients place little or no value upon, the program will not enhance the organization's performance and will simply add another bureaucratic record-keeping task.

The third prerequisite is that the organization must be open. Beckford states that benchmarking is "an exercise in organizational humility" (1998, 261). An organization must not think so highly of itself that employees fail to recognize they can learn from others, including organizations they may consider inferior. The second element to openness is a willingness to change. Recognizing that improvement can be made is only the first step; an organization must have a culture that is willing to accept the risk that accompanies change. Employees must be willing to learn new ways of doing things and change how they work.

Finally, the organization must understand its current processes, products and services, support services, and customer desires. Implementing change when one is unfamiliar with current practice is simply a random process with equal probabilities of improving or reducing outcomes. Benchmarking identifies a goal, but the third step of the process, determining how to achieve targets, requires clear ends-and-means thinking. What are the deficiencies in the current process, and what changes can be introduced to improve patient outcomes and satisfaction?

The primary goal of benchmarking is self-assessment: Is the organization performing effectively and efficiently? Effectiveness is producing a desired effect. Efficiency is maximizing output while minimizing inputs, or simply achieving maximum productivity from resources under the control of the organization. System effectiveness is measured by the outcome: Does a good or service satisfy the need or desire for which it was created? Efficiency concerns output: Did the expended resources produce the maximum amount of goods or services? Successful organizations must be effective and efficient; organizations that fail on either measure will lose customers to higher-performing providers.

The first question benchmarking should answer is: Are the desired results being achieved? If the desired results are being achieved, the second question is: Are the results being produced at the lowest possible cost? A successful provider must not only produce what patients want but produce the desired goods and services at prices patients and third-party payers are willing to pay.

Returning to Donabedian's structure-process-outcome paradigm, the starting point for benchmarking should be outcomes. Is the organization producing outcomes that meet established standards or satisfy the customer (or both)? The most obvious outcome measure is mortality rate; CMS Hospital Compare allows patients to access databases that compare risk-adjusted mortality rates across hospitals and medical conditions. Outcomes and effectiveness should be main topics of interest; we cannot expect patients to be concerned with issues of efficiency, process, or structure if health outcomes are less than expected. Table 14.3 provides a list of possible benchmarks for Donabedian's paradigm.

Efficiency standards often examine productivity issues, such as how many hours are required per patient encounter or how much revenue is generated per employee. Both of these measures deal directly with the productivity of resources and address structure and process concerns, for example whether there is adequate or excessive staffing and whether the employed manpower is fully utilized. Assuming a provider's mortality rates are lower than or equal to the rates of other providers, we still need to know if they are consuming an appropriate amount of resources to achieve this outcome. If the provider is consuming the average number of or fewer worker-hours per case, we may be satisfied with performance and outcome. If an excessive number of hours are consumed (unwarranted given the severity of the patient's treated) the result may be unacceptable. Could the same outcome be achieved by more fully using resources? Are employees idle or engaged in nonproductive or duplicate work? Is poor management of resources driving up the cost of health care?

Table 14.3 Benchmarking Structure-Process-Outcome

Structure	Process	Outcome
Ratio of patients to staff	Compliance with care standards	Mortality
Qualifications of staff	Length of stay	Morbidity
Scope of services offered	Readmission rates	Condition-specific measures: A1c, BP, LDL, etc.
Technology available	Infection rates	Return to work
Age of plant and equipment	Resource use (hours or cost per case)	Patient satisfaction

Table 14.3 displays other measures that can be used to benchmark and compare health care organizations. The structural variables measure resources in place and, according to Donabedian, having more, better, or newer resources should provide a foundation for quality care. The process measures are designed to determine whether generally accepted ways of delivering care are being followed and to determine performance on intermediate outcomes such as infection rates. Compliance with care standards could include a variety of measures that examine whether recommended tests and procedures were done and, if performed, whether they were delivered on a timely basis. Measures such as infection rates and length of stay

examine intermediate outcomes. For example, were there iatrogenic results from care? Is length of stay inappropriately short or long, are patients discharged prematurely, or are they in-house for extensive periods due to ineffective or inefficient treatment or care that harmed the patient?

General outcome measures, such as mortality rates and patient satisfaction, are frequently used to compare health care organizations, but their lack of specificity does not address questions for which patients seek answers. Patients want to know what they can expect from their medical condition and treatment. Condition-specific measures focus on the results of care for particular conditions, such as whether physiologic or functional markers are improved or within normal limits. For example, if a patient is being treated for hypertension, is the patient's blood pressure within the prescribed range at the conclusion of treatment? Return to work measures how rapidly a patient can resume productive activity after treatment. For example, one of the touted advantages of laparoscopic or minimally invasive surgery is smaller incisions that allow patients to heal faster and resume normal activities sooner.

The structure-process-outcome paradigm can be seen as a causal chain. If a provider discovers that it has substandard outcomes relative to its peers, the organization can attempt to drill down to determine the causes of the deficiency. Is the less-than-expected outcome the result of failure to follow generally accepted standards (process deficiencies)? Can the lower outcomes or the failure to follow generally accepted standards be the result of having too little investment in staff and equipment or the inability to provide comprehensive service (structural deficiencies)?

As mentioned before, the prerequisites of benchmarking include upper management commitment, openness, the selection of benchmarks that will enhance an organization's competitiveness, and understanding of current processes and products. Table 14.4 details the obstacles that can prevent successful implementation of a benchmark program.

The first obstacle is an excessive internal focus and the illusion of uniqueness. Excessive internal focus is the opposite of openness; organizations that see themselves or their processes as unique cannot imagine they can learn from others. The "not invented here" attitude dismisses the effectiveness of other organizations' processes or the ability of these processes to be applied to the organization's problems.

In one case, a hospital admitting department believed that their admission process was so unique that they could not use existing software systems but had to create their own system. Not only was their admitting process similar to that of the more than 5,000 other hospitals in the country, their admitting system also shared characteristics with the check-in function of

Table 14.4 Obstacles to Benchmarking

1.	Illusion of uniqueness: widespread belief that how others perform does not apply to our organization and we cannot learn or be compared with others.
2.	Poorly defined objectives: why undertaken and pursued? Inappropriate: increase quality, improve financial performance.
3.	Lack of employee buy-in: employees do not internalize goals or apply themselves to task.
4.	Insufficient top management support: if upper management refuses to devote itself to the program, lower-level employees will do the same.
5.	Poor team composition: team lacks skills to resolve issues that may arise, team must include physicians, managers and employees (operations), and quality management or IT (data analysis).
6.	Inappropriate benchmark objective: impossibility of attaining (too high, e.g., best in industry) or no challenge (too low, e.g., above average, half of providers will require no improvement).
7.	Unrealistic timetable for improvement: impossibility of rapid improvement (too little time) or lack of urgency and action (too much time).
8.	Overemphasis on process rather than goal: completion of reports supersedes data analysis and development of plans for improvement.
9.	Lack of data: required data not collected or easily assessable.
10.	Insufficient resources: when time is limited, employees will provide care, not paperwork.
11.	Physician opposition: given status and role of physicians, their opposition can stop a benchmarking program in its tracks.

the hotel industry. If the admitting staff could have seen beyond themselves, they would have learned that other organizations' admission and check-in processes moved patients and guests to their rooms in significantly less time and with less error. To address employee resistance to adopting methods developed by other organizations, Camp and DeToro emphasize that benchmarking is not simply the blind copying of the processes of other organizations. Benchmarking requires not only recognizing the superior results of other organizations but also the ability to creatively adapt another organization's processes to one's own operations (Camp and DeToro 1999, 12.19). Those who believe their uniqueness will be lost by using processes developed outside their organization miss the point of making comparisons. The point is to improve activities in which others have demonstrated superior performance while retaining those aspects of operations in one's own organization that have superior processes and outcomes.

The second obstacle is a poorly defined benchmarking objective. Often the benchmark goal is too broadly defined; poor goals include improving quality or increasing profit. While these goals summarize what the organization wants to achieve, their broadness fails to provide direction. Superior goals provide clear direction to employees and address issues important to patients and employees. Examples of superior benchmark targets would be reducing wait time by 10 minutes or missed OT treatments by 10%.

The third obstacle, little employee buy-in, is related to the second. Lack of buy-in may arise from poorly defined objectives or from targets that are not accepted or internalized by employees. Profitability objectives regularly fail to motivate care givers who see their jobs as improving patient health, so benchmarks must be formulated to appeal to the interests of employees. If employees see the process as adding another unproductive task to their workload without a corresponding reduction in other tasks or the addition of resources, they will be unlikely to embrace the improvement initiative. Employee commitment will parallel the commitment exhibited by upper management; if senior staff is detached from the process, this attitude will permeate all levels of the organization, the fourth obstacle.

The fifth problem is poor team composition. The benchmark team must include members who understand medical processes, patient needs and desires, and benchmarking goals and processes, and who have the authority to institute change. A mix of talent is essential to ensure that benchmarks are properly chosen, operations are examined from medical and process perspectives, and necessary actions are taken.

The sixth obstacle is that benchmarking objectives may be set too high or low. Setting a target too high may demoralize staff if the objective cannot be reached. An example of oversetting goals may be the use by a community hospital of benchmarks achieved by a teaching hospital. Differences in the structure and patient mix of hospitals may preclude one institution from matching the performance of another. Objectives can also be set too low and provide no challenge to employees and require no change. For example, if the benchmark is set at the industry average fully, 50% of hospitals already meet or exceed this target. Benchmarks should set targets that require improvement and that are challenging and obtainable.

A similar barrier is an unrealistic timetable: requiring too much change too quickly or setting too lax a schedule. In the first case, when multiple changes are required they should be phased in sequentially to ensure new behaviors are learned, incorporated into everyday routines, and produce the desired results before other changes are initiated. When an organization sets a goal of operating at the industry average it must recognize that given the distance it stands away from its target it may be months or years from achieving its goal. On the other hand, when too much time is given and too little action is expected, employees may lose sight of goals and the need to improve.

A common problem in many organizations is that the means—the program—becomes more important than the ends—the outcome sought. In benchmarking, this tendency manifests itself in an overemphasis on data collection rather than on process improvement. Organizations that lose sight of the goal of improving operations end up creating and filing reports but are unable to use the benchmark data to focus on areas of opportunity. Creating a benchmark report will have no impact if it is not used to evaluate processes, drill down to discover the source of performance gaps, and identify ways of enhancing operations.

Obstacles that are more apparent in health care than in other organizations include lack of information, insufficient resources to run a benchmarking program, and stakeholder opposition, the final three barriers shown in Table 14.4. Health care is data rich and information poor. One of the primary problems facing the health care industry is the lack of integration of information systems within an organization and the fragmentation of care between providers. As Codman ([1914] 1996) noted, the outcome that should be tracked is the patient's condition twelve months postcare, yet outcomes are often measured at discharge or discharge plus 30 days. These timeframes ignore common problems that arise after a patient is released from care. Health care organizations frequently employ different information systems for different tasks, precluding the ability to derive benchmarks. Providers often have different registration, medical record, clinical, inventory, payroll, billing, and accounting systems, which are not compatible with each other. Unintegrated systems complicate work for employees who must use information across platforms. Between providers, there is the problem of different and incompatible systems, making it impossible to compile a comprehensive record of patient care.

Unlike other organizations that have defined points at which quality is assessed and for whom quality assessment is the responsibility of multiple employees, the health care industry continues to rely on physicians to monitor quality. Physicians are powerful stakeholders, and their time is a valuable resource. As stated earlier, they receive little remuneration for quality assessment. As discussed in Chapter Thirteen, physicians continue to be skeptical of the validity of comparisons, given the lack of large samples and primitiveness of risk adjustment.

While the obstacles are daunting, Camp (1989) offers an engaging set of reasons why employees should embrace benchmarking. Camp makes it evident that internally focused organizations that refuse to utilize the benefits of benchmarking will make decisions on a severely restricted set of information. Internally focused organizations will often fail to identify critical pieces of information, so their decisions regarding customer desires, goals, and processes will often be suboptimal. In three critical areas—identifying customer wants, establishing goals, and measuring performance—internally focused organizations will be operating blind. Benchmarking forces an organization to look beyond itself and observe how other organizations are meeting customer demands, the goals they pursue, and the productivity of their workforce.

Camp (1989) presents a compelling case for moving beyond an organization's comfort zone to challenging employees to think about what they are attempting to achieve and how they perform their work. The goal of the externally focused, benchmarking organization is to identify and implement industry best practices. Only by focusing on objective data can an organization assure itself that it is providing customers with what they want (versus what employees think customers want) and operating efficiently and effectively. Benchmarking is a data-driven approach to process improvement that relies on identifying processes in which others have demonstrated higher performance. Benchmarks serve as stark examples that processes can be improved and as models for the types of changes that can be implemented to achieve improvement and maintain competiveness.

Benchmark Data Sources

One of the most challenging tasks in benchmarking is identifying appropriate benchmarks. Generic benchmarks can be obtained from the following three free and publicly available links:

CMS Hospital Compare: http://www.hospitalcompare.hhs.gov

AHA Chartbook: http://www.aha.org/research/reports/tw/chartbook/index.shtml

Dartmouth Atlas of Health Care: http://cecsweb.dartmouth.edu/atlas08/datatools/bench_s1.php

Proprietary organizations provide more specific measures, but subscriptions are generally required to access these databases.

One of the chief benefits of benchmarking is it signals that an organization is beginning to explicitly examine what it does and what it achieves. Rather than accepting the status quo, the organization is awaking to the possibility that it can improve its performance. After recognizing the possibility of improvement, benchmarking can establish expectations and goals. When goals are set based on results achieved by other organizations, especially when outcomes are achieved by rivals, they can provide strong motivation for change.

Benchmarking is not a one-time review of operations but a continuous process. Industries and rivals do not stand still, so performance must be continually assessed. This assessment should be directed toward identifying changes in performance as well as shifts in what measures are being tracked. Figure 14.1 demonstrates two of the potential benefits of benchmarking: identifying performance gaps and communicating goals and progress.

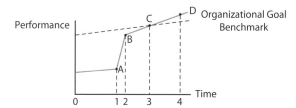

Figure 14.1 Improving Performance through Benchmarking

Source: D Goetsch and S Davis, 2010, *Quality Management for Organizational Excellence*, 6th ed., Pearson Prentice Hall, Upper Saddle River, NJ, 529.

Improvement from benchmarking occurs in three stages. The first stage is the recognition of a gap between the organization (the solid line in Figure 14.1) and the industry average or best-in-class performance (the dashed line). While the organization's and the benchmark's performance are improving (organizations that stand still will find themselves falling behind their improving competitors), the recognition of a large gap between the organization and the benchmark and the ability to capture low-hanging fruit through adoption of another's processes or methods may lead to dramatic improvement.

Between time 0 and 1, the organization is unaware that it is performing below the benchmark; recognition of the gap at time 1 leads to adopting new methods. Stage 2 documents the adoption of a new method and the period of refinement and adaption from time 1 through time 2. The movement from point B to point C documents the gradual refinement of the new method until the benchmark goal is achieved. The third stage is the result of employees' push toward higher performance after having achieved the first goal. Beyond point C, the organization may not have any model to follow and must rely on CQI or the PDCA cycle to propel it to superior performance or industry leadership at point D.

Benchmarking will be most effective if it is initiated and operated by the employees closest to the process who understand it best. The goal is to establish a system of self-management in which employees know the desired goals and can readily monitor their performance and initiate changes when they see fit.

Balanced Scorecards

Balanced scorecards were developed to communicate an organization's goals to its stakeholders and to define a plan for reaching these goals. The organization's goals and the means of achieving them are explicitly defined in measurable terms. The balanced scorecard may be viewed as a pyramid, as shown in Figure 14.2. The pinnacle, the *financial perspective*, defines the organization's goal of maximizing its value. Value in economic terms is created by maximizing the difference between an organization's revenues and expenses. The fact that consumers are willing to pay more for a good or service than the cost of the resources consumed in producing the product is prima facie evidence of the creation of value. The two paths to value maximization are revenue growth and cost reduction.

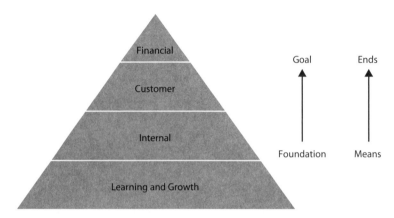

Figure 14.2 Kaplan and Norton's Balanced Scorecard

operational excellence
a means of satisfying customers through competitive pricing, meeting or exceeding quality expectations, timeliness, and broad product selection

As we move down from the pinnacle, we are faced with the question of how value is created. Returning to the generic definition of quality, value is judged by the customer. The second-highest level of the pyramid is the *customer perspective*, where the goal is to satisfy the customer, and where customer loyalty is the means to achieving the organization's financial goals. Customers who believe they are getting the most value from their purchasing dollars will provide a loyal base for maximizing revenue. How are customers satisfied? Kaplan and Norton (2000) identify three paths: achieving operational excellence, customer intimacy, and product leadership.

Operational excellence requires competitive pricing, meeting the customer's quality expectations, delivering product when the customer wants it, and providing a broad selection of product. Operationally excellent organizations minimize their costs to give customers competitive, if not the lowest, prices while meeting the organization's financial objectives. While minimizing costs, organizations must master the production process to ensure quality is the best it can be. Organizations must ensure that their resources are fully employed in value-creating activities; idle, unproductive, or wasted resources drive up cost and undermine quality. A high-quality, low-price product may not satisfy the customer if it is insensitive to what the customer wants or cannot be delivered at the time the customer desires. Organizations in tune with their customer base understand the many factors that determine customer satisfaction, and they monitor and control these aspects of their operations to ensure that the essential desires of customers are met.

A second means of achieving customer loyalty is the development of **customer intimacy.** Organizations that excel in customer intimacy are known for exceptional service and the completeness of solutions offered (Kaplan and Norton, 2000, 172). Poor customer service is characterized by phone trees, long wait times, frequent transfer, and inability to satisfy inquiries. Exceptional customer service involves creating in the minds of customers the perception that they are known and valued by members of the organization. This requires knowing customers' needs and delivering prompt resolution of inquiries. The idea of complete solutions requires an organization to be able to fully satisfy a customer's need or desire without requiring the assistance of other organizations. In health care, where multiple providers are often involved in care, completeness of solutions requires the principal care giver to identify other providers when necessary, facilitate the transfer of the patient across providers, and monitor and control care at each access point.

customer intimacy a means of satisfying customers by providing superior service, complete solutions for their needs, and demonstrating that customers are known and valued by members of the organization

The third way of building customer loyalty is through **product leadership.** Product leadership requires an organization to keep its goods or services one step ahead of the competition. Innovation is the key to product leadership when customers seeking cutting-edge goods and services flock to an organization with a reputation for delivering these types of products. Organizations should focus on providing expanded functionality and product features as well as superior performance to achieve a leadership position (Kaplan and Norton 2000, 172). Apple is an example of a company that epitomizes product leadership. Apple's continuous development of new products and enhancement of existing products has earned it loyal customers and placed it among the highest-valued companies on the NASDAQ.

product leadership a means of satisfying customers by providing products that are innovative and outperform and/or provide more features or functionality than the products of competitors

The third level of the pyramid, *the* internal perspective, identifies the organizational attributes that facilitate the achievement of its operational excellence, customer intimacy, and product leadership goals. The internal targets define how the organization expects to reach operational excellence to satisfy customers and achieve financial goals. Customer-pleasing internal characteristics are innovation, customer management processes, operation and logistic processes, and good corporate citizenry (Kaplan and Norton 2000, 168). Innovation requires the organization to be able to project what their customers will want in the future and create products that satisfy customers. A second aspect of innovation is the ability to target new customers. These could be untapped customers who reside in the geographic area in which the organization is operating, or they may be in markets outside an organization's traditional service area.

The second internal process to satisfying customers is to provide a higher level of service than expected. Organizations promote the idea of a supplier-customer partnership, versus simply supplying a product or service, but realizing this goal requires active customer management. Organizations seeking true partnerships with their customers must understand how their products and services are used and what the customer wants. In order for a supplier to bring value to a customer, it must know the customer-desired outcome and create a **customer relationship management (CRM)** system to track and respond to their needs and desires. In health care, partnership requires providers to understand their patients' life goals and develop treatment and rehabilitation plans that allow patients to realize these plans as fully as possible.

customer relationship management (CRM) a set of tools to collect and analyze interactions with customers to integrate design, marketing, sales, production, and service to optimize the value of goods and services in the eyes of the purchaser

An organization wanting to build customer intimacy seeks to provide prompt, efficient, high-quality responses to customer inquiries, guide employees through customer interactions, streamline operations and reduce manual processes, and provide consistent services, database connectivity, and workflow capabilities (McAvoy 1999, 26). Effective CRM systems track technical problems and breakdowns per customer, process, and time period to focus improvement processes; average time per process to improve timeliness; cost per service to evaluate resource allocation and revenue per customer; and after-sale transactions to direct sales (Curran and Ladd 2000, 260–261). The goal is to provide a complete picture of customer interactions to understand customers' needs and desires and to create a system that can more fully satisfy their expectations.

The third way to satisfy customers is by optimizing the organization's operation and logistic processes. Optimization centers on reducing cost, improving quality, decreasing cycle time, increasing asset utilization, and capacity management (Kaplan and Norton, 2000, 173). The term *value chain* is used to emphasize organizational characteristics that retain existing patients and attract new customers. Health care organizations must be concerned with their entire breadth of operations to consistently please patients. As we saw in Chapter Ten, Swayne, Duncan, and Ginter (2008) describe the health care value chain in two parts, in Figure 14.3. The service areas (the top half) deal directly with patients, and the support areas (the lower half) provide resources to the employees interacting with patients. The goal of both parts of the organization is patient satisfaction.

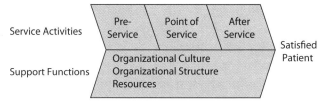

Figure 14.3 The Health Care Value Chain

The service activities of the organization are divided into three areas based on when employees interact with patients. The preservice activities involve marketing research, determining what customers want, and building a product and production system that can fulfill their desires. Organizations must first understand their customers before they can set targets that will have a significant effect on organizational success. Preservice activities involve determining what goods or services patients want (product), what patients are willing to pay (price), where products will be offered (place), and how potential patients will be made aware of the organization's products (promotion). The combination of product, price, place, and promotion form the organization's marketing mix and should guide it in its future operations. If the marketing research is accurate, it will define what patients want and provide the roadmap for point-of-service and after-service activities.

Point-of-service activities include what is done for patients and how they are treated. Point-of-service activities focus on the quality of care provided, the timeliness of treatment, and fulfilling the objective of the medical encounter. Point-of-service activities constitute the majority of the interaction between the provider and the patient, and while benchmarks and balanced scorecards track these encounters, the value chain emphasizes that point-of-service activities alone cannot guarantee patient satisfaction. Preservice, after-service, and support functions can enhance or destroy goodwill created at the point of service.

After-service activities focus on postcare interactions. Postcare interactions include follow-up activities where a provider contacts a patient to see how he is faring after being released from care. These contacts demonstrate that the provider is concerned about the patient and about the quality of care she delivered and views her relationship with the patient as enduring. Follow-up contacts attempt to identify other medical services the patient may benefit from based on his initial medical encounter. Follow-up can be used to expand the scope of services provided by attempting to meet all a patient's needs. Billing is another important after-service activity, as resolving bill and insurance issues often brings patients into direct contact with employees. Billing is a prime area in which patient goodwill can be lost. A patient may receive desired care in the desired manner but if his bill is incorrect and resolution takes weeks or months, he may choose another provider for his future medical needs.

Support functions provide resources to employees in direct contact with patients and should facilitate these interactions by providing the right resources at the right time. Swayne, Duncan, and Ginter divide support functions into three areas: culture, management structure, and resources. The organizational culture should establish expectations encouraging employees to put patients first, exercise initiative, function as a team, and seek continual improvement. The management structure should establish effective supervision of employees and facilitate rapid decision making. Resources recognize that service personnel must be provided with the necessary equipment and facilities and the human, informational, and financial resources to complete their tasks. The value chain emphasizes that all parts of an organization must operate in an effective and integrated manner to ensure that its goods and services will satisfy its customers. Failure in any area may make it impossible for point-of-service employees, however effective, efficient, and courteous, to prove to patients they selected the best provider for care (Swayne, Duncan, and Ginter 2008, 295).

The fourth means of satisfying customers is by effective stakeholder management and being a good corporate citizen. Following the mortgage crisis and the Deepwater Horizon oil spill, it is easy to see how customers can be lost through reckless, self-interested behavior. Kaplan and Norton recognize that organizations that go beyond their basic duties to customers, by diligently serving the larger communities in which they are situated, will often attract loyal customers and simultaneously undercut the need for public regulation that could diminish their latitude of action (Kaplan and Norton 2000, 174).

The foundation of the balanced scorecard pyramid rests on employees and infrastructure—the learning and growth perspective. Does an organization have employees with the requisite skills and motivation to drive its internal processes? Are the organization's equipment and facilities capable of producing the desired outcomes? Kaplan and Norton note that the foundation for effective processes lies in the core competencies of employees, technology in use, and corporate culture (Kaplan and Norton 2000, 175). The key to effective processes, satisfied customers, and achieving organizational goals is to build and continually improve employee skills and organizational capability. Organizations must invest in employee training programs and new equipment and facilities to ensure that service and support personnel have the proper resources to create a fully satisfying experience for patients.

Huang et al. (2004) applied the balanced scorecard framework to an emergency department and demonstrated improvement across all four perspectives. Revenue growth increased from 1.44% to 3.27%. Patient (customer) satisfaction increased from 3.05 to 3.47 while the rate of complaints fell from 0.28 to 0.10. **Internal perspective** was measured using the rates of incomplete lab tests and returns rates. The rate of incomplete biochemical, blood, and urine tests fell by 35.2% (12.8% to 8.3%), 65.9% (4.7% to 1.6%), and 69.6% (5.6% to 1.7%). The number of inappropriately returned tests fell from 3.5% to 2.1%. The organization used training to drive the improvements and documented a per-employee increase in the hours of continuing education from 4.3 to 9.7 per year. The program also documented an increase in staff satisfaction, from 2.83 to 3.29 as measured on a four-point Likert scale.

> **Internal perspective** assessment of the effectiveness and efficiency of an organization's processes

The goal of balanced scorecards is to set goals and determine how they will be achieved. Figure 14.4, based on Huang et al.'s work, demonstrates how the process should work. An organization must build employee skills through continuing education and create a working environment where they want to excel. When these two elements are in place, operations should run more smoothly, as seen in the substantial reductions in incomplete and inappropriately returned tests. Operational improvements reduce patient delays, hasten discharge or transfer, and increase patient satisfaction. The increase in patient satisfaction should cement the organization's status as the provider of choice and facilitate the achievement of its goals.

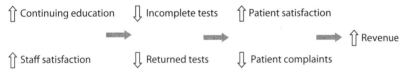

Figure 14.4 The Causal Chain Implied in the Balanced Scorecard

While the balanced scorecard is used extensively outside the health care industry, there are those in health care who see its formulation and main goal as problematic for a human service industry composed of non-profit or public organizations. Meliones et al. (2008) reorganized the traditional structure into one they see as more fitting for health care, as shown in Figure 14.5. Quality and safety are placed at the pinnacle, supported by the customer, finance, and work culture perspectives.

Meliones et al. see the primary goal of health care organizations as ensuring the quality of care and patient safety. In operationalizing these factors they focused on morbidity, readmissions, LOS, infection rates, and census. Their improvement program, based on the balanced scorecard, produced an unquantified reduction in morbidity, a 42.9% reduction in readmits (7% to 4%), a 0.6-day reduction in LOS, a 66.6% reduction in infection rates (3% to 1%) and a 9% increase in census.

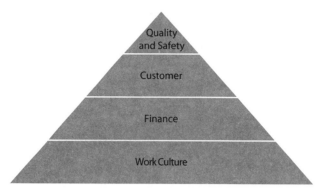

Figure 14.5 Reenvisioning the Balanced Scorecard for Health Care

customer perspective
assessment of the degree
to which the organization
satisfies its customers

Improvements in the **customer perspective** included higher-than-expected patient satisfaction scores when the target was set at the national mean, and a higher-than-expected rate of patients responding that the institution was "very good." Similar improvements were seen in finance. Financial measures included discharge time, pediatric intensive care unit (PICU) encounters, increase in contribution margin, and net margin. Discharge time improved 26%, PICU encounters increased 10%, and net loss was reduced from $7.4 million to $4.7 million over two years, a 36.5% reduction.

Several initiatives were instituted to improve the work culture, including improving communication processes for patient hand-offs, concerns, and reports and minimizing interruptions during team rounds. These changes produced improvements in staff's perception of teamwork (increased from 67% to 87%), use of briefings (63% to 84%), and identifying the proper channel for concerns (67% to 87%). While this program documented wide improvement, weaknesses included how it defined targets and an unclear cause and effect relationship. Their **financial perspective** focused on measures that reflected internal process (discharge time and number of patient encounters) rather than finance. It is questionable whether reducing the operating loss contributed to the improvement in patient satisfaction or quality and safety.

financial perspective
assessment of the degree
to which the primary
goals of an organization
are achieved, typically
the value created that is
the difference between
total revenue and total
cost

Balanced scorecards attempt to focus an organization's goals and give direction to its activities. By explicitly defining targets, balanced scorecards make employees aware of what behaviors are needed and what outcomes are sought. Balanced scorecards give energy to the saying "what gets measured gets attention." The Kaplan and Norton framework provides a clear cause and effect chain in which the organization's goals are pursued by ensuring customer satisfaction through running effective and efficient operations. The **learning and growth perspective** recognizes that effective and efficient operations can occur only if employees are provided with the necessary skills and tools to do their jobs. The duty of management is to identify and deliver the training and facilities needed by staff.

Dashboards

Dashboards, unlike balanced scorecards, which are often used to establish organization-wide goals and metrics, are focused on lower levels of activities, such as departmental activities or a single process. The beauty of dashboards is that they use departmental data, which may be easier for employees to understand, and they are designed to track activities that employees participate in on a daily basis. If departmental goals and dashboard measures are developed in partnership with employees, this should increase staff motivation and commitment toward achieving the targets. Of course, departmental goals must be consistent with what attracts patients and the larger goals of the organization.

Comparing a health care dashboard to an automobile dashboard is informative. A car dashboard is designed to provide key performance indicators (KPI) to drivers, such as speed, remaining fuel, and engine temperature, to improve their driving performance. Besides the constantly available displays, a series of indicators and lights appear when systems (such as turn signals, window defroster, and air conditioner) are in use. In addition, cars are equipped with a series of warning lights—check engine, oil pressure, charge, brake, low tire pressure, seat belt—that appear when relevant systems vary beyond acceptable parameters. Drivers are provided with a wealth of continually updated information to control the operation of the vehicle and alert them when service is needed. A car dashboard does not overwhelm drivers with details that could distract them and impair, rather than improve, their driving performance. Warning lights are a great example of economy of information. As long as systems function within set parameters, the driver is not alerted; the lights appear only on an as-needed basis.

Dashboards serve two distinct and interrelated purposes: reporting and management. Dashboards created for reporting typically involve aggregate data collected over a defined time period (day, week, month) and are designed to influence future behavior. If productivity is down due to a drop in cases, future staffing levels may be reduced. If the rate of infections shows a significant increase, staff may be reminded to redouble their attention to hand washing and gloving. Reporting-type dashboards are typically

learning and growth perspective measures the degree to which organizations provide employees with the knowledge and tools to work to their potential

paper based and distributed to employees or posted in prominent places in the unit.

Dashboards created for management purposes often aim at influencing current activity. This type of dashboard serves the same function as the warning lights in a car; they monitor systems and alert operators when immediate corrective action is required. This type of dashboard generally requires integrated information systems with drill-down capability such that users responding to a warning can access additional information to pinpoint potential causes of the deviation. Given the goal of affecting immediate action, this type of information is often fed into electronic displays in work areas.

The common components of a dashboard include the measures, their definition, and a description of how they are measured; the performance target; current performance (one or more periods); data sources; and the display and interpretation of performance (at, above, or below goal, as well as stable, improving, or worsening). Health care dashboard builders must identify the measures to be reported (or KPI) with economy. A rule of thumb is that a dashboard should include ten or fewer measures, to avoid overloading users. What measures should be constantly monitored, and what other factors should appear only when needed? Common measures include case load or backlog, productivity, technical quality and safety indicators, customer experience (satisfaction), and financial performance.

While it may seem that the definition of the measure and how it is measured are the same, they can vary. The definition provides a verbal or intuitive description of the measure, while how it will be measured provides a precise mathematical formula. For example, although defining late surgical starts appears straightforward, measurement requires knowing what constitutes the start of surgery and what is an acceptable or allowable deviation. The measurement formula should detail exactly what should be counted in the numerator and denominator when rates are calculated. This information might not be displayed on the dashboard, but all users should be familiar with the definition and measurement.

Establishing the performance target may be the most contentious part of establishing a dashboard. Targets should be challenging and obtainable, but people's interpretation of both terms varies. After targets are set, they must be clearly communicated to all personnel to ensure that everyone understands the goals to be pursued. The four primary choices for targets are prior period, industry average, rival, or best-in-class performance. While prior period is easiest to obtain, it does not provide much guidance as to the level of performance the organization should aspire to. Rival performance provides the most competitively relevant target—an organization should strive to outperform its competitors, but the competitors' performance may not establish what the organization should aspire to. Industry average provides an adequate initial goal but quality management holds that this goal is too low and organizations should strive for more. Best-in-class performance should be an organization's ultimate objective but could be disheartening to organizations whose current performance falls well short of this level.

Current performance is the critical piece of information, and the purpose of the dashboard will dictate whether current performance represents a single case or an aggregation of cases. If the dashboard is to help a surgical team with a particular patient, the relevant metrics would simply be that patient's allergies, respiration, heart rate, equipment and supply status, and case time (Egan 2006). When dashboards are tracking individual patient treatment, the only relevant targets are actual case time to scheduled time and vital signs. Dashboards for reporting purposes are designed to inform all employees of performance and identify areas where improvement is needed to meet targets. For this purpose, prior period data is necessary to demonstrate how performance is changing.

After the substantive decisions regarding what to report are made, data sources and report generators must be identified. Given the plethora of clinical and administrative systems in place, developers must determine where each bit of data will be drawn from and how it will be inputted into the dashboard. Management dashboards must have real-time interfaces to other systems to provide employees with up-to-date information to perform their work. Dashboards for reporting purposes could rely on paper reports, which are subsequently manually entered into the dashboard generator. Excel is a competent report generator, if a manual reporting dashboard will meet a user's need. The trade-off is clear: a dashboard reporting information for aggregate events can be developed and produced on a PC, but it will require continual manual input. An integrated management dashboard could reduce ongoing manual input and provide drill-down capabilities, but its development cost will be extensive.

The display and interpretation of performance is the bottom line of the dashboard: Is action required or should the system be left alone? Information is typically displayed in run graphs or tables. When graphs are used, employees received multiperiod displays of performance and targets. Figure 14.6 relays two important bits of information. The first is that the target of 80% of surgical cases starting within five minutes of the scheduled start time is not being met; late starts appear to be a problem from February through April and September through November. The other takeaway is that 2011 performance has improved relative to the prior year.

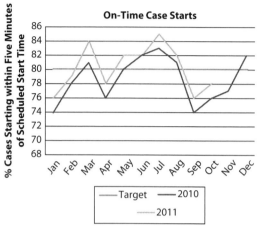

Figure 14.6 Dashboard Run Chart

When tables are used to display information, a verbal interpretation of performance is included and is frequently color-coded to facilitate visual identification of important trends. The color coding frequently parallels the red, yellow, and green indicators of traffic lights. Red is often used to identify significant negative variance or the failure to meet performance expectations, yellow indicates an early warning of potential performance failure, and green is used for performance that is meeting or exceeding established targets. Color codes and their meanings are established by users and may vary from the definitions given above.

An article in *OR Manager* (2011) reported on the operating room dashboard used by the Indiana University Hospital, which displays information on nine metrics: full-time equivalent (FTE) utilization, first-case starts, case cancellation rate, post anesthesia care unit (PACU) admission delays, turnover time, PACU LOS, OR utilization, number of cases, and number of surgical hours. Information is displayed in a table and includes the metric definition, how it is measured, the data source, performance target, the last three months of performance, status (met/did not meet target and improved/worsened), and a color-coded interpretation of performance (achieved target, target not achieved but improvement, and target not achieved but decreased improvement). Table 14.5 is a modified example of the dashboard used at Indiana University Hospital.

Table 14.5 Operating Room Dashboard

Metric	Definition	Measure	Target	Performance	Trend
FTE utilization	Staffing levels above flexed budget	Comparison between actual and flexed budget	1% or less	2.02%	Not achieved but improving
First-Case Starts	Patients in room at scheduled time for first case	% of cases in room within 5 minutes of scheduled start	80%	72.0%	Not achieved and reduced performance
Case Cancellations	Number of canceled cases	Number of cancelled cases ÷ total cases	2%	1.5%	Achieved
OR Discharge Delays	Occurrences and minutes patient is held in OR	Occurrences and total minutes patients are held in OR	0 cases, 0 minutes	2 cases, 49 minutes	Not achieved and reduced performance
Turnover time	Time between patients	% of cases turned over in 30 minutes or less	95%	86.0%	Not achieved and reduced performance
LOS in PACU	Time from recovery room admission to discharge	Minutes between recovery room admission to discharge	90 minutes or less	45 minutes	Achieved
OR utilization	OR hours used ÷ total OR hours available	OR hours used ÷ total OR hours available	85%	65%	Not achieved but improving

Source: OR Manager, 2011, Tracking Data, Changing Behavior, *OR Manager* 27 (2): 11.

Table 14.5 is easy to interpret and highlights performance. The shading highlights areas meeting objectives (dark), areas not meeting objectives but improving (medium) and those not meeting target and moving in the wrong direction (light). As mentioned earlier, these could also be color-coded green, yellow, and red. The report is produced on a monthly basis using Excel, and its objective is to continually remind employees what the department values and wants to achieve. Employees, through a brief glance at the report, can see that case cancellations and PACU LOS are meeting targets and that FTE and OR utilization are not meeting targets but show improvement. First-case starts, PACU admission delays, and turnover time are not meeting and are moving away from target; the light-colored cells indicate employees need to immediately address the causes for these trends.

Park et al. (2010) focus on the use of OR supplies with drill-down capability to the physician level. Their dashboard attributes sought to align incentives, provide accurate and contextual data in intuitive informational displays, be timely, establish a hierarchy of information, be assessable, and increase employee willingness to use data. Park et al. demonstrate how dashboards can be tailored to address a wide range of management issues including staffing, supply, scheduling, space, quality, outcome, and finance.

While Park and his colleagues reviewed an OR dashboard at the departmental level, others have taken the idea to the level of a single patient, demonstrating how a dashboard can be used to provide information to a surgical team during surgery. Egan (2006) describes the purposes of a dashboard for a patient as integrating data from disparate systems, rapidly assimilating clinical data, and facilitating the hand-off of patients at shift change. This use of dashboards derives from the clinical monitoring systems used in ICUs that continually monitor patient vital signs and sound alarms when patients become unstable. Unlike systems that focus on a single physiological measure, dashboards attempt to draw information from many sources and provide a single source of information to care givers.

Morgan et al. (2008) reported on the use of dashboards to track the number of unsigned radiology reports. The dashboard was designed to integrate a picture-archiving and communication system in which films are read with a radiology information system that incorporates the report-signing function. The study documents a statistically significant reduction in report signing time, from 22.5 hours prior to implementation to 17.7 hours with an integrated dashboard that allowed radiologists to launch the report-editing application. Two primary benefits of this initiative were system linkage and continuous status updates. Users knew how many records were incomplete and could sign off on reports without logging into another system.

Dashboards address the simple need of workers to know the goals toward which they are working and their progress. Dashboards identify what is measured (things that can be changed and that, if improved, will advance the organization's goals), define the measure and how it will be measured, identify where the data will be drawn from, establish targets, and determine how the reports will be produced and distributed. Where these challenges have been met, organizations have produced an effective management tool that enhances communication and performance. Serb (2011) reports that Cleveland Clinic has instituted dashboard monitoring systems to track the use of information and found departments that frequently access information have better performance than less-frequent users.

Implementation Strategies

The text has emphasized how to use quality tools, but these abilities will be of little use if the holders of these skills cannot convince their fellow employees to act on the knowledge produced. Successful implementation of a quality improvement program is based on planning, execution of the plan, and postexecution control.

The *planning* phase requires understanding of the quality issue to be tackled, since different problems require different staff and resources. The execution phase requires that the prerequisites for change be in place. Table 14.6 notes that this includes top management support, the resources and infrastructure to complete the task, and successfully communicating the need for the change to employees. Establishing the case for change requires convincing people who may be content with their current work that they can do things better, which will improve patient satisfaction and enhance their job satisfaction.

Table 14.6 Prerequisites for Successful Implementation

1.	Need for change
2.	Top management commitment
3.	Resource commitment
4.	Receptive and able culture
5.	Explicit plan
6.	Communication
7.	Execution

Making a case for change to medical staff may emphasize clinical outcomes (high mortality or morbidity rates) or treatments costs that are out of line with comparable institutions. Patient and payer demands or regulatory and accreditation requirements may also be cited to encourage employees to embrace new ways of doing things. Perhaps the most effective method of encouraging change is to focus on areas in which the medical staff believes improvement is needed and start with these initiatives.

Effecting change in administrative areas—registration, transportation, housekeeping, dietary, medical records, accounts receivable, and so on—requires building a compelling rationale based on data. The quality management staff may emphasize the financial cost of the current process, or the degree of error produced. The number of errors and the costs they create should be pointed out; for example, how much product must be discarded due to poor performance, or how much work must be redone or corrected?

The desires of patients, regulators, and accreditors may also be referenced to convince employees of the need for change. Regardless of whether a clinical or an administrative change is sought, those seeking change must consider the cost of implementing it and the probability of the change successfully being carried through. It makes little sense to undertake a quixotic goal that will yield little and consume employee goodwill.

Assuming upper management supports the quality program and has committed to providing resources to carry through the initiative, another component is organizational climate. Are employees likely to embrace the need for change and be capable of changing? A need for change, upper management support, and additional resources are insufficient to produce improvement. In *Bureaucrats in Business*, the World Bank (1995) noted the difficulty in implementing change to state-owned enterprises in third world countries. They identified three criteria as being essential to change: **political desirability**, **political feasibility**, and **credibility**.

Political desirability results from an economic crisis that makes it impossible to continue operations as they functioned in the past. Political feasibility requires securing the support of stakeholders whose cooperation is vital to success. Finally, credibility addresses whether management has in the past followed through on its pronouncements. According to the World Bank, if any condition is absent, the probability of change is small. These three conditions pertain as much to health care organizations as they do to other organizations; employees will resist change if they do not see a compelling reason for change or if they do not believe management will follow through. Thus political feasibility is concerned with how to encourage employee buy-in. Table 14.7 details some of the methods used to induce change. The World Bank emphasizes that change occurs only if there is a pressing need for change, if resisters can be brought on board, and if management has a track record of carry-through on initiatives.

Once the organization is set to move forward, the initiative must be planned. The plan consists of assembling the project team (who and what skills), researching the initiative (what quality tools have been used to study the phenomenon, what changes have been used to improve outcomes, what level of performance is achievable), identifying the key activities to be implemented, identifying where the initiative will be introduced, designating a point person who will assume primary responsibility, establishing a time schedule for completion and for how and when results will distributed.

Once the plan is set, it must be communicated to all affected parties. After starting the program, no one should be surprised by what is being

political desirability
an economic crisis that makes it impossible for an organization to function as it did in the past

political feasibility
the ability to secure the support for change from essential stakeholders

credibility
the reputation of management for following through on plans with action

Table 14.7 Inducing Change

Traditional Methods	
1.	Education
2.	Input
3.	Feedback
4.	Administrative barriers
5.	Positive feedback
6.	Negative feedback
Newer Methods	
1.	Incentive methods
2.	Compensation: capitation, risk pools, and the like
3.	Profiling
4.	Recognition
5.	Leadership opportunities
6.	Economic credentialing
7.	Equity

Source: DB Nash, JB Coombs, and H Leider, 1999, *The Three Faces of Quality*, American College of Physician Executives, Amelia Island, FL.

done or why it is being done. Lack of communication is a prime reason for mistakes in everyday activities; lack of communication when planning new behaviors can be fatal for new initiatives.

Execution is carrying the plan into action and dealing with any contingencies that arise. The first step in executing the plan is to establish a baseline by collecting and analyzing data (if this was not done in the planning phase). The second step is to initiate changes as required. New procedures should be written and distributed, and employees should be trained on their new procedures. If new equipment is needed, it should be in place and employees trained on its use prior to the expected start date. After the start date, the point person and management should be on site to assist employees with any questions or difficulties they may encounter with the new procedures and ensure that new work patterns are implemented. The duty of management is to facilitate employee work; their involvement and visibility in the early stages of the program is essential to the success of the plan.

The results of the changes should be fed back to the work group as soon as possible to reinforce the importance of the change. The results will allow the work group to experience the satisfaction of their efforts if outcomes and satisfaction improve, or to adjust the plan if results are less than expected. Continual feedback and reinforcement is essential to ensure that desired changes become a normal part of employees' daily activities.

Postexecution control requires continuation of the reporting initiated during the execution phase. The goal of quality management is to permanently improve how an organization operates. To achieve long-lasting improvement, employees must see fundamental and sustained changes in the organization. Quality initiatives must be followed through, employees must receive continual feedback on performance to reinforce the point that quality goals are not a passing fad, and workers must have a personal interest in achieving targets.

We have discussed the components of the plan and organizational culture, but is the organization appropriately designed to succeed (or to derive maximum benefit from its resources)? *Organizational architecture* encompasses two concepts. One concerns physical space, and the other deals with responsibility for decision making, performance incentives, and monitoring systems. We are concerned with the organizational architecture as it pertains to human action. Brickley, Smith, and Zimmerman, hold that decision-making rights, reward systems, and performance evaluation must reinforce each other and that the absence of, deficiency in, or misdirection of any factor will undermine the achievement of organizational goals (1997, 173).

According to Brickley, Smith, and Zimmerman, employees must be given the authority to make decisions in their areas of expertise. The goal is to make timely decisions and provide rapid service to customers; this requires delegating decision-making rights to the lowest appropriate level. These decisions include purchasing, input mix (what resources are used to produce product), product mix (what products are produced), pricing, promotion, and capital investment. However, delegating decision-making rights creates an opportunity for employees to act in self-interested ways that could harm the organization and its customers.

The ability to make self-interested decisions calls forth the necessity to evaluate performance. The job of management is to ensure that employees are acting in the best interest of the organization and customers. The role of the performance-monitoring system is to determine whether good or bad decisions are being made and to assess the appropriateness of the actions that arise from these decisions. If poor decisions are being made, they need to be stopped; conversely, organizations need to promote decisions and actions that add value: Is the organization measuring and monitoring the right things?

Another component is to establish incentive systems that align the goals of the organization with the goals of individual workers. Employees whose activities create value should share in the value created; that is, they should see their pay increase or receive bonuses. The organization should drive its own goals by establishing a compensation system that taps an individual's desire for self-betterment. The beauty of organizational architecture can now be fully seen. Individual employees should have the authority to make value-adding decisions and undertake value-adding activities, have a personal stake in reaching organizational goals, and be effectively monitored to ensure targets are met. Successful organizations understand that decision-making rights, performance monitoring, and incentive systems must be properly structured and mutually reinforcing to achieve their goals.

The absence of any component will undermine the performance of a system. Assume an employee lacks authority. He may know what to do, have an incentive to do so, and be effectively monitored but cannot initiate change, and so nothing gets done. In the absence of a value-sharing compensation system, an employee may have authority and be monitored but have no incentive to introduce change, so opportunities may be left uncaptured. The lack of an effective monitoring system may perhaps be the most dangerous. An employee with decision-making rights working under a compensation system that rewards self-interested behavior could undertake actions that damage the organization but enrich himself. A common example of this is when salespeople in a sales commission system sell the products that provide them with highest sales commissions rather than those that provide the organization with the highest profit or those that the customer needs. The Canadian health care system provides a second example. Canadian hospitals are reimbursed on occupancy, and their average LOS in 2006 was 7.3 days, compared to 5.6 in the United States (OECD 2009). Supplier-induced demand parallels this situation; physicians have the ability to order tests and procedures that increase health care expenditures but may provide little to no benefit to patients. Conflicting incentives is a dilemma, and no reimbursement system to date has been able to reconcile the convergent interests of patients, payers, and providers.

The preceding discussion addressed broad issues of organizational design. However, quality improvement initiatives are most frequently undertaken at a departmental level, where a variety of approaches are available to enhance the receptivity of the care givers and to increase the odds of successful implementation. Ellrodt et al. (1997) defined a number of tactics to increase providers' willingness to change their practice patterns and adopt evidence-based guidelines and pathways. The first approach recognizes that providers are busy people working under severe time constraints. Short manuals and executive summaries that provide a synopsis of evidence and expected benefits are preferred because they respect providers' time constraints. The second approach addresses who communicates and how requests for change are communicated to providers. The use of respected peers (also known as champions) often increases the willingness of providers to consider change. The use of one-on-one sessions rather than large, impersonal groups has been shown to be effective in changing practice patterns.

A third factor that increases the probability of successful change is concurrent feedback and reinforcement. People want to see that their efforts were successful; the ability to demonstrate that the change has produced the desired results is essential to reinforce the change. Without feedback, people will often return to their prior ways of doing things. Feedback can be made more effective and immediate if it can be incorporated into clinical information and reminder systems by which providers will be alerted to desired behaviors that improve patient care.

A last method to induce change is incentives. Table 14.7 includes a variety of options that attempt to align the incentives of providers and employees with the objectives of the organization. These incentives are both nonmonetary and monetary. Nonmonetary incentives include recognition and leadership opportunities. Monetary compensation includes salary, bonuses, and equity positions. Third-party payers can also encourage change through their use of preferred provider networks by including in the network providers who meet quality standards. The power of preferred provider networks is their ability to direct covered patients to network providers by using patient financial incentives, such as lower copays for in-network providers.

Summary

This chapter expands the quality horizon by emphasizing benchmarks. Benchmarks are simply comparing one set of results against another. Benchmarking is frequently performed across organizations, with superior results in another organization spurring the benchmarking organization toward improvement. The goal of benchmarking is to ensure that best practices are utilized across an industry. In health care, the goal of every organization should be the best possible care for their patients, and this goal cannot be accomplished in isolation. Health care providers must compare their outcomes with those of other organizations to ensure they are doing all they can for their patients.

Balanced scorecards and dashboards are two tools used to communicate performance and goals to employees. Balanced scorecards provide an organization perspective on goals and how the organization expects to meet their goals. Balanced scorecards recognize that employee skills and organization resources are the bedrock of performance and that improved performance requires nurturing of employees and resources. Skilled and motivated employees working with the appropriate resources will be able to complete their tasks effectively, efficiently, and in a way that pleases customers. Customer satisfaction and loyalty become the means to achieving the organization's objectives.

Dashboards are designed to guide department actions. Dashboards may track key performance indicators that follow patient outcomes or resource use. These reporting dashboards compile information on a periodic basis to influence future performance. Dashboards have also been designed for use at the patient level, where real-time information on patient vital signs and team performance can be displayed to influence current action. Dashboards should tie department objectives to the larger goals of the organization.

Finally, a plan is only as good as its implementation. Those implementing change must have a clear idea of what they want to achieve and determine whether the organization culture is receptive to change. If the organizational culture is unreceptive, the first step is to convince employees of the necessity of change. After persuading employees, the team must carefully define what it wants to achieve and how to create employee buy-in. It is essential that any improvement plan contain clear statements of what behavior and goals are sought, define responsibilities, set timetables for achievement, and establish reporting systems by which employees can see the results of their efforts. Postimplementation control must continually emphasize the commitment of the organization to long-term change, and performance assessment will be a standard part of future department operations.

KEY TERMS

Balanced scorecard

Competitive benchmarking

Credibility

Customer intimacy

Customer perspective

Customer relationship
    management (CRM)

Dashboard

Financial perspective

Functional benchmarking

Industry benchmarking

Internal benchmarking

Internal perspective

Learning and growth perspective

Operational excellence

Political desirability

Political feasibility

Product leadership

REVIEW QUESTIONS

1. What are the benefits of benchmarking?

2. What are obstacles to the use of benchmarking?

3. Using CMS Hospital Compare, locate benchmarks for a hospital in your area. How does its performance compare to that of its two closest competitors?

4. Develop a balanced scorecard for the organization you work in.

5. Develop a dashboard for the department you work in.

6. What is the role of balanced scorecards, value chain, and dashboards in achieving organizational goals?

7. Discuss the three phases of implementation.

8. What can managers do to encourage change?

References

Beckford J, 1998, *Quality: A Critical Introduction*, Routledge, New York, NY.

Brickley J, Smith C, and Zimmerman J, 1997, *Managerial Economics and Organizational Architecture*, Irwin, Chicago, IL.

Camp RC, 1989, *Benchmarking: The Search for Industry Best Practices That Lead to Superior Performance*, ASQC Quality Press, Milwaukee, WI.

Camp RC and DeToro IJ, 1999, Benchmarking, in *Juran's Quality Handbook*, 5th ed., edited by JM Juran and AB Godfrey, 12.1–12.20, McGraw-Hill, New York, NY.

Codman EA, (1914) 1996, *A Study in Hospital Efficiency*, Joint Commission on Accreditation of Healthcare Organizations, Oakbrook Terrace, IL. Citations refer to JCAHO edition.

Curran TA and Ladd A, 2000, *SAP R3 Business Blueprint*, Prentice Hall PTR, Upper Saddle River, NJ.

Egan M, 2006, Clinical Dashboards: Impact on Workflow, Care Quality, and Patient Safety, *Critical Care Nursing Quarterly* 29 (4): 354–361.

Ellrodt G, Cook DJ, Lee J, Cho M, Hunt D, and Weingarten S, 1997, Evidence-Based Disease Management, *JAMA* 278 (20): 1687–1692.

Goetsch D and Davis S, 2010, *Quality Management for Organizational Excellence*, 6th ed., Pearson Prentice Hall, Upper Saddle River, NJ.

Heizer J and Render B, 1996, *Production and Operations Management*, 4th ed., Prentice Hall, Upper Saddle River, NJ.

Huang S, Chang W, Chen P, Lee H, and Yang M, 2004, Using a Balanced Scorecard to Improve the Performance of an Emergency Department, *Nursing Economics* 22 (3): 140–146.

Juran JM and Godfrey AB, 1999, *Juran's Quality Handbook*, 5th ed., McGraw-Hill, New York, NY.

Kaplan R and Norton D, 2000, Having Trouble with Your Strategy? Then Map It, *Harvard Business Review* (September–October 2000): 167–176.

McAvoy J, 1999, Make a Difference with CRM Solutions, *Health Management Technology* 20 (8): 26.

Meliones J, Alton M, Mericle J, Ballard R, Cesari J, Frush K, and Mistry K, 2008, 10-Year Experience Integrating Strategic Performance Improvement Initiatives: Can the Balanced Scorecard, Six Sigma, and Team Training All Thrive in a Single Hospital? in *Advances in Patient Safety: New Directions and Alternative Approaches*, edited by Henriksen K, Battles JB, Keyes MA, Grady ML, vol. 3, *Performance and Tools*, 13 pages, Agency for Healthcare Research and Quality, Rockville, MD.

Morgan M, Branstetter B, Lionetti D, Richardson J, and Chang P, 2008, The Radiology Digital Dashboard: Effects on Report Turnaround Time, *Journal of Digital Imaging* 21 (1): 50–58.

Nash DB, Coombs JB, and Leider H, 1999, *The Three Faces of Quality*, American College of Physician Executives, Amelia Island, FL.

OECD (Organisation for Economic Co-operation and Development), *OECD Health Data 2009*.

OR Manager, 2011, Tracking Data, Changing Behavior, *OR Manager* 27 (2): 10–11.

Park K, Smaltz D, McFadden D, and Souba W, 2010, The Operating Room Dashboard, *Journal of Surgical Research* 164: 294–300.

Serb C, 2011, Effective Dashboards: What to Measure and How to Show It, *Hospital and Health Networks* 85 (6): 42–46.

Swayne L, Duncan WJ, and Ginter P, 2008, *Strategic Management of Health Care Organizations*, 6th ed., Jossey-Bass, San Francisco, CA.

World Bank, 1995, *Bureaucrats in Business*, Oxford University Press, New York, NY.

CHAPTER 15

THE FUTURE OF QUALITY MANAGEMENT IN HEALTH CARE

Introduction

Valentin Bondarenko died March 23, 1961, of extensive burns. At the time of his death, Bondarenko was on his way to becoming the most famous man in the world. Bondarenko was the cosmonaut chosen to man Vostok 1. Had he lived, he, and not Yuri Gagarin, would have been the first man in space.

Bondarenko died as a result of a fire in the oxygen-rich pressure chamber in which he was training. News of his death did not reach the West until 1980. Bondarenko's death is important to quality management as it highlights the need for dissemination of error. On January 27, 1967, a fire started in Apollo 1 as it sat on its Florida launch pad, killing its three-man crew. The cause was a fire in an oxygen-rich environment, similar to that which killed Bondarenko (Teitel 2012). Had his death been publicized, the deaths of Virgil Grissom, Edward White, and Roger Chaffee might have been avoided. The lack of disclosure stems from two sources. First, the Cold War was on, and one can understand Soviet reluctance to share information which could have helped an opponent. Second, those in power too often resort to silence and cover-up when they do not want to have their mistakes publicized.

Public disclosure is essential to ensure that knowledge gains are not the result of learning by error but rather learning from others. When we learn from others, we do not have to repeat their mistakes. Others note that NASA had experienced an oxygen fire in 1966, and the U.S. Navy and Air Force had experienced three other fires under similar circumstances that took two lives in the five years

LEARNING OBJECTIVES

1. Review the history, philosophy, and goals of quality improvement and the impact of variation on performance

2. Reiterate the role of process analysis tools and SPC in quality improvement

3. Understand the role of practice policies; case, disease, and outcomes management; and reporting systems

4. Increase the value of health care services to patients

5. Speculate regarding the future of quality management in health care and understand the conditions required for reform

denial

refusal to accept the fact that failure has occurred or attempt to conceal the failure from others

repair

actions designed to address the symptoms of a failure rather than address the cause of the failure typically involving local fixes and/or public relation efforts

reform

comprehensive system actions designed to eliminate failure or reduce their severity when elimination is not possible

encapsulation

attribution of a failure to a particular set of circumstances unlikely to reoccur, typically to rationalize away the need for action

suppression

deliberative attempts to prevent knowledge of a failure from achieving widespread recognition

preceding the Apollo 1 accident. While knowledge of Bondarenko's death may not have changed NASA's actions, it certainly would have heightened their awareness of the danger they faced.

Disclosure is the basis for Joint Commission's sentinel events policy, the third goal of which is "to increase the general knowledge about sentinel events, their contributing factors, and strategies for prevention" (Joint Commission 2011, SE1). Reason notes that there are three major reactions to failure: **denial**, **repair**, and **reform** (1990, 211). Denial refuses to accept the fact that failure has occurred or attempts to conceal the failure from others. Reason labels the first response **encapsulation**. The failure was the result of a particular set of circumstances unlikely to reoccur, a freak accident. Categorizing events as freak accidents frequently results in no corrective action being taken, as people rationalize that the set of circumstances will not reoccur. The second response is **suppression**. If the error is not known, then it is as if it did not happen. Corrective action is often not taken when errors are suppressed, as activity may raise the question as to why processes are being changed. Change runs counter to the old adage, "if it ain't broke, don't fix it."

Repair leads to public relations and local fixes. Public relations repair is designed to improve the image of the organization rather than how it works. Typical PR responses include advertising campaigns, such as "We Care." As seen after the Deepwater Horizon spill in the Gulf of Mexico, BP attempted to provide information on the magnitude of the accident, when the oil flow would be stopped, and the impact on the local environments and economies. BP hoped to impress local citizens, legislators, and regulators that they were being forthright in their handling of the situation and would accept responsibility for damages caused. On the other hand, some failures are met with attempts to shift blame to others ("it's the subcontractor's fault") or change the subject ("we did bad, but look at all the jobs we provide to the local community"). A second response is local repair. Local repair attempts to fix a problem at the point of occurrence but does not extend corrective actions to other locations. The introductory case provides an example. Fires in high-oxygen areas occurred at NASA and in the Navy and Air Force, but no one recognized that these types of accidents had occurred in different locations and that a comprehensive solution was needed to address all areas at risk.

Reform is the best response to failure because it seeks effective and comprehensive solutions to problems. Reform requires dissemination of information on failures to all parties that could be affected and requires reorganization of processes. People are often unwilling to admit failure and be subjected to scrutiny, or to admit a lack of understanding of current process or error-reduction methods; this is why many organizations take the path of denial and repair. True reform of processes requires time, knowledge, and an ability to change the organization. All three are in short supply, and since all three are required to improve processes and outcomes, it is easy to see why reform often flounders.

Reason provides a seven-part system for reform, shown in Table 15.1. Reason's reforms depend upon building simplified operational models in which actions, effects, and goals are understood by all. The actions, effects, and goals are observable, ensuring accountability. If action, effects, or outcomes are not as expected, they will be recognized and improved as soon as possible. Systems should be standardized and flexible. Systems should never depend on a single person; rather, others should be able to step in to perform duties necessary to produce the desired goal. The system itself should be designed to reduce the likelihood of failure through the use of constraints and to allow rapid identification of error and minimization of harm when error occurs (Reason 1990, 236).

Table 15.1 Reason's System Reforms

1.	Reconcile theoretical and real-world information into an operational model
2.	Simplify the process
3.	Make execution and evaluation visible: what needs to be done, and what outputs or outcomes are produced?
4.	Establish mappings between:
	a. intentions and action
	b. actions and effects
	c. actual system state and perceived system state
	d. system state and needs of user
5.	Utilize natural and artificial constraints and safeguards
6.	Establish error detection and recovery systems
7.	Standardize the process

Source: J Reason, 1990, *Human Error,* Cambridge University Press, New York, 236.

Bringing It All Together

The recommended quality management structure should now be clear. The structure parallels the Three Faces of Quality advocated by Nash, Coombs, and Leider (1999). Quality management is designed to ensure that a desired goal is consistently achieved and must be built on a solid foundation of theory and tools. After a goal is selected, employees must precisely define it and decide how it will be measured. Measurement is the next step: Is the process meeting expectations or does it require improvement? If improvement is desired, a plan must be developed that can produce the desired results. Continuous monitoring must take place to ensure that processes meeting expectations continue to do so and, when change is needed, that improvements produce the desired outcomes.

If quality improvement is to be successful, it must start with the desire to improve outcomes and processes. This desire may emanate from a charismatic, inspirational leader motivating an entire organization, or it may arise from the mind of a single individual capturing an opportunity to improve the lives of his or her patients. Those initiating quality management actions must always keep in mind that the purpose is to improve lives, not to achieve the appearance of improvement or meet bureaucratic objectives.

Once a goal is selected, Figure 15.1 shows how the quality improvement team can move toward the realization of the goal. Changing established processes should not be undertaken without understanding the system and the continuous quality improvement (CQI) philosophy. Quality management holds that improvement is a continuous process and defines the relationship between workers and management, and between workers and systems. Backstopping this understanding is statistics; the concepts of central tendency and variation provide the key elements necessary to evaluate the performance of systems. Is performance predictable, or is it not? Obviously, an organization faces different problems if it can or if it cannot predict what it will produce. Understanding human behavior, why people err, and reengineering—how systems can be improved to reduce error—are critical information to possess before attempting to improve a process.

Goal	Theory	Tools	Outcome	Realized Goal
Improve patient outcomes	TQM/CQI philosophy	Process analysis	Evidence-based medicine	Better care and outcomes
	Human behavior and error	Statistical process control	Practice policies	
	Reengineering	Physician profiles	Case management	
		Disease management		
		Outcomes management		
		Benchmarks		
	Foundation	**Means**	**Ends**	

Figure 15.1 Bringing It All Together

Statistics, human behavior, and reengineering provide the foundation for analyzing the performance of systems. Process analysis tools and statistical process control (SPC) provide the means to document and evaluate performance. Is a particular system stable or unstable, and is it meeting targets? If a system is stable and meeting its target, is it reaching its potential? Benchmarking and other tools are used to compare outcomes across individuals and organizations. Employees and organizations should strive for excellence. Knowledge of how others perform may establish a goal, but in the end an organization's objective should be to surpass this target.

Measuring performance and setting targets is fine, but the true challenge is to create a plan to get there. Disease and outcomes management define systems designed to guide treatment to desired results for patients afflicted by certain diseases and to establish outcome standards and build care around meeting or exceeding these targets. When improvement is desired, it is essential that employees be provided with new ideas, supplies, tools, and processes. As Albert Einstein noted, insanity is doing the same thing over and over again and expecting different results. Improvement will occur only if fundamental change occurs within individuals and systems. The goal of Part III, the section on medical practice management, is to provide information on systems that have yielded better outcomes in multiple health care settings.

Quality management seeks to reduce variation in care and improve patient outcomes through knowledge and appropriate use of tools and standards. When there is clear evidence of superior outcomes arising from a certain path of care (evidence-based medicine) and patients overwhelmingly favor the treatment in full knowledge of its expected benefits and costs, then practice should adhere to the standard. Clinical practice guidelines attempt to define the preferred path of care and supply information to care givers to simplify clinical decision making and allow everyone involved in care to understand what should happen and when. Not every case can be managed to a standard, so case management ensures that patients with complex conditions and multiple complications or comorbidities are individually handled.

Foremost, the goal of quality management is not the creation of a system but the improvement of patient health. When quality management goes off track, as it frequently does, the means becomes the end and documentation and the idea of management supersedes the goal of improvement. Care givers must always remember that quality management ideas and tools are only one way to achieve the goal of improving patients' health. When properly used, quality management tools will improve patient health and enrich the jobs of health care workers.

Quality and Variation

Quality is a key to keeping customers happy, and the first hurdle that must be cleared is to define what quality is. In 1931 Shewhart recognized the vagueness of the common usage of the term *quality* in his classic book, *Economic Control of Quality of Manufactured Product*. Shewhart declared, "Without exception every conceptual 'something' is really a group of conceptions more elementary in form" ([1931], 1981, 38). We must first recognize what these more elementary concepts are. We can neither measure nor control something we cannot define.

Quality, like the words *strategic* and *sustainable*, is a word that people use rather loosely with the implicit assumption that it imparts a common meaning. However, it is quite clear when people discuss quality health care or quality education that everyone is not talking about the same thing. Although we all prefer a quality product or service to one that fails to meet basic expectations, this simple truism does nothing to advance us toward producing better goods and services.

Quality encompasses both what is produced and how it is produced and delivered. Consumers have different expectations of what a product or service should deliver and how they wish to be treated during the consumption process; there is no common measure of quality. In Chapter One, a product was assessed based on the characteristics of the good or services offered, selection and choice, how the product was provided to the consumer, timeliness of delivery, the attributes of the environment in which the product is transacted, and the price of the product. The five Ds of health care quality—death, disability, disease, discomfort, and dissatisfaction—remind us that there is more to the creation of a valued patient experience than simply addressing a medical condition.

The second hurdle, after we create an operational definition and quality measure, is to collect data. Semmelweis, Nightingale, and Codman demonstrate the power of data collection. By accumulating and analyzing data on deaths due to puerperal fever, in military field hospitals, and under anesthesia, they were able to dramatically reduce mortality rates. In each case, the importance of the deaths had been minimized and accepted as inevitable by those in positions of authority due to their lack of understanding of the magnitude of the problem and unwillingness to have their performance scrutinized. Semmelweis, Nightingale, and Codman all achieved dramatic local improvements and, more importantly, laid the foundation for systemic reform. Their devotion and work continues to be a beacon for those seeking to improve health care outcomes for all patients.

While the pursuit of quality improvement continued in the 20th century, its stature received a tremendous boost from Donabedian's structure-process-outcome framework and the analyses of John Wennberg. Wennberg and others focused on differences in utilization of medical services, demonstrating that similar patients were regularly treated differently.

While differences in treatment (and cost) would be acceptable if they led to improved outcomes, Wennberg and others have been unable to conclude that higher utilization of services leads to better outcomes.

The inability to document better outcomes from more intensive treatment and the failure to provide basic care have led to greater scrutiny of health care. Is society receiving an appropriate return for its investment in health care? The clearest example of this movement is the recent changes in Medicare reimbursement that deny payment for hospital-acquired infections and that give incentives for meeting Medicare quality indicators (and reimbursement reductions for hospitals that do not reach specified thresholds). Health care, while rapidly incorporating new technologies and achieving stunning advances in life expectancy, has yet to fundamentally alter its administrative and organizational practices, so differences in practice styles and patient outcomes continue to characterize present-day medicine.

Quality Management Tools

Semmelweis, Nightingale, and Codman had to develop their own measures and tools to accomplish their goals. Today we are blessed with a variety of tools that can be applied to health care processes. Other industries discovered after their products gained widespread consumer acceptance that their customers wanted better products, thus ushering in the era of process improvement. Starting with Shewhart, process improvement has dramatically improved goods and services through an intensively analytical approach to defining what customers want, how production is performed, and how products perform in the hands of customers.

The goal of health care should be to incorporate the CQI mindset and process analysis tools and SPC into treatment in a manner that adds value and does not multiply work. Quality management tools will add value if they can improve patient outcomes and the efficiency of practice. It is unreasonable to state that these tools will reduce what we ask care givers to do. The more important question is, will it reduce workload? This is the idea behind "do it right the first time." Can we reduce what we have to do by working smarter? If we deliver the right care at the right time in the right setting, can we improve outcomes while reducing the number of tests, treatments, and procedures?

The answer is an unequivocal yes. Quality management will change what we ask care givers to do. Physicians, instead of managing patients, must manage patient care systems. Physicians often do not need to manage day-to-day treatment but could provide more value to their patients and the health care system by building effective and dependable processes and focusing on exceptions. It is easy to see that health care systems can be improved by physicians reorienting themselves to higher-order decision making, such as, how do treatments perform across patients, are treatment processes working as they should, and does an individual patient require special attention? Is the standard treatment appropriate, or can it be improved? Like random clinical trials, standardized treatment provides a control group to compare alternative approaches without having to worry if the outcome is the result of an innovation or changes in other treatment variables.

The question is: How do we get there? Health care education, whether designed to train physicians, nurses, allied health personnel, or managers, does not devote enough attention to quality management tools, so care givers must learn these tools in a haphazard way while accomplishing other duties. Health care education at all levels must focus on instilling knowledge of quality management tools into their graduates if patients are to receive maximum benefit from their treatment.

The text explored tools to identify problems, their causes, and potential solutions, and to monitor corrective actions to determine their effectiveness. The logical chain exemplified by these four tasks forms the basis of quality improvement. First, a worker must identify a less-than-acceptable or less-than-desired outcome. After identifying the opportunity for improvement, the worker must understand the system and why superior outcomes are not produced. Of course, the worker could be wrong about the problem and its cause, which complicates the identification of solutions. This third task is the least quantitatively based.

Once a problem and its cause are correctly identified, there is the challenge of picking a solution from a catalog of possible improvements. But choosing a solution will be limited by knowledge and availability of resources. What can be done given the situation and culture? Choosing a solution often comes down to arriving at a consensus among the assembled group. To improve the solution choice, the quality improvement team should thoroughly review the literature to see who else has faced a similar issue, what they implemented, and what was achieved. The probabilistic nature of identifying an effective solution requires monitoring performance after the corrective action is implemented.

efficacious

having the power to produce the desired effect in ideal circumstances

A solution may be effective (able to perform in typical operating conditions); it may be **efficacious** (capable of performing in ideal circumstances) but ineffective; or it may be inefficacious. The quality improvement team cannot assume that a correction will be effective but must monitor outcomes to ensure that the selected solution works and continues to work. Quality management does not provide a one-time, quick-fix solution but only yields significant rewards to those prepared to devote continuous attention to desired outcomes.

Root cause analysis (RCA) and failure mode and effects analysis (FMEA) techniques were reviewed to introduce the reader to investigative techniques. RCA and FMEA can be used to fulfill the goals sets forth by the Joint Commission in their sentinel events and leadership or continuous quality improvement standards, these chapters introduce the reader to the larger issues of the relationship between unsafe practices and problems, investigative tools, and prevention and recovery techniques.

SPC provides the icing on the cake for investigative techniques and statistical tools. SPC is driven by the goal of the quality improvement team and can be applied to processes and outcomes. What was done, what occurred, and is it acceptable? SPC seeks to identify processes experiencing major change and epitomizes the idea of **freedom through control**. Workers are left free to do their work as long as a process is capable (achieving the desired outcome) and stable (operating within its historical parameters). When expectations are not met or significant change is observed, employees must discover the cause of lower-than-desired performance. SPC is built on identifying whether change is a normal part of the operation of a system or the result of new factors affecting performance. By recognizing the difference between natural and special cause variation, employees do not have to waste time exploring routine fluctuations. It is only when special causes arise that investigation and possibly correction are required. SPC should be applied to critical processes where failure may have adverse effects on outcomes; Chapters Six through Eight reviewed a variety of case studies demonstrating the improvements that resulted from the use of SPC.

freedom through control
the idea that workers should be left free to perform their work as long as the work equals or surpasses defined standards

Deming (1986) is well known for his assertion that 94% of all problems are due to management, that is, due to the failure of management to control the system in which employees are working. It is the duty of management to design systems that minimize the chance of failure and to monitor systems to determine whether they are meeting expectations. This duty can be fulfilled only if management understands the system and is willing to take on the difficult and sensitive job of addressing performance. In unstable systems, managers must identify the cause of variation and correct it. In stable systems that fail to produce desired outcomes, managers are responsible for determining why the system does not perform better. Systems belong to managers, and it is their duty to create systems in which workers can be successful. History provides a long record of the failures of organizations that could not manage their processes and allowed more nimble competitors to draw their customers away.

Quality improvement does not need to be a top-down affair in which upper management (or external parties) decide objectives and how they will be pursued but rather can be decentralized to every department and employee. Employees closest to a process have the greatest opportunity to identify potential improvements, understand how processes can be changed, and introduce change. It is the job of management to impart organizational goals and build employee skills so performance can be "owned" at the local level and so we can see greater employee commitment and ongoing improvement.

It is easy to see how a different distribution of functions can release physicians from mundane tasks, enrich the jobs of nursing and other personnel, and improve patient care and satisfaction. By focusing on systems (rather than individuals), physicians will have more control and more time to devote to exceptional cases. Other health care workers will have greater latitude to perform their duties without oversight (as long as measures fall within defined limits), and patients can be incorporated into the medical decision-making process and monitoring the progress of care.

Medical Practice Management

In medicine, diagnosis is only the starting point for treatment. The effectiveness of treatment is dependent on identifying the cause of a medical condition, but cure is determined by the ability to carry out a plan of action. Similarly process analysis and SPC provide the means to identify suboptimal performance, but this ability will be of little use if effective improvement plans cannot be implemented. Medical practice management tools move the discussion from tools and techniques that can be applied across industries to interventions specific to health care. Chapters Eleven through Fourteen explore clinical decision making, evaluating medical effectiveness, and specific tools to manage, monitor, and measure treatment. While process analysis tools and SPC can identify systems that are not meeting expectations, health care presents special challenges and requires unique interventions to improve patient outcomes. Chapter Eleven explores the standardization of treatment through practice policies and demonstrates that the applicability of practice policies depends on the evidence base on which they rest and the unanimity of patient preferences.

Chapter Twelve provides examples of how care can be standardized using case, disease, and outcomes management. These patient care management techniques target different populations (high risk, similar medical conditions) and pursue different ends (processes versus results) but use similar assessment, planning, education, implementation, coordination, monitoring, and evaluation methodologies to improve care.

Chapter Thirteen explores the sensitive area of how care givers should be evaluated and whether performance should be publicly reported. When making comparisons across providers, it is essential that patients be similar or that differences in patients be quantified and considered when assessing performance. Risk adjustment details the difficulty in achieving valid comparisons and highlights how patients' clinical and nonclinical factors and random events, in addition to treatment, affect the clinical and nonclinical outcomes of care. Risk adjustment will remain an imprecise science, so comparisons should be considered tentative.

Statistics reminds us that small differences in outcomes may not be significant and that we should focus on large differences. When large differences in outcome are observed, we must recognize that issues other than treatment choice and performance may explain the difference. Large differences provide the starting point for examination and discussion; they do not supply necessary information to draw conclusions.

Chapter Fourteen moves away from the more contentious issues of individual comparison toward the measurement of organizational and departmental performance. The advantage of comparing large groups of patients is that we can expect differences among patients to average out and organizational comparisons are less sensitive than individual comparisons. The ability to compare results against other groups or individuals is essential to improvement and allows employees to understand where an organization wants to go in terms of performance and demonstrates that others have been able to achieve better outcomes.

Balanced scorecards revisit the idea that organizations must explicitly state their goals and establish a roadmap of how they intend to achieve their goals. The balanced scorecard reinforces the idea that goals are achieved by instilling the necessary skills into the workforce and providing employees with the tools and equipment they require. Dashboards demonstrate how departmental and patient objectives can be monitored through the consolidation of information from disparate sources. It is always worth remembering that the purpose of comparison is not to make one group or individual look good or bad but rather to demonstrate examples of superior performance that others may emulate to improve patient outcomes.

Theory is well and good, but the real test of quality management is to restructure processes and institute a new way of thinking and performing among employees. Implementation of new processes is the key to improvement and runs the gamut from establishing a case for change to introducing incentives that align employee objectives with organizational goals. The success or failure of quality management can be judged only by the degree of improvement it achieves.

Shewhart (1981) noted that "the limit" of a system is the level of performance it is capable of producing; it is the job of management to recognize when other systems are capable of higher performance. Deming emphasizes that better performance cannot be expected when an organization continues to use the same resources and processes. Management must recognize when performance failures are the result of poor design of products or services or the result of obstacles to performance, poor instruction, poor supervision, lack of standards or measurement, supply or machinery problems, unsuitable procedures, or environmental factors (Deming 1986, 336–337). Deming's point, like Einstein's, is that improvement cannot arise from doing things in the same way they have been done in the past. Improvement requires substantive changes in people, supplies, equipment, processes, and environments and management is the primary force that can muster organization-wide change.

Value and What an Employee (or Manager) Should Do

Besides holding that 94% of problems and opportunities for improvement are due to systems and are the responsibility of management, Deming (1986) believes that people want to do a good job. When we think about why people work, it is obvious we hold jobs to earn money to purchase things, but it is also obvious we seek a sense of satisfaction or identity through our work. In health care, populated by highly educated people seeking to improve the health and lives of others, it is easy to see the truth in Deming's idea.

Health care workers want to improve the lives of their patients; they want to take actions that are instrumental in improving lives. The goal of quality management is to increase the value of health care goods and services, and this goal pertains equally to patients and care givers. Quality management can be a means by which employees find increased meaning in their work. Health care workers do not want to simply produce exams, tests, and procedures; they want to see their work improve patients' health and lives.

A quality management orientation allows employees to see the results of their work and ask: How can I do this better? Ensuring that exams, tests, and procedures contribute to better outcomes addresses job satisfaction, while the ability to analyze present practice and offer improvements leads to job enrichment. For patients with terminal conditions in which no improvement in health can be expected, it is still easy to see health care workers striving to improve the final moments of their patients' lives by relieving uncertainty and loneliness through providing information and compassion.

Poorly functioning systems deny employees the pride in workmanship they seek. Quality management, with its explicit recognition of means and ends and monitoring of outcomes, provides a means for employees to find value in their work. *Value* is another term, like *quality*, that is used loosely. An explicit measure of value will clarify thought and illuminate definitive ways of increasing value. A big-perspective formula for value is

$$\textbf{Value} = \textbf{satisfaction} \div \textbf{price} \qquad \textbf{15.1}$$

This formula uses the all-encompassing goal of satisfaction in the numerator and the price consumers pay to obtain the good or service in the denominator. Consumers buy goods to meet a need or desire, so anything that increases satisfaction or reduces the price they pay to acquire a product will increase value. The formula demonstrates that value can be increased by increasing satisfaction, decreasing price, increasing satisfaction by a greater amount than the increase in price, or decreasing satisfaction less than the decrease in price. Since decreasing customer satisfaction is not a strategy typically invoked, we will concentrate on increasing satisfaction and reducing price.

The formula leads us to ask: How can we increase patient satisfaction? There is a multitude of ways to increase a person's satisfaction in any field. In health care, satisfaction can be improved by increasing the effectiveness of care, reducing discomfort and the time required for treatment, handling patients with greater courtesy and respect, and improving the physical characteristics of the patient care facility, among other approaches.

The other primary means of increasing value is to reduce price. The ability to cut prices is constrained by the need of the organization to generate sufficient revenues to cover its resource use and reinvest in its operations. Formula 15.1 presents one way of thinking about value. A second formula presents a narrower perspective of value. The second formula presents a more objective measure of why products are purchased for those uncomfortable with the ambiguity of the term *satisfaction*. The second formula (Porter 2010, 2477) for value holds:

$$\textbf{Value} = \textbf{outcome} \div \textbf{cost} \qquad \textbf{15.2}$$

This formula is called a small-perspective formula because, unlike 15.1, where satisfaction is affected by events throughout the value chain and an individual worker may be relatively powerless to increase total patient satisfaction or reduce prices, it focuses on more controllable measures. Formula 15.2 places outcome in the numerator. It is easier to subdivide outcome because any health care encounter will include multiple intermediate outcomes, and an individual employee can see his or her contribution in one of these sub-outcomes. Similarly, employees have little control over the price charged for a product but can affect the cost of services they deliver.

Formula 15.2 places the concept of value squarely within the control of individual workers. Employees can increase or decrease value by their effect on outcomes (or sub-outcomes) and costs. To increase value, an employee must improve outcomes, decrease cost, or improve outcomes by a greater amount than the increase in costs. Again we will ignore the option of reducing costs by a greater percentage than outcomes. Outcomes move away from the subjectivity of satisfaction to a more objective measure. While two people may differ on the value of more personalized care or even the desirability of less pain or an extended life expectancy, no one can argue against an outcome, such as increase in life expectancy, an increase in functionality, less pain, or lower use of future health care services that is documented as a result of treatment. While satisfaction is subject to debate, a focus on documentable outcomes provides a clear cause and effect relationship that employees and patients can observe.

While individual employees may be unable to alter the entire treatment process or the overall attractiveness of a large medical facility, they can implement change within their sphere of influence. We have all experienced the joy of an employee who goes the extra mile by brightening their work area by bringing flowers from their garden, taking more time than necessary to visit with a patient, or doing things off-the-clock for patients. These employees create value for patients by providing service beyond what is expected, and they exemplify how we want to be treated and how we want our organizations to perform.

The shift from price to cost similarly represents a change from something an employee may have zero control over, price setting, to an area to which every employee can contribute. The means to reduce cost include increasing the efficiency of resource use (increasing productivity and decreasing waste), eliminating unvalued or low-value activities, and seeking the best priced (not necessarily the cheapest) resources. Under the DRG system, where reimbursement for inpatient services is determined by the patient's age, comorbidities and complications, and the care he or she receives, it is easy to say nothing that an employee does or does not do will change what the patient or Medicare pays, but instilling in employees the fact that everything they do consumes resources that must be recovered in one manner or another is vital. The costs of poorly performed work or of expenditure of resources that produce little or no benefit must reduce the resources that could be employed in activities that patients and payers would value and pay for.

The ramifications of poorly utilized resources include the inability to provide care to those unable to pay; lower profits, which could hamper reinvestment in the organization; and stagnant or declining incomes for employees. It is vital that workers see expenditure of resources in uses that do not produce value as a loss for society. Individuals may believe that poor resource use does not directly affect them, and they could be right, but all poorly used resources must reduce the benefits a society may have enjoyed.

Quality management provides a vehicle to pursue higher quality health care and to give employees what they want from a job: the ability to make a contribution to others. Quality management, when effectively implemented, should improve care and patient outcomes, increase patient satisfaction, reduce malpractice suits, raise employee morale, and lower costs.

Any of the benefits detailed in Table 15.2 should provide sufficient motivation to employees. These benefits, taken as a whole, should be the goal of all employees and managers.

Table 15.2 Expected Outcomes of Quality Improvement

1.	Improve care and patient outcomes
2.	Increase patient satisfaction
3.	Reduce malpractice suits
4.	Increase employee morale
5.	Lower costs

The Future of Health Care and Quality Management

It is widely reported that U.S. health outcomes are less than those in other countries. The World Health Organization ranks the United States 29th in life expectancy at birth and 43rd in infant mortality rate (WHO 2012). Beyond these rankings, it is clear that health care outcomes have improved dramatically in the United States over the last 50 years. Tables 15.3 and 15.4 (*Statistical Abstract of the United States,* 2012) demonstrate the continual increase in life expectancy and fall in infant mortality rates. Health care has played a role in both trends, as have improvements in the economy, technology, nutrition, and other areas.

Total life expectancy has increased by 8.1 years (11.6%) since 1960 while infant mortality rates decreased by 5.8 per 1,000 births (−46.0%).

Table 15.3 Expectation of Life at Birth

Year	Total	Male	Female
1960	69.7	66.6	73.1
1970	70.8	67.1	74.7
1980	73.7	70.0	77.4
1990	75.4	71.8	78.8
2000	76.8	74.1	79.3
2001	76.9	74.2	79.4
2002	76.9	74.3	79.5
2003	77.1	74.5	79.6
2004	77.5	74.9	79.9
2005	77.4	74.9	79.9
2006	77.7	75.1	80.2
2007	77.9	75.4	80.4
2008	77.8	75.3	80.3

Table 15.4 Infant Mortality Rates

Year	IMR
1980	12.6
1990	9.2
1995	7.6
2000	6.9
2001	6.8
2002	7.0
2003	6.9
2004	6.8
2005	6.9
2006	6.7
2007	6.8

While preliminary estimates indicate that life expectancy dropped by 0.1 year in 2008, long-term forecasts indicate that life expectancy will increase through 2020.

What will the future look like? Will health care remain close to its roots or will it transform itself into an industry that fully utilizes quality control methods developed over the last 200 years? It is apparent that improvements in health care technology will continue. The question is, will we accept the current level of error in the system or will we take decisive actions to make the system safer? Will we accept the level of waste (poor performance and unnecessary tests) in the system, or will we demand more for our money?

Three Conditions for Reform

Reforming health care will require three major changes: sophisticated data analysis, teamwork, and new incentives. The health care industry has resisted previous change; the shift to DRG reimbursement designed to encourage efficiency was met with unbundling of services and up-coding. The desired change did not occur. When managed care began to affect medical practice in the 1990s, the effort was short-circuited by legislative changes that restricted the ability of insurers to set standards, restrict access to services, and limit physician participation in preferred provider networks. As a result, health care spending continues to grow faster than the economy, foreshadowing a major crisis within the next 20 to 30 years.

To evolve toward better quality, health care must move toward sophisti-cated use of data rather than simply documentation. In addition to the cur-rent emphasis on documentation to guide a particular patient's treatment and to adjudicate payment, data analysis must be developed that allows all participating and affected parties to know what they should expect from treatment. Better data systems are required to determine how treatment performs across groups of patients over longer time horizons, to identify underuse, overuse, and misuse of care, and to evaluate the effectiveness of new treatments.

The Medicare Quality Initiative must be seen as only a start. Medicare's concentration on process measures and limited outcome measures fails to address the bigger issues of whether treatment improves patient lives. These measures only scratch the surface of what distinguishes one health care provider from another. One can see that there may not be any distinguish-able differences between organizations in the tests they run or the outcomes they achieve, but there may be substantial differences in how patients view these organizations. More successful organizations will understand that their job is to manage the entire patient experience, while others may see their job as simply providing medical treatment. The organization that commits itself to creating the best patient experience, all other things con-stant, will clearly enjoy greater patient loyalty.

The second major change is cultural. Health care must more fully incor-porate all health care workers into the treatment process. While physicians will remain the captain of the ship, other health care workers must provide another set of eyes on patient care. Other industries have found that workers far from the point of production can make valuable contributions toward improving products and services. Salesmen inform companies of what their customers want, while service technicians provide valuable information on postproduction performance. Health care must evolve into an industry that is more willing to share information and more fully incorporate non-physician employees into the treatment process. Health care workers at various points in the treatment process can identify what should and should not be done and evaluate whether treatment is effective. To get to this point, a more open system must develop in which treatment choice and clinical performance are democratized. HIPAA regulations and the threat of litigation have moved us away from information sharing and will require policy and legal reforms before we can assure ourselves that mistakes made in one location can be used to improve patient safety in other locations.

To drive these two changes, health care providers must receive payment for results, rather than for actions. Providers must be incented to use resources intelligently and produce quality care. Payment cannot be limited to successful action, given the factors other than treatment that affect outcomes, but it is clear that payment should be tied to performance.

Simplified reimbursement systems such as charges, cost per case, and capitation have failed to achieve the goals of ensuring safe and effective care, encouraging long-term tracking of patient outcomes, coordinating care across providers, and minimizing the use of resources. Quality management may provide the vehicle to pursue each of these goals, but it will require us to move beyond our current level of understanding and accept that we, as health care professionals, are only one component of the system and that the evaluation of care must be broadened within health care and extended to patients and payers. Acceptance of the changed roles will be easier once we recognize that the goal of change is improvement in patient health and that treatment is only one element that affects health outcomes.

Summary

Health care has achieved significant successes in the last 150 years and stands on the cusp of larger gains due to genetic engineering and the potential of quality management. Quality management has succeeded in creating better products and services and reducing variation in other industries but remains underused in health care.

Quality management has a variety of tools for monitoring and evaluating performance and a proven track record of success. The sooner the health care industry fully embraces quality management philosophy, tools, and objectives, the better we will be as patients and health care workers. Patients will see a safer and more effective health care system, and care givers will receive greater satisfaction from their work. While every worker has a role to play in this transformation, the greatest challenge lies with managers, who must provide the climate and tools necessary to accomplish this change.

This text has introduced a definitive plan for quality management based on a theoretical foundation, a means for evaluating performance, and a desired end. The central idea of the text, introduced in Chapter One, was:

No Measurement → No Management → No Mission

Without objective measures of performance, organizations cannot know where they stand or whether changes are required. Not only must actions be measured, but knowledge of performance must be widely distributed to ensure that opportunities for improvement are recognized and acted on. Closely held information will not meet the goal of quality management, as those possessing the information will be able to determine what is focused on and their choice may be based on personal interest rather than on the necessity of improvement.

Without measurement there can be no management. Managers changing systems without information cannot know when a system requires correction or if the correction had a positive or negative impact on system performance. Management is a difficult job; few people relish the duty of telling others how their work can be improved. Providing direction is easier when measurement identifies underperformance or inconsistency in performance. Objective data reduces arguments and defuses interpersonal conflict by focusing attention on particular issues. The job of management is not simply to tell people to improve but requires managers to identify the means to improvement. Managers must identify what skills or tools are needed to improve performance and coach employees in their use. Employees cannot be expected to achieve better results if they continue to work under the same conditions that produced substandard outcomes.

The mission of health care providers and individual employees is to facilitate the best possible health among their patients. This mission can only be achieved with measurement and management. Organizations without purposeful action and direction will be unable to compete with organizations that know how they are performing. The ability to measure and manage performance will determine which organizations thrive and which wither and die. To achieve success, everyone must understand that the purpose of quality management is not to record the past but to improve the future.

KEY TERMS

Denial

Efficacious

Encapsulation

Freedom through control

Reform

Repair

Suppression

References

Deming WE, 1986, *Out of the Crisis*, Massachusetts Institute of Technology, Cambridge, MA.

Joint Commission, 2011, Sentinel Events, http://www.jointcommission.org/assets/1/6/2011_CAMH_SE.pdf, accessed June 12, 2013.

Nash DB, Coombs JB, and Leider H, 1999, *The Three Faces of Quality*, American College of Physician Executives, Amelia Island, FL.

Porter M, 2010, What Is Value in Health Care? *New England Journal of Medicine* 326 (26): 2477–2481.

Reason J, 1990, *Human Error*, Cambridge University Press, New York, NY.

Shewhart WA, (1931) 1981, *Economic Control of Quality of Manufactured Product*, Quality Press, Milwaukee, WI. Citations refer to ASQ edition.

Teitel AS, 2012, Apollo 1: The Fire that Shocked NASA, January 27, 2012, http://blogs.scientificamerican.com/guest-blog/2012/01/27/apollo-1-the-fire-that-shocked-nasa/.

WHO (World Health Organization), 2012, *World Health Statistics 2011*, http://www.who.int/gho/publications/world_health_statistics/2011/en/index.html, accessed April 13, 2012.